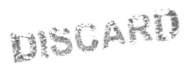

The Voice
and its
Disorders

The Voice
and its
Disorders

Margaret C L Greene
FCST

J. B. Lippincott Company
Philadelphia   Toronto

Third edition 1972

ISBN 0–397–50300–8

Library of Congress Catalog Card Number 72–560

Distributed in the United States and Canada by
J. B. Lippincott Company
Philadelphia and Toronto

Made in Great Britain at The Pitman Press, Bath

G2—(01.1213.81:11)

Preface to the
Third Edition

It is over eight years since the second edition was prepared and during that time voice science has continued to extend the boundaries of investigation and its body of knowledge. Information is mostly recorded in learned articles not readily available to clinical speech pathologists and many articles on superficial inspection do not appear specially relevant to their work. As author of an established textbook with a world-wide distribution, I have the responsibility of keeping it up to date and when I find students quoting 'Professor Greene' as gospel in their examinations I feel it is time for me to adopt once again the role of alchemist and to endeavour to transmute the baser products of research into pure gold for the speech clinician. In addition, seeing so many relevant connections between the work and reading I have carried out since the last edition and its application in the clinical field, I am impelled to set these down on paper in the hope that they will prove as exciting, interesting and provocative to the student as they have appeared to me.

This new edition reflects my further experience in teaching students over the period of almost a full six years as Director of Studies of the Speech Therapy Department at the Central School of Speech and Drama, where I rode uneasily over traditions laid down by Elsie Fogerty and Joan van Thal. For the past eight years too I have had the inestimable advantages of holding the appointment of Senior Speech Therapist at St. Bartholomew's Hospital, with its tradition of service to the poor and the sick of the City of London since the Prior, Rahere received the Royal Charter from Henry I in 1133. Here I have qeen able to work with colleagues of outstanding ability engaged in research projects many of which have had a direct bearing on speech pathology and treatment of voice disorders. Although I am grateful to all my colleagues and friends, I must single out a few who have given time to correcting errors of fact and judgement and provided constructive suggestions. These are Mr R. F. McNab Jones and

Mr J. L. Dowie in the Ear, Nose and Throat Department; Professor Linford Rees, Department of Psychological Medicine; and Dr B. Watson, Department of Medical Electronics. The final text has not been scrutinised by any of my colleagues and to save them any possible embarrassment I can but quote the words in the preface of the Second Edition: 'While acknowledging the help received, I take full responsibility for the errors of fact and opinion which are my own and to which it is hoped my readers will in due course draw my attention so that they may be corrected.'

My aim, as indicated above, has been to examine new discoveries and to apply these to voice therapy, with improved understanding of function and diagnosis. This renders possible the selection of therapeutic attitudes and exercises with the confidence and enthusiasm without which no exercise or therapy will prosper. The reader who turns the pages for discovery of more exercises and new treatment will be disappointed because Chapter 10 is the least revised of all. The basic principles of voice training remain unchallenged despite newly coined terms of reference such as 'air-flow rate', since they are established on the unchanging anatomy and physiology of the human instrument. What is new is the knowledge recently acquired concerning structure and function and their relation to performance. This is of great importance and it is this above all that has made a revised edition necessary, since we must re-examine some old ideas, decide whether these are valid (and mostly they are), and discard them if not. The work of Zenker and of Kirchener and Wyke on the structure and reflex intrinsic sensorimotor mechanisms of the vocal cords is a case in point, needing to be viewed in relation to the known amazing versatility of the voice, the extreme irritability of the larynx in vocal abuse and the prolonged vocal effects following stripping of the vocal cords in microsurgery. Discoveries concerning embryological development of the larynx lead to new surgical approaches in management of laryngeal carcinoma, all of direct concern to the speech pathologist. The use of teflon injections is another new development in the management of dysfunction of the cords, perhaps enabling the services of the speech therapist to be dispensed with for this. The recommendation that amplifiers should be used extensively as teaching aids for their value in speeding up hearing training and speech monitoring is a very important new method of treatment discussed; so is the recommendation of the early use of vibrators to assist laryngectomees in the acquisition of voice.

In the First and Second Editions I felt considerable dissatisfaction with the section dealing with hysterical voice disorders, while lacking the confidence and experience to break away from the views of the psychiatrists with whom I was working at the time. I feel much happier with the present account, which is influenced more strongly by the psychosomatic concept of dysfunction. The distinctions between anxiety, anxiety hysteria and frank hysteria, and their overlapping in varying degrees of interaction between inherited personality and environmental stress, provide a basis for a more acceptable hypothesis for treatment of such anxiety-prone individuals.

There are many new case histories and of those in the last edition I have retained only those which were too instructive and reminiscent of old friends to throw out. The Index is more detailed and will make rapid reference that much easier. The Bibliography is referred to in the text no longer by anonymous numbers but via the names of the actual authors, which will familiarise students with the names of distinguished workers in their area of study; this leads inevitably to some repetition but appears preferable to the infuriating need to trace an *op. cit.* in back pages. Finally I am happy to say that, as with so many new fashions, the life of 'vocal fold' has terminated and 'vocal cord' again holds sway.

Throughout the year of revision and reading I have been accommodated for days on end in the reading room of the Royal National Institute of the Deaf Library and been given unstinting help by the staff headed by Miss M. Plackett, the Librarian. The free facilities provided by this unique specialised library is all the more appreciated since in England the status of a speech therapist is such that it debars her from the untrammelled use of the London medical libraries!

WINGRAVE   MARGARET GREENE
1971

Contents

Preface to the Third Edition   v

List of Illustrations   xiii

Phonetic symbols used in the text   xv

Part One NORMAL VOICE

1 The vocal instrument   3

   Voice in speech, as expression of personality. Physics of speech:
   pitch, volume, resonance. Musical instruments, including the voice

2 Respiration and phonation   19

   Anatomy and physiology. Breathing for speech. Research
   studies. Techniques in voice production

3 Larynx and phonation   32

   Anatomy and physiology. Phonation. Registers.
   Research studies into structure and function of vocal cords

4 Articulation and resonance   55

   Anatomy and physiology of oral and pharyngeal resonators.
   Linked resonator system. Articulation and resonance.
   Balanced resonance. Singing voice. Voice training

5 Vocal synthesis   82

   Muscular co-ordination and relaxation.
   Rhythm, pace, inflection, intelligibility

6 Normal voice mutation: infancy to senescence   92

   Infant vocalisation. Growth of larynx. Pitch changes in
   childhood and adolescence. Ageing of the voice

Part Two VOICE DISORDERS

7 Hyperkinetic dysphonia: vocal strain   109

   Assessment of dysphonia. Causes. Organic and psychogenic
   factors. Hoarseness in children. Asthma. Myasthenia laryngis

                                                                 ix

8 Hyperkinetic dysphonia: vocal abuse   122

Vocal nodules. Personality and environmental factors.
In children and pop singers. Contact ulcers, causes and treatment

9 Rehabilitation of hyperkinetic dysphonia   144

General considerations. Role of Laryngologist. Endolaryngeal
microsurgery. The case history. Speech assessment

10 Treatment of hyperkinetic dysphonia: exercises   155

Exercises in relaxation, breathing, phonation and
expression. Rehabilitation of asthenic voice

11 Psychogenic disorders: anxiety and hysterical states   180

Personality of anxiety-prone persons. Management.
Hysterical personality. Laryngeal signs. Speech
therapy. Spastic dysphonia. Intractibility

12 Disorders of pitch: abnormal voice mutation   219

Endocrine disorders. Structural abnormalities.
Psychogenic disorders. Female pitch disorders. Myxoedema

13 Disorders of nasal resonance   238

Insufficient and excessive nasality. Palatal insufficiency.
Adenoidectomy. Neurological disorders. Exercises of
palatopharyngeal incompetence. Nasal obstruction.
Speech exercises

14 Dysarthrophonia   277

Upper and lower motor lesions. Extrapyramidal lesions.
Parkinson's disease. Amplifiers. Cerebellar lesions.
Cerebral palsy

15 Laryngeal palsy   309

Peripheral lesions of recurrent laryngeal nerves.
Types of paralysis. Thyroidectomy. Personality
factors. Laryngeal trauma. Neuritis

16 Inflammation, stenosis and benign neoplasms   341

Tuberculosis, arthritis, structural abnormality.
Hyperplastic laryngitis. Multiple papillomata in
children and adults

17   Laryngeal carcinoma: partial and total laryngectomy
and pseudo-voice   358

*Laryngofissure. New approaches in surgery.
Pharyngo-laryngectomy. Oesophageal carcinoma and
colon transplants. Psychological considerations.
Oesophageal voice*

18   Speech rehabilitation after laryngectomy   387

*Factors impeding oesophageal voice. Use of artificial
larynx and amplifier. Teaching methods. Exercises.
List of available local aids and suppliers' addresses*

Bibliography   424

Author Index   447

Subject Index   453

List of Illustrations

Fig.

1 The vocal instrument 2
2 The ear 7
3 Wave forms of different intensity but same pitch 9
4 Tuning-fork: constant pitch, varying volume 10
5 Sound waves in visual form shown by a cathode-ray oscilloscope 14
6 Spectrographs of vowels [aː] and [iː] and of [s], [ʃ] 15
7 The skeleton of the thorax 19
8 Diagrams illustrating enlargement of the thorax during inspiration 21
9 The laryngeal cartilages 33
10 The laryngeal skeleton 35
11 Some extrinsic muscles of the larynx and the nerve supply 36
12 Front of the neck, showing suprahyoid and infrahyoid muscles 37
13 Intrinsic muscles of the larynx 40
14 *A*: Transverse view of laryngeal cartilages and muscles
 B: Scheme of action of laryngeal muscles on vocal cords 41
15 Coronal section of the larynx 43
16 Laryngoscopic view of the larynx 44
17 Positions of vocal cords in action 45
18 Diagrams of laryngoscopic and coronal views of vocal cords 47
19 Saggital section through nose, mouth, pharynx and larynx 56
20 Oral view of palate and pillars of the fauces 57
21 Dissection of the pharynx showing muscles of soft palate in relation to tongue and larynx 58
22 The muscles of the nasopharyngeal isthmus and Passavant's muscle 60
23 Site of contact of the elevated velum with the posterior pharyngeal wall in speech 61
24 Changes in oral and pharyngeal cavities as seen in lateral X-ray photographs 64
25 Lateral X-ray photographs of normal soft palate positions in speech 66

26	Labelled lateral X-ray tracing for orientation	67
27	Diagrams made from lateral X-rays of soft palate	68
28	Vocal nodules	122
29	Contact ulcers and pachydermia	135
30	Diagram illustrating bellows action of lungs in expiration and inspiration	166
31	Lateral X-ray tracings before and after Hyne's pharyngoplasty	250
32	Lateral X-ray tracings of child with adenoids	252
33	Lateral X-ray tracings of patient before and after repair of palate	263
34	Lateral X-ray tracings before and after pharyngoplasty	264
35	Diagram of double connection from both hemispheres of upper neurones with bulbar nuclei	278
36	Sample of Parkinson patient's writing and copying of patterns	285
37	Posterior view of the larynx showing distribution of left and right laryngeal nerves	310
38	Vocal cord palsies: lines of orientation	315
39	Positions of vocal cords in various types of paralysis	319
40	Coronal view of larynx showing partial laryngectomy	360
41	Respiratory tract before and after laryngectomy	364
42	S. G. Brown amplifier and Pacific head set	392
43	S. G. Brown amplifier, hand microphone and table loudspeaker	392
44	S. G. Brown contact microphone worn on spectacle frame and on throat	393
45	Patient using Sama minielectronovox and telephoning	406
46	Dutch polythene reed type vibrator	414
47	Mark 5 Western electric vibrator, Aurex Neovox, and Sama minielectronovox	421

(The author's thanks are due to the Governors of St Bartholomew's Hospital for permission to reproduce Figs. 1, 2, 41, 44, 45 and 47.)

Phonetic Symbols
Used in the Text

Vowels

[i]   as in it

[i:] as in eat

[ɛ]   as in bed

[a]   as in at

[a:] as in arm

[ə:] as in her

[ə]   as in supper

[ʌ]   as in cut

[ɔ]   as in not

[u:] as in pool

Diphthongs

[au] as in house

[ei] as in day

[ai] as in lie

Consonants

[m] as in me

[n]   as in no

[ŋ]   as in sing

[p]   as in pea

[b]   as in bat

[t]   as in to

[d]   as in day

[k]   as in cat

[g]   as in go

[f]   as in fit

[v]   as in vim

[θ]   as in think

[ð]   as in that

[r]   as in red

[j]   as in yet

[s]   as in so

[z]   as in zoo

[ʃ]   as in shoe

[tʃ] as in chat

[dʒ] as in jam

[ʒ]   as in leisure

[h]   as in he

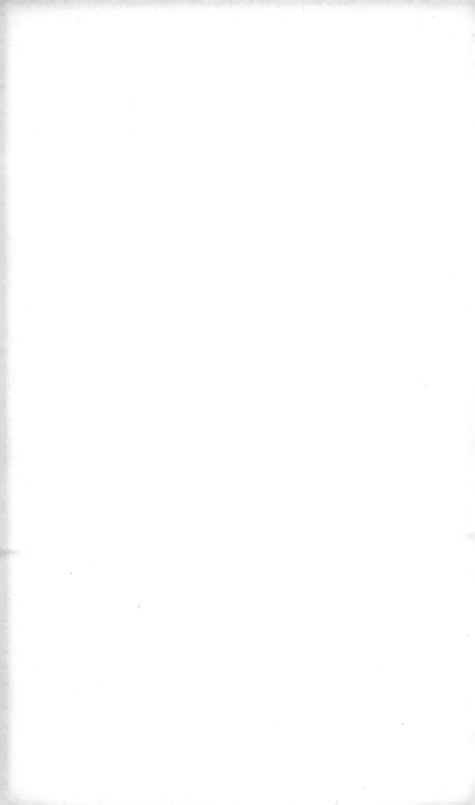

Part One
Normal Voice

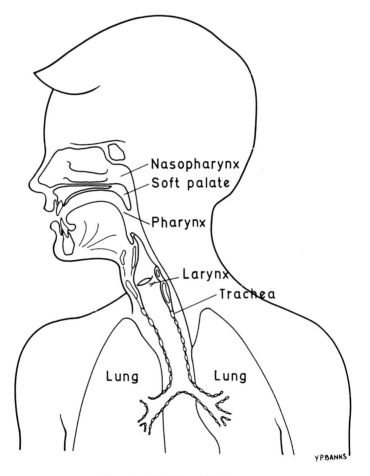

Fig. 1   The Vocal Instrument

1 The vocal instrument

Voice is the musical sound produced by vibration of the vocal cords in the larynx by air from the lungs. This process is known as phonation. In the language we tacitly acknowledge voice to be an exclusively human attribute. Birds cheep, chirp, twitter, cry, call, trill and sing, but we do not speak of birds having voices. Ducks quack, doves coo, geese honk. As to animals—lions roar and growl, cats purr and mew, dogs bark, horses neigh and whinny, donkeys bray. The rich vocabulary which is available to denote the noises produced by creatures of the land, sea and air has arisen out of the need to avoid placing these in the same category as the human voice, which not only provides an all-important vehicle for communication but conveys intrinsic linguistic and grammatical features of stress and intonation in speech so that voice and speech are exclusively human attributes.

The linguistic features of voice we will not be considering to any great extent in the following pages, but largely the voice as the vehicle *per se* of communication by the spoken word. To emphasise the distinction it is useful to contrast whispered speech with voiced speech and to consider what we lose from whispering a message as compared with speaking it aloud. Provided we are near enough to hear the speaker we will have no difficulty in understanding what is said. We will be able to judge the educational, social and regional background by the choice of vocabulary, grammar and semantic features. We will be able to detect whether the speaker has an Oxbridge type of accent or speaks a dialect showing that he comes from Wales, Scotland, Ireland or America. This information is conveyed chiefly by the vowels and diphthongs, which have clear resonance characteristics even when the voice is silent. The speed, stress and rhythm of utterance also carry information concerning dialect, and combined with variations in force of the whisper these features may also convey a little of the emotional content of the message. An urgent warning may be hissed, a loving remark whispered softly, a furious aside be tense and staccato. If the face of the speaker is concealed, the emotional aspects of the message will be less clear because the expression of

3

the face, the lips and especially the eyes speak volumes, if the voice cannot.

Whispered speech therefore is a pretty effective form of communication and on first examination the voicing of speech has seemingly but one overall advantage—that of imparting greater audibility by increasing carrying power. On closer examination however it becomes apparent that voice plays a far greater role than this in speech. Pitch, for example, indicates the sex of the speaker, whether male or female, and the maturity of the speaker's voice can be heard: the childish treble compares with the voice of the older child. Pitch variations account also for the intonation patterns and melody of speech. Bloomfield (1933) speaks of 'pitch phonemes' which constitute separate or secondary phonemes and carry their own meanings independent of the words of a sentence. Fry (1968) goes farther and refers to inflection as prosodic phenomena having an important grammatical function in language structure.

Besides pitch and volume, the voice has subtle qualities which convey the personality of the speaker. The timbre of the voice is linked with the physiognomy, build, facial expression, habits of dress and movement of the individual so that a total impression is built up by the appearance a man presents to the world. However, if we hear a voice without seeing the speaker, we gain a certain impression of his personality. This is best illustrated by 'radio personalities', some being far more successful than others, and popular on account of some generally intangible but sympathetic quality of voice. Pear (1931) in his work on voice and personality, long before the days of television, describes an interesting experiment carried out in 1927 on the BBC in which listeners were invited to fill in a form answering questions on nine anonymous readers of a set passage. Unfortunately the questions asked were not directly related to voice and personality but concerned age, sex, occupation, leadership and locality of birth. Listeners evolved very definite impressions on these aspects of the readers despite the reception which, on the wireless sets of those days, was poor and infinitely more distorted than over modern radio sets and especially very high-frequency channels. Listeners were asked to indicate in their replies whether they listened on a crystal set or valve set, with head-phones or loudspeaker. It would be interesting to conduct a similar experiment now with modern equipment and the psychologist's research laboratory expertise of the present day.

Every mature voice has unquestionably a unique character dependent upon the structure of the head, neck and face of the individual. Just as no two faces are the same, neither are two voices. Voices of members of the same family are frequently very similar because of the genetic and environmental resemblances but the voices of identical twins one would expect to be identical and probably are in childhood. Ostwald *et al.* (1962) reported inconclusively on the matter after analysing the cries of 16 pairs of twins, some of whom were uniovular in the first month. Gedda *et al.* (1960) on the other hand found considerable similarity in the voices of identical twins before puberty. The ordinary individual infant born with no language but a cry has individual and personal vocal characteristics which machines may not recognise but mothers can often identify from the voices of other babies even in the first few days (Formby, 1967; Valanne *et al.*, 1967).

In the adult, voice delineates the personality of the speaker as much as or more than the words he speaks. It is generally recognised that it is not WHAT is said but HOW it is said which really counts. The 'edge' to the voice precipitates misunderstanding. We say one thing but mean another (Uris, 1960). Nothing so betrays a man as his voice. The subtle variations of timbre, speed, inflection, stress and volume all contribute to the impression made by speaker on listener and convey his emotional attitude to the situation and to the 'other one'. Subtle innuendo, the loud voice of anger, the low soft tones of love, the high and rapid speech of anxiety and the monotonous tones of depression are recognisable. The voice conveys a kaleidoscope of emotional undercurrents such as joy, excitement, tranquillity, irritation, suspicion, true sympathy or lack of it, humour which softens the sly thrust, and the venom of hate. Thus emotions 'colour' the voice (Wyllie, 1894), giving infinite shades to meaning which defy interpretation by modern methods of electro-acoustic analysis.

Paul Moses (1954) was the first to emphasise the importance of the voice in neurosis and the emotionally distressed individual. Latterly even phoneticians and linguists have become interested in the qualities of voice as an indication of biological, psychological and social characteristics of the speaker. Laver (1968) refers to these features as the 'indexical' information of voice quality. Abercrombie (1968) includes tones of voice among the paralinguistic features of speech which comprise also gesture, posture, facial expression and interjections. Ruesch (1959), interested from the psychiatric standpoint, speaks of the importance of the 'metalanguage' of verbal speech conveyed in the tonal qualities of the voice, gestures and patterning of speech.

Normally the voice plays the musical accompaniment to speech, rendering it tuneful, pleasing, audible and coherent, being essential to efficient communication by the spoken word. A bizarre or harsh and ugly voice can be a serious handicap and embarrassment to the speaker if he is aware of its repercussions on his audience. It may at least make him ill at ease in company and at most induce him to shun social contacts and to isolate himself.

Control of the voice, therefore, quite apart from the words chosen to express thoughts, is an essential component in the individual's ability to adjust to social situations, to make good contact and maintain equilibrium in relation to the audience, whether it be one or many. When the voice deteriorates as a result of strain or actual disease the whole personality suffers with it, giving rise to feelings of inadequacy and insecurity. No consideration of voice can omit the psychological and socio-economic implications involved. Voice disorders and vocal strain in those who depend upon good speech for a living—the teacher, salesman, actor or singer—produce quite obvious anxieties on account of the serious professional and economic hazards involved. Another side of the problem, however, is the personality which produces this voice disorder, for example, the highly strung and hyperactive individual. Thus cause and effect react one upon another and this interplay and the psychosomatic aspect of voice disorder has to be taken into account in every programme for vocal rehabilitation. The personality of the individual and its reflection in the sick voice, whether the cause be primarily psychological or purely organic, must not be underestimated, and speech therapists need to be trained to listen for the vocal signals of distress which may carry a different message from that contained in the words spoken

THE VOCAL MECHANISM

It is axiomatic that before any deviation from normal function can be understood, normal function must be studied. The aetiology, diagnosis and treatment of voice disorders are no exception to this rule. They must be soundly based upon psychological principles and a knowledge of the anatomy and physiology of the vocal mechanism, besides some knowledge of the physics of sound and modern methods of instrumental investigation and analysis.

The voice is classified as a musical sound, and the human mechanism which produces it can be compared to a musical instrument. For this reason it is generally considered helpful to know something about the vibration of a musical note by an inanimate instrument of human manufacture before embarking upon the study of the complexities of the human vocal instrument. Such knowledge unquestionably contributes to the better under-standing of the mechanics of voice production, besides being of use when explaining the acoustic properties of the voice to patients.

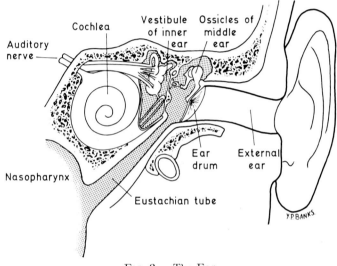

FIG. 2   The Ear

The propagation of a musical sound requires an exciter, a vibrator and a resonator. The vibrator has to be set in motion or 'excited' by some source of energy (a blow or blast of air). The sound waves generated by movements of the vibrator are differ-entially emphasised by the resonator. The sound thus created has the PSYCHOLOGICAL characteristics of pitch, volume and quality. We thus distinguish between high and low notes (notes of different pitch); loud and soft notes (notes of different volume); mellow or harsh notes (notes of different quality).

The propagation of sound is dependent upon the vibration of air particles producing waves of alternately compressed and rarefied air. The vibrations reach and excite the ear drum or tympanum, travel through the middle ear via the ossicles, and thence pass on to the fluid of the inner ear. A part of the vibratory energy of the outer air is thus eventually transferred to the fluid of the cochlea which pulsates in sympathy, stimulating the nerve endings of the organ of Corti. These stimuli then travel via the auditory nerve to the brain. The interpretation of sounds, their recognition and their meaning is dependent upon cortical function. The intelligence and emotional state and awareness or attention of the individual listener are also important aspects in determining what is heard or listened to at any particular moment.

PHYSICS OF SOUND

Pitch and Volume

Apart from the speed of sound which remains constant and need not concern us here, sound waves have two variable and measurable features. These are the rate or speed at which the wave oscillates, known as its frequency, and the size of the wave, known as its amplitude. This means the pitch of a sound is dependent upon the frequency of the sound wave; and the loudness of a sound upon the amplitude of the wave. It is difficult, perhaps, to imagine the manner in which sound waves travel through the air since they are invisible, and it is helpful to consider a similar phenomenon which takes place in a visible medium. If a brick is thrown into a pond the water is at first thrown aside and compressed and then rushes back into the cavity torn in its surface: thereafter the water at this point continues to move up and down, and it can be seen that fresh oscillations radiate outwards in ripples from the original point of disturbance. Should a stick be stuck upright in the water it is possible to measure the time it takes for one complete undulation to pass by, and the total number which pass by in one second. The size of the undulations can also be gauged by measuring the height the water rises and falls in relation to the stick. Thus the frequency and amplitude of the waves are known. In the case of air waves, one undulation executed by the air particles is called a cycle and the number of cycles occurring in one second determines its pitch in psychological language and its frequency in physical language. The size of each wave, and the amplitude of the movements of the air particles in one cycle, determine the loudness or amplitude of the sound heard. A sound wave always travels at a constant rate but its size varies according to its loudness. At its point of origin it has a maximal size, but as it travels away through the air it loses energy and, therefore, loudness. It encounters resistance from the particles of the atmosphere and the energy associated with the sound is gradually dissipated. People standing at different distances from the source of sound will therefore hear the same pitch but at different levels of intensity as the sound wave loses strength and amplitude (Fig. 4).

Fig. 3 shows two sound waves oscillating at the same frequency of 256 cycles per second but at different intensities. The wave represented by the continuous line is less loud than that represented by the broken line, but both are of the same frequency, the pitch of middle C (C_3). The exact pitch of any sound can be measured in this way in terms of cycles per second. As pitch rises,

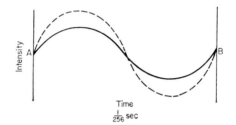

Fig. 3   Wave forms of different intensity but same pitch

the frequency of cycles per second increases proportionately. Thus, the frequency of notes that rise at intervals of an octave will be 64; 128; 256; 512; 1024; 2048; 4096 cycles per second (c.p.s.).

The pitch of a vibrator, that is the number of cycles per second of vibration it can execute, is dependent upon its size, shape, elasticity and mass. As long as these factors remain constant, the pitch never varies however strongly the vibrator is set in motion. The vibrating force, whether it be a blast of air or a blow, only changes the volume of the sound. For instance, a pendulum keeps up the same number of movements to one side and then the other of the mid-line and so does a swing, however strongly or lightly it is pushed and however far it travels in these excursions. A straight spring or a tuning fork tuned to the pitch of middle C will always pass back and forth past the mid-line at a rate of 256 c.p.s., whatever the amplitude of vibration and therefore of the sound waves generated.

All musical sounds are characterised by sound waves which form a recurring pattern and occur at regular intervals. The sound waves of noises, however, follow an irregular and jagged course of considerable complexity and they do not occur with any recognisable regularity.

A cathode ray oscilloscope presents sound waves in a visual form. In Fig. 5 the oscillograms (*A*) and (*B*) show the complex waves produced by vowel [a:] and vowel [i:], which constitute musical notes; (*C*) and (*D*) show the oscillograms of [s] and [ʃ] which are noises.

The physical properties of noise are difficult to classify and to measure. Bangs, taps, hisses, shrieks and squeaks are all noises

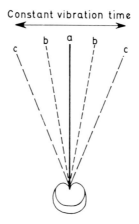

Fig. 4   Tuning-fork: constant pitch, varying volume

a: tuning-fork
b–b: note of small volume
c–c: same note of greater volume

and are mainly sounds to which no definite pitch can be attributed. Practically all types of sound which are not classified as vowels or musical notes are noises. The fricative and plosive consonants of speech are noises as opposed to vowels and diphthongs which constitute the musical aspects of speech on which the linguistic vocal melodic or inflectional pattern is based.

Resonance

Before we discuss resonance or the quality of sound it is necessary to dispose of the confusion which exists in the common usage of the words 'tone', 'note' and 'quality'. For example, 'tone' may refer to a pure sound of particular pitch (with no overtones), such as its use in 'pure-tone audiometry'. Or 'tone' may refer to notes of particular pitch, e.g. the semitones of the chromatic scale. Or again, 'tone' may refer to tone of voice such as 'a nasty tone' meaning quality, overtones or resonance.

In this text 'note' will be used exclusively to denote pitch, while vocal tone and quality will refer to resonance, now to be described.

The question of a single sound wave or pure note having the characteristics only of pitch and amplitude seldom occurs in nature. Either a complex tone is produced directly by complex vibrations generated by the vibrator, or a pure note is changed into a complex tone by the cavities and resonators associated with it which modify the fundamental note. Thus a complexity of waves varying in amplitude and frequency can be produced. It is this complexity of sound waves which gives musical sound its quality or resonance. The original sound wave generated in the complex sound is the loudest in the group and determines the pitch or fundamental of a note; the superimposed abundance of component frequencies supplies the overtones, harmonics, quality, timbre, or resonance. For the resonant sound to remain a musical and harmonious one, there must be a definite mathematical relationship between the various frequencies which compose it, otherwise dissonance and noise result. In fact a harmonic may be defined as a note of which the frequency is an exact multiple of the fundamental.

The movement of the vibrator determines the pitch of the note. But at the same time—depending upon its elasticity, whether a vibrating string or column of air—different sections of the vibrator may vibrate at different frequencies, giving rise to subsidiary sound waves which impart overtones or harmonics to the fundamental and lowest note imparted by the vibrator. If one observes a violin string vibrating it can be seen that it not only vibrates along its whole length, but that its two halves vibrate independently, executing a figure-of-eight in both the horizontal and the vertical planes. A skipping rope held between two people can be made to swing from side to side and wriggle like a snake at the same time.

Every note propagated by the vibrator or generator determines the fundamental pitch which predominates by reason of its greater energy in relation to the overtones created by the vibrator and the assortment of harmonics which sympathetic vibration of the resonator adds to it. Resonance energy can be clearly demonstrated by comparing the thin and quickly deadened note produced by bowing a violin string when pegged at each end to a simple board of wood, which acts as an inefficient sounding board, with the rich and full resounding note from the same string when attached to the body of the violin itself. The greater the range of frequencies compounded in a musical note the richer will be the quality or resonance.

The strict definition of a resonator is a selective body designed to respond to one particular frequency which is known as its resonance frequency. The term resonator, however, is more commonly used with reference to objects which are more or less 'universal resonators' capable of reinforcing a certain range of tones.

The effective frequency range of a resonator is known as its 'band-width'. The sound which excites the resonator is known as the 'input' and the sound which the resonator produces is its 'output' (Ladefoged, 1962).

The resonators of musical instruments respond either to a particular resonance frequency, as in the case of the various pipes of an organ, or to a certain frequency range or band-width such as with the violin, viola or double bass, the bodies of which are suited to the high, middle and low registers respectively. The band-width of frequencies (or harmonics) with which a resonator responds to a particular note is known as the 'formant'. If the formant of a selective resonator is in the region of middle C, for example, and a note of this pitch is sounded in its vicinity, the air within will respond sympathetically and 'speak' more loudly than for any other note which is divergent from this particular resonance frequency. When a resonator fulfils this function it is said to act as an acoustic filter—a filter being a resonator which passes on sound but is selective and capable of transmitting one frequency range more efficiently than any other. Vibrations which are passed on less efficiently and die away quickly are said to be 'stopped' by the resonator or filter.

Helmholtz, the father of physiological acoustics and the founder of the fixed-pitch theory of vowel tones in his *Sensations of Tone* (1862), described his experiments with the design of selective resonators whereby he analysed and synthesised the quality of vowel sounds.

A Helmholtz resonator consists of a hollow brass sphere having an opening for admission of sound and another for holding to the ear. The enclosed sphere of air, having a particular fundamental frequency of its own, picks this up and intensifies it by resonance whenever this note is introduced (Everett, 1907). A simple laboratory experiment is often used to demonstrate how a resonator acts as an acoustic filter. If water is poured into a measuring cyclinder and a vibrating tuning-fork is held over its mouth, it will be found that as the water rises and the column of air in the measure obtains the ideal proportions suited to resonate or 'tune into' the pitch of the fork, it will suddenly amplify the sound by vigorous resonation. Then as the air cavity is reduced by the continued flow of water the sound diminishes and dies away. A tap dripping into a bottle also changes in resonance pitch as the bottle fills.

PHYSICS OF VOICE

Vowel Formants

In man, voice is produced by vibration of the vocal cords, the fundamental note thus created being modified instantaneously in the cavities of throat, nose and mouth. The vocal tract in fact acts as a series of acoustic filters which stop or reinforce the original and fundamental note. These linked filters or resonators are capable of assuming an infinite variety of differently shaped cavities with varying sizes of orifice. The articulation of the vowels of speech changes the shape of the pharyngeal and oral cavities; the tongue, palate and jaw movements involved thus produce the characteristic formants which distinguish one vowel from another. Each vowel has two characteristic formants which show up very clearly on the spectrum produced by a spectrogram. The vowel [a:] for example produces characteristic frequency bands in the region of 800 c.p.s. and 1100 c.p.s. The formants of vowel i: are in the region of 280 c.p.s. and 2500 c.p.s.

The sound spectrograph was originally invented at the Bell Telephone Laboratories in order to throw a display of 'visible speech' (Potter *et al.*, 1947) upon a screen, with the purpose of teaching the deaf. It has not been used much for the purpose for which it was originally devised but is a most useful tool for phoneticians and acoustic physicists.

The 'Kay Sonograph' machine instead of throwing a spectrum of sound waves upon a screen translates these into graphic form and provides a permanent, in place of a fleeting, visual record of the frequency spectra of speech signals. The instrument contains a recording device and an analyser consisting of built-in filters covering a range of 0–8000 cycles per second which respond to the

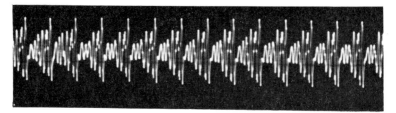

A: [a]

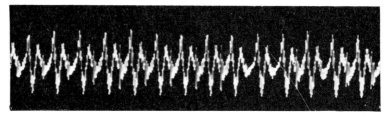

B: [i]

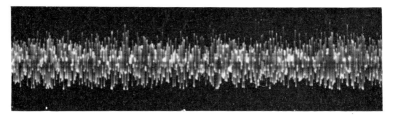

C: [s]

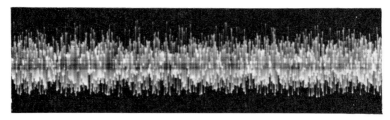

D: [ʃ]

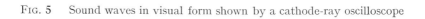

FIG. 5   Sound waves in visual form shown by a cathode-ray oscilloscope

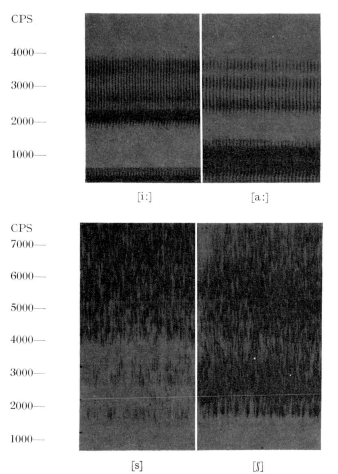

CPS

4000—

3000—

2000—

1000—

      [i:]   [a:]

CPS
7000—

6000—

5000—

4000—

3000—

2000—

1000—

      [s]   [ʃ]

Fig. 6

Spectrographs of vowels [iː] and [aː] and of [s] and [ʃ]
(From *An Introduction to the Pronunciation of English* by A. C. Gimson.
Reproduced by permission)

frequency and intensity of the sounds fed into it. The analysis is
converted into ink tracings which eventually issue from the
machine on a strip of paper. The length of speech it is possible to
analyse in this way per spectrograph is limited to 2·4 seconds.
This, of course, imposes limits on its use in the analysis of connected speech. Fig. 6 shows samples of spectrograms.

The spectrograph shows frequency on the vertical axis, duration
of sound on the horizontal axis, while the intensity of the sound

is shown by the degree of blackening produced by the tracing pens. The fundamental pitch of the voice is shown either by the temporal separation of successive vertical striations in the case of a wide band-width analysis, or by the frequency separation of successive horizontal harmonic lines when a narrow band analysing filter is used (Petersen, 1954).

The enhancing of fundamental notes by resonance is obviously a very important factor in production of musical tone and of the human voice. It is often stated in the teaching of good voice production that resonance 'amplifies' the voice. This is not strictly true by standards of physical measurement of amplitude since clearly resonant components of the note cannot be louder than the fundamental. Nevertheless the human ear or auditory cortical analyser may register a resonant booming voice as more conspicuous than a thin reedy one. Resonance adds significance to the voice and perhaps energy. It is well known that a singer may, by singing the right note very loudly and clearly, actually shatter an empty wine-glass by the violence of the vibrations set up within it. If one of two identical tuning-forks of the same pitch is struck and set beside the other, the stationary fork will begin to vibrate in unison and will continue to do so even when the original fork is removed. The second fork takes some time to build up energy and to sound loudly. The displaced air particles in the region of the second fork move back and forth and act as small blows which have a cumulative effect on the fork and gradually increase its oscillations and therefore the volume of sound produced. In an enclosed air space such as a wine-glass or cavity of the throat and mouth the build-up of resonance frequencies is quicker.

In the case of a hollow resonator, the complex mixture of resonance frequencies generated depends upon the size and shape of the enclosed air space, the size of its orifices and the composition of its walls. Minute variations in these factors can appreciably alter the quality of the sound produced. It has never been possible, for example, to reproduce the beautiful mellow resonance of the old Stradivarius violins despite the most faithful imitation of construction and use of materials. This fact is attributed to loss of the secret art of varnishing these instruments known only to the old master violin-makers. The factor of ageing materials must also play a part. Notes of identical pitch are therefore found to vary considerably in quality in accordance with the materials used in construction of any instrument. A silver flute differs from a wooden one and a silver trumpet from a brass. Differences in tension in the elastic and muscular walls of the throat and mouth cavity change the flexibility of the human resonators and influence vocal tone. It is the minute changes in size, shape and texture of the vocal cavities which interpret the emotions and flicker over the tone of voice reflecting fleeting expression as surely as the eye 'mirrors the soul'.

TYPES OF MUSICAL INSTRUMENTS

Musical instruments are classed according to the type of vibrator, whether wind, string or percussion. Stringed instruments include the harp, piano and violin, the strings being plucked, hammered or bowed. The size and tension of the strings affect pitch primarily and may add some overtones to the sound as has already been described. The frame of each instrument is responsible for resonance. Wind instruments are subdivided according to the nature of their vibrators. The mouthpieces of the oboe and clarinet are fitted with reeds which vibrate under the pressure of the breath; the fingering applied to the holes in the pipe regulates the length of the vibrating column of air, and its pulsations working back to the mouthpiece regulate the speed at which the reed vibrates and therefore the pitch of the note. The energy of the enclosed air affects the walls of the tube, and resonance is imparted to the note. The flue mouthpieces of organ pipes merely excite the air stream and each pipe is tuned to a single pitch, hence the need for an enormous number of different pipes of varying size. Percussion instruments, cymbals, xylophones and drums, scarcely come within our field of interest since they have little resemblance to the vocal instrument and contribute little to our understanding of it.

VOCAL INSTRUMENT COMPARED TO MUSICAL INSTRUMENT

The vocal instrument has something in common with both wind and stringed instruments: with wind, by virtue of the exciting force of air from the lungs and the resonating air column above the glottis, and with strings, by virtue of the laryngeal regulation of pitch. The pitch of a note played upon a violin string is dependent upon the tension of the string (regulated by the turning of the peg); on the thickness of the string (the violin having four strings of different thicknesses and range of pitch); and on the length of string which is allowed to vibrate when regulated by stopping with the fingers. The vocal folds being elastic and vibrant, vary in length, thickness and tension according to the

action of the laryngeal muscles and therefore have a little in
common with string vibrators. True comparison, however, of the
vocal instrument with any other muscial instrument is impossible
because the living mechanism is incomparably more versatile
than any instrument of human manufacture can ever be.

THE VOICE

Voice is the result of breath under pressure from the lungs causing
the approximated vocal cords to perform the rhythmic excursions
of separation and closure. In this way, air escapes through the
glottis in pulses. The alternate compression and rarefaction of the
stream of air particles thus created is responsible for the sound
waves which determine the fundamental pitch of the vocal note
produced. The whole process is called phonation. The cavities
of the chest below, and the pharynx, mouth and nose above the
larynx provide a universal resonator for all speech sounds. The
human vocal instrument is most remarkable for the versatility
of the supraglottic resonators. The infinite variety of modifications
in size and shape provided by movements of the tongue render
possible their use as selective resonators (acoustic filters) for the
production of the various vowels and for noise-making in the
consonants of the language.

The vocal instrument was primarily designed for the purposes
of mastication, deglutition and respiration (Negus, 1959). The
adaptation of vital reflex functions to the purposes of speech is
one of the most remarkable features of human evolution. The
primitive and vital functions of the speech apparatus are of great
interest and importance to the speech therapist. When the
secondary voluntary speech function is impaired for organic or
psychological reasons, movements involved in involuntary reflex
functions may be utilised either to restore the lost voice or to
supply an adequate substitute for it. Thus the exercise of coughing
may restore the voice in a case of hysterical aphonia or improve
the function of a paralysed cord. Expulsion of air from the
oesophagus may compensate for total loss of voice due to excision
of the larynx (laryngectomy).

Our broad survey of vocal and instrumental sounds is now
completed and in the following chapters we can turn to a detailed
study of the anatomy and physiology of the vocal instrument.
Respiration, phonation, articulation and resonance will be
examined, also the contributions made by these separately and
collectively in the production of normal speech and voice.

2 Respiration and phonation

THE ANATOMY OF THE THORAX AND THE PHYSIOLOGY
OF RESPIRATION

The skeleton of the thorax consists of the sternum or breast bone
in front, the spine behind and the ribs at the sides. These bony
structures form a strong but elastic cage housing the lungs and
heart and also give attachment to the muscles of respiration.

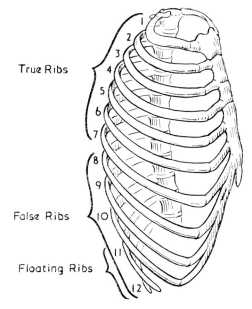

True Ribs

False Ribs

Floating Ribs

FIG. 7   The skeleton of the thorax

Posteriorly twelve pairs of ribs articulate with the transverse
processes of the thoracic vertebrae by means of the synovial
costovertebral joints which permit gliding movements. Anteriorly
the attachments of the ribs vary according to their relation to the
sternum through the intervention of the costal cartilage at their
tips. The first pair of ribs is joined directly to the sternum by

cartilage and is immovable. The second to seventh pairs of ribs form synovial sternocostal joints with the sternum and are there-fore, mobile. The eighth to tenth pairs are not attached directly to the sternum but each is attached by an interchondral joint to the costal cartilage above, and they are dubbed 'false ribs' for this reason. The false ribs follow the movement of the seventh pair in respiration. The last two pairs, the eleventh and twelfth, are known as the floating ribs because they are not even indirectly attached to the sternum; they do not float adrift, however, but are firmly anchored to the abdominal wall by fascia.

The lungs, which lie on each side of the mediastinum, are roughly pear-shaped, broad at the bases where they are in contact with the diaphragm, and narrow at the apices where they extend to the level of the clavicle. The lungs are composed of elastic, non-muscular tissue surrounding the alveoli or air cells, which are profusely supplied with blood vessels. The lungs are capable of expansion and contraction only by intervention of the respiratory movements activated by the muscles of respiration. Air enters the lungs through the passages of the nose, pharynx, larynx, trachea and bronchi. In the lungs the process known as the diffusion of gases takes place. Oxygen is absorbed from the air by the blood circulating through the capillaries of the air-sacs, while at the same time carbon dioxide passes from the blood into the air-sacs to be exhaled during exhalation. This is the vital purpose of respiration essential for the maintenance of life.

THE MUSCLES OF RESPIRATION

The chief muscles of respiration are the external and internal intercostal muscles and the diaphragm. The accessory muscles of expiration are the external oblique, rectus abdominis and latissi-mus dorsi (Ladefoged, 1960).

1. *The External Intercostals* originate in the external inferior border of one rib and are inserted in the external upper border of the rib below, thus filling in part of the intercostal spaces. They elevate the ribs upon contraction and assist inspiration.

2. *The Internal Intercostals* form an internal muscular layer below the external intercostals, and they originate in the internal inferior border of one rib and are inserted in the internal upper border of the rib below. They assist in lowering the ribs in expiration.

3. *The External Oblique Muscle,* forming the lateral interior part of the abdominal wall, arises from the lower border of the

lower eight ribs and is inserted in the iliac crest. It assists expiration.

4. *The Rectus Abdominis Muscle* arises in the pubic crest and is inserted in the cartilages of the fifth, sixth and seventh ribs. It forms the whole front wall of the abdomen. It assists expiration.

5. *The Latissimus Dorsi* is a broad flat muscle covering the lower part of the chest and loins. It originates in the lower vertebrae and lower ribs. It is inserted in the bicipital groove of the humerus. It assists expiration.

6. *The Diaphragm* divides the thoracic cavity from the abdominal cavity. Its fibres originate in the circumference of the

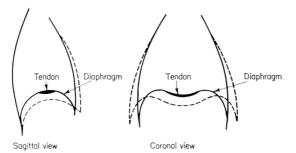

Sagittal view   Coronal view

FIG. 8.   Diagrams illustrating enlargement of the thorax during inspiration

thoracic outlet—the sternum in front, the ribs on each side, and the vertebral column behind. These muscle fibres are inserted in a trilobed central tendon. The diaphragm is dome-shaped when relaxed, but upon contraction it flattens and increases the vertical dimension of the thorax. The muscles of the abdominal wall move in sympathy with the rise and fall of the diaphragm and can, therefore, be accessory muscles of respiration. As the diaphragm descends, the viscera below are compressed and the abdominal muscles relax to accommodate them and the stomach wall moves forwards. Then, as the diaphragm ascends, the upper abdominal wall contracts exerting a gentle pressure upon the viscera, indirectly assisting the rise of the diaphragm. The external intercostals and the diaphragm only are used in quiet breathing, but after violent exercise various other muscles are brought into action: the trapezius, levator scapulae and sterno-mastoid which haul the thoracic cage upwards and enlarge the cavity.

VITAL RESPIRATION

Respiration is a co-ordinated muscular act whereby the volume of the cavity of the thorax is alternately increased and decreased in the perpetual rhythmic movements of inspiration and expiration. As the thorax is enlarged by the elevation of the ribs and descent of the diaphragm, a partial vacuum is created and air rushes in to equalise the thoracic air pressure with that of the atmosphere. As the diaphragm ascends, the external intercostal muscles relax and the ribs descend so that the air in the lungs is compressed and expelled (Fig. 8).

When the ribs are elevated the movement at the sternocostal and costovertebral joints is inconsiderable but each rib behaves like the handle of a bucket: the excursion of the ribs with each breath is considerably greater at the periphery than at the axis, and materially increases the circumference of the thorax.

The chest is so constructed that there is a far greater possibility of lung expansion in the area below the seventh pair of ribs than in the area above this level. The ribs of the upper thorax being attached before and behind enclose the lungs in a fairly rigid encasement. The eighth to twelfth pairs of ribs, being unattached in front to the sternum and confronting each other across a muscular expanse, permit in this region considerable expansion of the lungs. These are larger at their bases than their apices and in expansion are able to push the mobile lower ribs outwards in a forward and lateral direction. Added to this, the flexibility of the abdominal wall permits the full descent of the diaphragm. In speech and song the thoracic air reservoir must be increased by three or four times over and above the 500 c.c. of tidal air which is adequate for the purposes of normal quiet breathing. A greater volume of inspired air is necessary to activate the vocal folds and to sustain their vibration throughout protracted phrases. The admirable anatomical structure of the thorax in the diaphragmatic and lower costal region is, accordingly, utilised in obtaining this increase in phonic air capacity.

BREATHING FOR SPEECH

In the past there has been much disagreement over the question of which muscles are used in respiration for speech and the exact roles individual muscles play in inspiration and expiration.

The research of Draper, Ladefoged and Whitteridge (1959) has apparently settled many controversial points. The antagonistic action of the external and internal intercostals during inspiration and expiration respectively, for some time under question, is now confirmed. The *active* role of the diaphragm in expiration is now in some doubt.

The instrumental techniques employed in this research in the department of physiology at Edinburgh University are worth describing briefly in order to impress the student with the advanced nature of Speech Science.

A cathode ray oscillograph was used for registration of sound wave forms which were photographed and analysed. A meter measured vocal volume. Electrodes were inserted (by a surgeon) in the respiratory muscles of the subjects examined and electro-myographs obtained. Subglottal air pressure was measured by inserting a small latex balloon at the end of a catheter through the nose into the oesophagus. The catheter could be connected either to a tambour system and kymographic records obtained, or an electronic transducer system might be used if a more rapid frequency response was required. Nor is this all. Volume recordings of lung air were measured by the experimental subjects being placed in a body plethysmograph—an air-tight container from which head and neck only protruded. When the lungs were inflated the volume of air displaced from the plethysmograph was recorded by a spirometer which made ink tracings.

The results of examining 18 university lecturers in this way showed that to maintain a relatively constant loudness level, the air pressure below the vocal folds has to remain practically constant. In order to mainta'n the subglottal air pressure in ordinary conversation, after a deep inspiration and elevation of the ribs, the external intercostals remain in action by regulating the air pressure and preventing descent of the cage.

As speech continues and volume of air in the lungs decreases, sub-glottal air pressure is maintained by gradual relaxation of the external intercostals. Then the internal intercostals come into action with gradually increasing intensity. When the volume of the air in the lungs is slightly less than that at the end of normal expiration, the accessory muscles of expiration (external oblique, rectus abdominis, latissimus dorsi) contract and help maintain sub-glottal air pressure. The diaphragm, traditionally held to be of the utmost importance in controlling pressure in expiration, was found to play a mainly passive part, rising as the central tendon relaxed, assisted by the abdominal muscles. The diaphragm's function in *inspiration* of course remains unquestioned.

RESEARCH IN PHONIC RESPIRATION

Yanagihara and Koike (1967) carried out an important investigation into the air flow rate in the sustained phonation of notes of differing pitch by subjects wearing a pneumotach-mask. By 'sustained phonation time' is meant the time a subject can hold a note comfortably at a given pitch after taking a deep breath. The research was designed in order to clarify the relation between vital capacity and the total amount of air volume necessary to sustain notes of different pitch. The subjects were 11 male and 11 female adults who were not professionally trained singers. The subjects were measured for air flow rate, total air volume, vocal duration, pitch and intensity when producing a note of medium pitch, and highest and lowest notes in chest register sustainable without special effort. The authors found physiological differences in their subjects. The air volume available for maximally sustained phonation varied in proportion to the vital capacity of air available and this was specific to sex, height, age and weight of individuals, which are significant factors. A greater flow rate was necessary to achieve increase in vocal volume at higher pitches, but at low and middle pitches the flow rate had little relation to voice intensity. This was an unexpected finding but confirmed the findings of Isshiki (1965).

Yanagihara and Koike conclude that maximum sustained phonation is achieved by three physiological factors which are as follows:

1. Total air capacity available for voice production
2. The expiratory power
3. The adjustment of the larynx for efficient air usage, i.e. the glottal resistance

Hirano, Koike and Von Leden (1968) have also used maximum phonation time as a means of assessment of vocal function and this would appear to be a useful and practical means of judging vocal disorders in the speech clinic.

Rubin, Le Cover and Vennard (1967) studied vocal intensity, subglottic pressure and air flow in three singers—a baritone, a bass and a soprano. A needle was introduced into the trachea to measure subglottic pressure, a close-fitting mask was applied over the face to measure air flow and a microphone in front of the mask recorded sound intensity. The complexity of such operations imposes limits naturally upon the number of subjects it is possible to test and the number willing to be tested. The authors observe that singers do not lend themselves kindly to puncture of their tracheas and it was essential that experiments be conducted with a minimum of delay! On the basis of this restricted study, Rubin *et al.* concluded that air flow is not the major factor in supporting a tone of increasing loudness and that glottal resistance is far more important. Further observations were as follows:

1. Subglottic pressure measurements do not necessarily reflect sound pressure levels
2. Vocal inefficiency in the form of laryngeal constriction or breathiness exerts a markedly disturbing effect on flow pressure measurements
3. Poor breath control and inadequate breath support impair vocal quality by causing *secondary* interfering glottal tension

Although the human voice is being examined systematically by refined research techniques for its essential physical components, the best judge of its artistic quality is still the human ear. Werner-Kukuk, Von Leden and Yanagihara (1968) also stress that laryngeal efficiency is based chiefly on this sensitive balance between the two opposing physical factors of subglottic pressure and glottic resistance.

Van den Berg (1964) has made the important discovery that man's larynx would be much more efficient if he had a shorter, narrower trachea. An excised human larynx was mounted on a short subglottal system which comprised about one-third of the volume of the normal system. It appeared that the flow of air needed to actuate the larynx with this short system was about one-third of the flow needed with the normal subglottic system. The mean subglottal air pressures in both systems were comparable but with the short systems the sound level was much larger. This discovery has obvious implications in assessing the vocal efficiency of speakers and singers. The shorter the neck and dead volume in the trachea of the professional singer or speaker the longer time he will be able to hold a note with the given amount of available air. This also explains the extraordinary efficiency of children's voices issuing from small frames and the quite remarkable volume of sound babies are capable of producing.

These highly complicated aerodynamic and acoustic studies carried out in speech science research laboratories are of great value to ordinary speech pathologists in their clinical work. They provide insight into remedial methods and indicate a rather different emphasis in traditional teaching of good voice production with its great stress on breathing technique and adequate volume of phonic air. The fact that air pressure levels are not correlated exactly with sound pressure levels in middle and lower ranges of the voice is a new finding and relevant in teaching of singing. Air volume needs to be thought of as dynamic energy controlled by the respiratory muscles it is true, but air pressure levels and air flow are equally controlled by vocal cord resistance. The muscular co-ordination of respiratory muscles has to be developed through kinaesthetic and auditory training. The reflex control of muscular tension within the vocal cords is also of major importance in producing the desired note and the pitch, tone and volume (Wyke, 1969).

PHONIC BREATHING METHODS

Tarneaud (1961) describing the best breathing technique says 'to breathe well for phonation, a rapid inspiration and a measured expiration is necessary, and we add that the expiration time must be regulated, flexible, and match the vocal effort needed, and that this results from the regulation by the subject of the return movement of the thorax and abdominal walls'. He also draws attention to the errors and dangers of over-stressing the need for large volumes of inspired air in singing and quotes Thooris: 'l'air en excès étouffe le chanteur'. This observation is valid in speech as well. In clinical experience the patient in the first stages of treatment often complains of feelings of breathlessness and suffocation. There should be no exaggeration of abdominal or thoracic movement, but inspiration and expiration should be easy, smooth and effortless and tension of the vocal cords adequate, but not exaggerated, when a vocal note is produced.

BREATHING TECHNIQUES IN SPEECH

The most efficient method of respiration for vocal purposes is considered to be that known as the intercostal diaphragmatic method, or 'lateral rib swing', which may be considered as a 'central' type of breathing (Aikin, 1951) and is distinct from other less efficient methods. One of these is the lower and 'abdominal' type of breathing in which the intercostals play a negligible part and the diaphragm is used almost exclusively, accompanied by obvious sympathetic movements of the abdominal wall. In men, according to Last (1960), abdominal movement is greater than in women, especially as the years go by.

In women and many children the thoracic movement is greater than the diaphragmatic. The ordinary simultaneous rib and diaphragmatic movement can be so balanced that the abdominal wall does not move at all. This is known generally as 'thoracic' breathing and is not necessarily inadequate for the ordinary purposes of conversational voice production.

Luchsinger (1965) confirms that abdominal respiration pre-dominates in males, whereas 'pectoral' respiration with marked elevation of the upper front of the chest is typical for the female sex. He suggests that this physiological sex difference may be due to interference with abdominal respiration during pregnancy. Lower thoracic breathing with lifting of the ribs he terms, rather quaintly, flank respiration and agrees with the generally accepted view that the most efficient breathing pattern for all physical effort including phonic is a combination of abdominal and lower pectoral.

An aberrant form of breathing is that known as 'clavicular' or upper thoracic breathing during which the external intercostal and accessory thoracic muscles are utilised as in forced inspiration (page 29). With elevation of the upper ribs, the diaphragm is elevated and the abdominal wall is sucked in passively. This latter method of breathing, if habitual for speech, can be injurious to the voice, since it is accompanied by the expenditure of much muscular tension and a disproportionate amount of energy which does not assist in increasing the volume of air inspired nor its control in expiration for phonation. Tension will also overflow into neck and laryngeal muscles. Clavicular breathing is never taught as a method in connection with voice production but is sometimes taught by physiotherapists when dealing with chronic bronchial catarrh and 'postural drainage' of the lungs. Upper thoracic breathing frequently develops in especially tense and nervous individuals and is encountered in patients suffering from vocal strain. It is also common in asthmatic patients as a direct result of dyspnoea and the effort to ventilate the lungs which accompanies contraction of the muscles of the bronchioli and difficulty in expiration.

In the correct and desirable intercostal diaphragmatic or central method of respiration for phonation the volume of inspired air and the control of expiration can be achieved voluntarily and without effort or strain. The movement downwards of the dia-phragm which contains no proprioceptive nerve endings and contraction of the intercostals cannot be felt consciously, but awareness of movements of the ribs and abdominal wall can be felt under the hands and the individual may thus learn voluntary control of the required respiratory movements. Aikin (1951) describes the regulation voluntarily of the upper abdominal muscles in the area above the umbilicus while the lower region of the abdominal wall remains passive but supporting the abdominal organs. Deliberate forward and backward movement of the upper abdomen in conjunction with rise and fall of the costal margin is utilised in teaching central breathing technique.

A different method of breathing is advocated by teachers of singing and acting in order to give added support to the voice. This is known as 'die Stütze' (hold) in German (Luchsinger, 1953) and 'appui' (support) in French (Tarneaud, 1961). These terms appear to be synonymous with 'rib reserve' in English, which refers to the anatomical and physiological process of obtaining the required breath support and strength to the voice, and not the subjective sensations experienced by the singer implied in the terms 'Stütze' and 'appui'. Tarneaud in discussing this problem says that whatever the process which produces the entirely subjective experience of support to the voice and its increased resonation, its existence is unquestionably in evidence from the improved voice when support is achieved. It gives the voice a precious element of stability and solidity. These sensations are phonetically and artistically indispensable although apparently indefinable physiologically since they include the sum total of both respiratory and phonatory technique. The feeling of thoracic support and tension would seem to be evoked by the opposing actions of the external intercostals and the diaphragm as described by Last (1960) who points out that as the ribs elevate the diaphragm is lifted by reason of its attachment to the ribs and as the diaphragm is pulled down by the central tendon it pulls downwards against the upward pull of the ribs.

The breathing technique which brings about 'die Stütze' and is incorporated in the 'rib reserve' method encompasses two different breathing techniques about which there has been and remains much confusion and disagreement. This concerns control of expiration during phonation. In one method the diaphragm must remain flattened in the inspiratory position while the chest wall (ribs) descends as air is utilised in voice. In the other method the ribs are held in elevation and in the inspiratory position while the diaphragm ascends and the abdominal wall is gradually retracted as air is utilised in voice. This latter method is, it seems, the more popular in England, and the rationale for its use appears the more logical. It presumably ensures a more effective universal resonator for the voice than the intercostal diaphragmatic method in which expansion of the chest is steadily reduced in expiration and phonation. Another advantage is that when the diaphragm has risen to the maximal height, the ribs may be allowed to descend by relaxing the external intercostals and tensing the internal intercostals, thus providing a supplementary supply of air when the emergencies of a long aria or recitative necessitate, without recourse to inspiration and interruption of the note held.

The rib reserve technique is not advocated for teaching public speakers; being very difficult to master it is generally confined to the teaching of actors and singers, for whom the experts consider it essential.

Luchsinger (1965) gives a well-documented historical survey of the theories relating to phonic breath support in speech and particularly song.

Lieberman (1967) is to be recommended for a clear account of the subglottal system and respiration and an introduction to the scientific measurement of variables in production of pitch, volume, length of phrase and breath group.

THE DUAL CONTROL OF RESPIRATION

Respiration is chiefly controlled by the respiratory centre in the medulla from which impulses reach the striated voluntary muscles of respiration by way of the spinal nerves, which can also be regulated by the cerebral cortex. Respiration in this way is under both involuntary and voluntary nervous control and can function independently or in conjunction with the will as required by the needs of the individual at any particular moment.

The respiratory centre is sensitive to the amount of carbon dioxide in the blood and the rate of respiration is adjusted automatically to retain the proper ratio between carbon dioxide and oxygen. Hence it is that after strenuous exercise, when the muscle tissues have consumed oxygen and discharged an excess of carbon dioxide, we pant and puff to correct the balance. The centre is also responsive to the secretions of the endocrine glands and of hormones, such as adrenaline, into the blood in times of stress. Then nervousness and fear are experienced psychologically, with accelerated breathing as a somatic concomitant. The autonomic nervous system, as Walter (1953) puts it, is responsible for the 'domestic chores' of the body and is in charge of respiration when we are not thinking about it, in sleeping, unconsciousness and preoccupation. Respiration, however, can become a voluntary operation, and this makes possible the development of a breathing technique for vocal purposes. Like all voluntary motor habits, breathing habits for speech and singing may be so well learned that they become practically automatic; but they still retain a voluntary aspect since it requires volition to switch from quiet breathing for speech or singing and to maintain this adjustment in spite of primitive and vital breathing patterns. However, when the respiratory centre and central nervous system come into conflict it is always the former which triumphs. One may deliberately indulge in over-rapid breathing during which carbon dioxide is excessively exhaled and the normal chemical stimulation of respiration is removed. After a period of apnoea, however, carbon dioxide again collects sufficiently in the blood to stimulate the respiratory centre, and breathing recommences. (Pearce, 1959.)

In the following table comparison of the physiology of quiet breathing with that of breathing for speech demonstrates the extent and nature of the voluntary control which can be obtained over respiration in the development of breathing techniques for speech.

DUAL CONTROL OF RESPIRATION

A Comparative Table

Respiration for quiet purposes	*Respiration for speech*
1. Respiration for sole purpose of absorbing O_2 and excreting CO_2	1. Respiration for phonation
2. Involuntary	2. Voluntary
3. 500 c.c. air inspired	3. 1,500–2,000 c.c. air inspired for speech and 3,000–4,250 c.c. in singing
4. Minimal movement of respiratory muscles and passive role of accessory muscles	4. Increased movement of all muscles of respiration and active role of accessory muscles
5. Average of 15 inspirations per minute	5. Considerably fewer than 15 inspirations per minute
6. Inspiration and expiration time equivalent	6. Expiration time greatly exceeds inspiration time
7. Breathing through nose	7. Breathing through mouth
8. Respiratory tract uninterrupted	8. Respiratory tract interrupted by movements of vocal folds and organs of articulation

9. Expiration uninterrupted

10. Air pressure in expiration at a constant level

9. Constant pauses in expiration to meet the needs of phrasing and punctuation

10. Considerable variations in subglottic breath pressure and glottic resistance to regulate the volume and pitch of voice

3 Larynx
and phonation

The larynx, which contains the vocal cords, is situated in the neck at the level of the third to sixth cervical vertebrae. It forms a continuous tube with the trachea or windpipe below and opens into the laryngeal portion of the pharynx above. It consists of a skeletal framework of articulated cartilages, bound together by ligaments and membranes and activated by the intrinsic laryngeal muscles. The extrinsic laryngeal musculature is responsible for maintaining the position of the larynx in relation to the other structures in the neck, and its elevation and depression in swallowing, speaking and singing. The larynx is suspended from the hyoid bone which is in turn suspended from the back of the tongue. Movements of the back of the tongue therefore influence the position of the larynx.

THE SKELETON OF THE LARYNX

The larynx consists of nine cartilages; the thyroid and cricoid cartilages and the epiglottis are single cartilages; the arytenoid, corniculate and cuneiform cartilages are paired.

1. *The Thyroid Cartilage* (Fig. 9, diagram 1) is the largest cartilage and consists of two quadrilateral plates having superior and inferior horns projecting from their outer corners; the plates are fused together in mid-line at an angle which forms the laryngeal prominence or Adam's apple.

2. *The Cricoid Cartilage* (Fig. 9, diagram 2) is fashioned somewhat like a signet ring with the signet facing to the back, and is deep behind and narrow in front. Its lower edge is horizontal and forms the base and circumference of the larynx; it is attached by the criocotracheal ligament to the first ring of the trachea. The sides of the cricoid slant upwards, and the back forms the posterior wall of the larynx. It has two small facets on its external posterior and lateral surface with which the inferior horns of the thyroid cartilage articulate. At the back, and on the upper crest, there is a notch in the mid-line, on either side of which depression is presented a convex oval surface for articulation with the base

of each arytenoid cartilage. In front, the cricoid is connected to the thyroid by the cricothyroid ligament.

3. *The Arytenoid Cartilages* (Fig. 9, diagram 3) are roughly pyramidal in shape. The concave base of each articulates with the articulatory facet of the cricoid cartilage, forming a mobile synovial joint. The apex articulates with the claw-like corniculate cartilage. The medial surface is smooth and flat and confronts the cartilage of the opposite side. From the apex, an angular crest

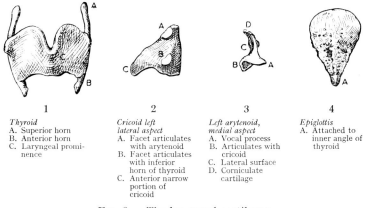

1	2	3	4
Thyroid	*Cricoid left*	*Left arytenoid,*	*Epiglottis*
A. Superior horn	*lateral aspect*	*medial aspect*	A. Attached to
B. Anterior horn	A. Facet articulates	A. Vocal process	inner angle of
C. Laryngeal promi-	with arytenoid	B. Articulates with	thyroid
nence	B. Facet articulates	cricoid	
	with inferior	C. Lateral surface	
	horn of thyroid	D. Corniculate	
	C. Anterior narrow	cartilage	
	portion of		
	cricoid		

Fig. 9   The laryngeal cartilages

projects downwards and inwards into the laryngeal cavity, terminating in a point, the vocal process. The lateral angle is a rounded prominence projecting backwards and sideways, and it forms the muscular process which gives insertion to the posterior and lateral cricoarytenoid muscles (page **41**). The vocal cord is attached to the vocal process of the arytenoid and to the inner aspect of the angle of the thyroid. Movement of the arytenoid is therefore responsible for alteration in the position of the vocal cord.

4. *The Corniculate Cartilage* (Fig. 9, diagram 3) or the cartilage of Santorini, is a minute cone-shaped cartilage articulating with the apex of the arytenoid and sometimes fused with it. The corniculate projects into the aryepiglottic fold.

5. *The Cuneiform Cartilage* (Fig. 9, diagram 3) (cartilage of Wrisberg), is a tiny club-shaped cartilage placed in the aryepiglottic fold where it shows as a whitish bump beneath the mucous membrane just beside the corniculate (see Fig. 16). The cuneiform cartilage acts as a passive prop and helps to maintain the upright

position of the aryepiglottic fold when pulled and stretched by movement of the arytenoid.

6. *The Epiglottis* (Fig. 9, diagram 4) is a leaf-shaped cartilage which projects obliquely upwards from the interior of the larynx past the thyroid to the base of the tongue. The stalk is attached to the thyroid cartilage by the thyroepiglottic ligament, a little below the thyroid notch in the interior angle of the laryngeal prominence. The epiglottis helps to close the larynx in swallowing. Negus (1949) thought that the epiglottis was a residual vestige of an earlier developmental stage in animals when a funnel of cartilage extended to the soft palate and was useful in olfaction but that the epiglottis in man today serves no useful function in swallowing. Ardran and Kemp (1967) basing their opinion on the evidence of radiographic studies state that the epiglottis performs an essential function in protecting the larynx and airway in swallowing. The epiglottis is pulled backwards over the laryngeal entrance, the sides are bent downwards and food or liquid is deflected down the lateral food channels on either side of the larynx.

MUSCLES OF THE LARYNX

The muscles of the larynx are classified according to their position and function as extrinsic and intrinsic laryngeal muscles. The extrinsic muscles, the supra- and infrahyoid muscles and the cricopharyngeal muscle exert a steadying influence on the larynx, performing the functions of anchorage, elevation and depression. The intrinsic muscles are attached to the laryngeal cartilages and are concerned with movement of the vocal cords.

The Extrinsic Muscles of the Larynx

The cricopharyngeus muscle is composed of the lower fibres of the inferior constrictor of the pharynx. It arises from the lateral plates of the cricoid cartilage and encircles the junction between the hypopharynx and the oesophagus (Fig. 11). It anchors the cricoid and, therefore, the whole larynx against the pharyngo-oesophageal wall (Negus, 1949). Its fibres also form the oesophageal sphincter which normally closes the gullet but relaxes on swallowing when it allows the sphincter to open and the larynx to ascend. The steadying influence of the cricopharyngeus on the larynx during phonation is of importance. It is particularly active in production of notes of low pitch: by pulling the cricoid forward it shortens the vocal cords (Zenker, 1964a).

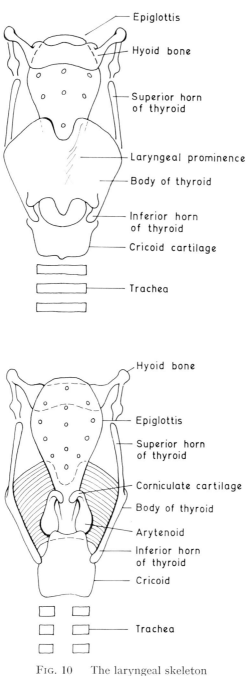

Epiglottis

Hyoid bone

Superior horn
of thyroid

Laryngeal prominence

Body of thyroid

Inferior horn
of thyroid

Cricoid cartilage

Trachea

Hyoid bone

Epiglottis

Superior horn
of thyroid

Corniculate cartilage

Body of thyroid

Arytenoid

Inferior horn
of thyroid

Cricoid

Trachea

FIG. 10   The laryngeal skeleton

The suprahyoid muscles elevate the hyoid bone and therefore the larynx through the intervention of the thyrohyoid muscle which connects the larynx with the hyoid (Fig. 12). The suprahyoid muscles are chiefly used in swallowing and elevation of the

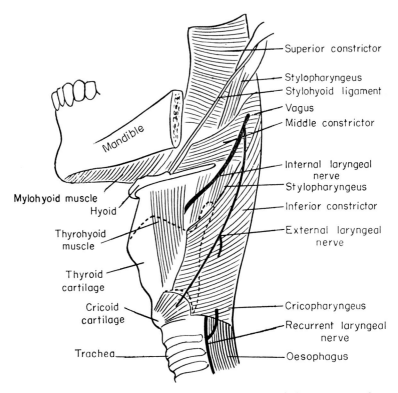

Fig. 11   Some extrinsic muscles of the larynx and the nerve supply

tongue. The chief muscles are the stylohyoid, mylohyoid and geniohyoid (Fig. 19).

The infrahyoid muscles or 'strap' muscles anchor, depress or elevate the larynx by exerting a pull on the hyoid bone or larynx. The omohyoid and sternohyoid depress the hyoid after it has been elevated in deglutition or the production of high notes in singing. The sternothyroid draws the larynx down after elevation. The thyrohyoid depresses the hyoid bone or raises the larynx. In production of very low notes contraction of the muscles depressing the larynx takes place. Vocal cord length is smallest for low tones, but the shortening of the cords with decreasing pitch cannot be due to active inner tension alone and for the lowest as well as highest notes the help of the extrinsic muscles of the larynx is necessary. Sonninen (1968), in examining what he calls 'the external frame function' in the control of pitch in the human voice, demonstrates how the action of the sternothyroid is antagonistic to the pull of the cricothyroid and active in singing at both extremes of the vocal range. His diagrams illustrating the pulls and stresses on the laryngeal cartilages by the various muscle forces and 'functional chains' are of great clarity. Sonninen made sonographic records of singers while taking cine radiographic films. He used calcified areas in the laryngeal cartilages

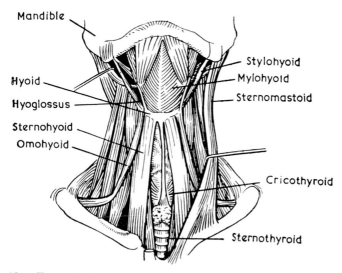

Fig. 12   Front of the neck, showing suprahyoid and infrahyoid muscles

(which became more sharply defined with increasing age) as reference points or landmarks for gauging cartilage position.

Faaborg-Andersen and Nykøbing (1965) examined the action potential of the extrinsic laryngeal muscles electromyographically. They found there was pronounced activity in the sternothyroid muscle in low- and high-pitched phonation but a decrease in the middle pitch. The mylohyoid on the other hand showed pronounced activity in the middle of the tone scale and decreased in low and high pitch.

The position of the hyoid bone and larynx is determined to a large extent by the balanced tonus of the supra- and infrahyoid groups of muscles (Last, 1960).

The Intrinsic Muscles of the Larynx

The intrinsic laryngeal muscles are attached to both the inner and outer surfaces of the larynx. Unlike the extrinsic muscles they do not affect the spatial relations of the larynx but are responsible for movements of the cartilages, sphincteric closure of the larynx in swallowing, and adduction and abduction of the vocal cords in phonation.

The vocal ligaments are formed by the upper free margins of the conus elasticus (cricovocal membrane) which consists of thickened fibrous and elastic connective tissue lying over the vocalis muscle. The fibres of the vocalis muscle form the medial portion of the thyroarytenoid muscle. The conus elasticus actually provides the origin of the vocalis muscle. (Negus, 1957.) (Fig. 13, diagrams *A* and *B*.) The vocalis muscle fibres are inserted into the vocal process of the arytenoid from which the fibres fan out into the cricovocal membrane.

The vocal cords extend from the middle of the angle of the thyroid cartilage or Adam's apple to the arytenoids behind (Fig. 14, diagrams *A* and *B*). The cords are therefore fixed in front but follow the movements of the arytenoid cartilages behind and thus form the lateral boundaries of the glottic aperture. This is triangular in shape when the arytenoids are abducted, but is closed forming a slit when the arytenoids are adducted for phonation (see Fig. 17).

The intrinsic laryngeal muscles are of importance on account of their functional relationship to the varying positions of the vocal cords. The muscles are named after the cartilages to which they are attached. The chief muscles are the criocothyroid muscle, the thyroarytenoid, the posterior cricoarytenoid, the lateral cricoarytenoid and the transverse arytenoid. The transverse arytenoid is a single muscle, the rest are paired.

1. *The Cricothyroid Muscle.* This muscle, which is fan-shaped, originates in the outer anterior and lateral surfaces of the cricoid cartilage and is inserted in the lower border of the plate and inferior horn of the thyroid cartilage (Fig. 13, diagram *D*). When the muscle contracts the cricoid is tilted up in front and down behind, thus increasing the distance between the arytenoid and the angle of the thyroid and so lengthening the vocal cord. The approximation of the anterior upper border of the cricoid towards the thyroid is compared to the action of a visor upon the cricothyroid joint by Ardran and Kemp (1966).

The lengthening of the vocal fold which takes place does not necessarily mean an increase in its tension. Last (1960) expresses it clearly and simply when he explains the action of the cricothyroid thus: 'the vocal fold consists of a felted membrane of fibro-elastic tissue whose strands run in all directions. Squares of this network are converted into diamonds by increased length of the vocal folds without an increase in tension'. The cricothyroid with the cricopharyngeus is active in production of low notes.

The cricothyroid muscle is innervated by the external branch of the superior laryngeal nerve and is the only muscle not to be supplied by the recurrent laryngeal nerve (Fig. 11).

2. *The Thyroarytenoid Muscle.* This muscle originates in the internal aspect of the angle of the thyroid cartilage, the crico-thyroid ligament and the wing of the thyroid, and is inserted in the anterior and lateral surfaces of the arytenoid cartilage. The relation of the thyroarytenoid to the vocal ligament is described above and illustrated in Fig. 13, diagrams *B* and *C*.

The thyroarytenoid is innervated by the recurrent laryngeal nerve.

The vocalis muscle forms the medial and outer portion of the thyroarytenoid muscle (page 38). The thyroarytenoid muscles when contracted oppose the lengthening of the vocal cords brought about by the action of the cricothyroid muscle and determine the degree of tension and the bulk of the main body of the vocal cords. The vocalis muscle when it contracts bunches up the conus elasticus and thereby increases the vertical depths of the opposing surfaces of the cords, which is an important factor in producing low vocal notes (Fig. 18).

On account of its elasticity the thyroarytenoid is often called the 'internal tensor' of the vocal cords by laryngologists who refer to 'bowing' of the vocal cords due to internal tensor weakness in patients with dysphonia.

3. *The Posterior Cricoarytenoid Muscle.* This originates in the broad depression of the posterior and outer surface of the cricoid and is inserted in the muscular process of the arytenoid (Fig. 13, diagram *E*). It consists of both vertical and oblique fibres. The vertical fibres brace the arytenoid back against the pull of the thyroarytenoid, while the lateral fibres also pull the cartilage outwards and laterally. Traditionally it is considered to be the sole abductor of the vocal cord.

Stroud and Zwiefach (1956) point out that the chief function of this muscle is to pull the arytenoid back, whereas its action as

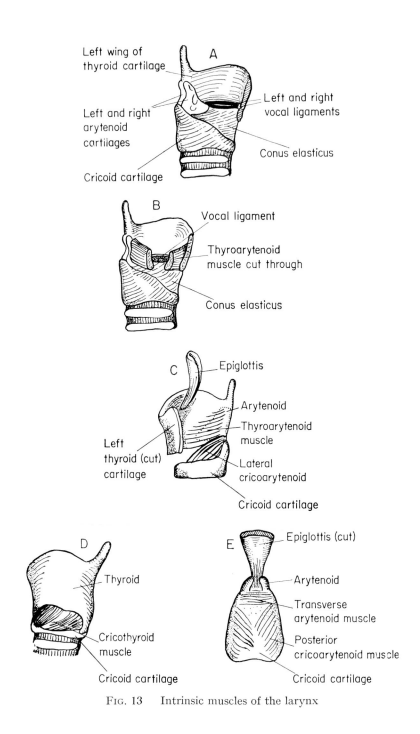

FIG. 13   Intrinsic muscles of the larynx

abductor and external rotator of the vocal fold is weak. It is innervated by the recurrent laryngeal nerve.

4. *The Lateral Cricoarytenoid Muscle* arises from the superior margin of the cricoid cartilage and passes back obliquely upwards

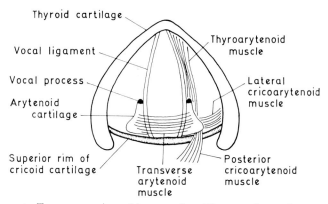

A: Transverse view of laryngeal cartilages and muscles

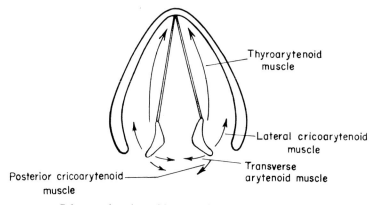

B: Scheme of action of laryngeal muscles on vocal cords

Fig. 14   Transverse view of laryngeal muscles with scheme of their action on the vocal cords

to be inserted in the anterior border of the muscular process of the arytenoid cartilage (Fig. 13, diagram *C*). According to classical anatomy this muscle adducts the vocal folds by rotating the arytenoid cartilage internally and drawing it forwards as in Fig. 14*B*. Stroud and Zwiefach (1956) draw attention to the

fact that the lateral fibres are almost in line with the long axis
of the cricoarytenoid joint so that their contractions must pull the
cartilage laterally and *outwards*. The more medial fibres of the
lateral cricoarytenoid muscle may draw the arytenoid forward
and rotate the cartilage *inwards*, in which case the lateral cricoarytenoid and posterior cricoarytenoid muscles act as synergists
maintaining the arytenoid cartilage sensitively poised. At times,
however, both muscles may act as abductors when the action of
the oblique fibres of the lateral cricoarytenoid predominates. The
lateral cricoarytenoid is innervated by the recurrent laryngeal
nerve.

   Ardran and Kemp (1966) in their study of the movements of
the arytenoid cartilages question the validity of accepted teaching
which describes the arytenoids as rotating about a vertical axis
or gliding towards or away from each other. (Gray, 1946; Negus,
1949.) Closure of the glottis, they find, is dependent upon apposition of the vocal processes which is brought about by a rocking
movement of the arytenoids on the cricoid border with an internal
rotation of the whole arytenoid about a vertical axis of about 10
degrees. Von Leden and Moore (1961) investigated the mechanics
of the cricoarytenoid joint and describe gliding and rocking
movements. Broad (1968) following up this investigation explains
that the gliding and rocking movements of the arytenoid are
determined by the geometry of the articular interface. The rocking
movement is utilised in vibration of the whole cord in low notes.

   5. *The Transverse Arytenoid Muscle.* This muscle connects the
posterior and part of the medial surfaces of the arytenoid cartilages
(Fig. 13, diagram *E*). Contraction of the muscle draws the arytenoids up over the shoulders of the cricoid and approximates
them without rotating them. It is the one intrinsic muscle of the
larynx whose action is unequivocal and solely that of adduction
of the vocal cords. It is innervated by the recurrent laryngeal
nerve from both sides.

The Aryepiglottic Folds

Two bands of muscular fibres pass over the transverse arytenoid
from the back of the muscular process of one arytenoid to the
apex of the other forming an X and constitute the oblique arytenoid muscles. Some of the fibres continue round the lateral
margin of the apex of the arytenoid cartilages and are prolonged
into the aryepiglottic folds and constitute the aryepiglottic
muscles. The oblique arytenoids and the aryepiglottic muscles

bring the aryepiglottic folds together and approximate the arytenoid cartilages to the tubercle of the epiglottis. They are active in swallowing and in tense abnormal phonation.

THE CAVITY OF THE LARYNX

The cavity of the larynx extends from the inlet, which is bounded by the aryepiglottic folds, to the outlet which is continuous with the trachea. The cavity is divided by two pairs of folds, the

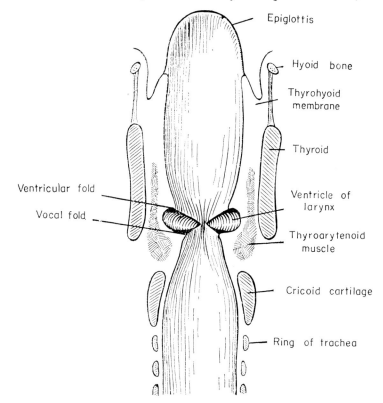

FIG. 15   Coronal section of the larynx, the anterior section being viewed from behind

ventricular and the vocal. 'Each thyroarytenoid fold is divided by a lateral recess or ventricle into an upper division or ventricular band and lower division known as the vocal fold' (Negus, 1949). (Figs. 15 and 16.)

The vocal fold or cord extends from the vocal process of the arytenoid to the middle of the angle of the thyroid and its free edge is banded by the vocal ligament formed by the upper expanded and lateral portion of the conus elasticus as already explained (page 38). The vocal ligaments are white in colour in contrast to the muscular folds which are pink.

The ventricular folds, also called the vestibular or false cords, are red in colour and plainly distinguishable in a laryngoscopic view from the white ligaments. The space between the upper and lower folds of the thyroarytenoid muscle is known as the sinus of

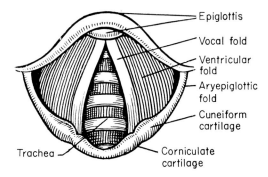

Epiglottis
Vocal fold
Ventricular fold
Aryepiglottic fold
Cuneiform cartilage
Corniculate cartilage
Trachea

Fig. 16   Laryngoscopic view of the interior of the larynx

the larynx or ventricle (of Morgagni), and the triangular aperture between the cords is the glottis.

The laryngeal cavity is covered by ciliated mucous membrane continuous with that of pharynx, nose and trachea, and supplied by sensory fibres of the internal branch of the superior laryngeal nerve. The vocal ligaments are covered by squamous epithelium to withstand friction. The larynx is well supplied with mucous glands especially in the region of the ventricle, so that the surfaces of the folds are constantly bathed in mucus and lubricated to prevent friction.

FUNCTIONS OF THE LARYNX

The primary function of the larynx is to close the air passage by means of the sphincteric action of its muscular folds. The vocal cords and ventricular bands close together in swallowing and prevent the entry of food into the trachea and lungs. Coughing is also preceded by forceful closure of both true and false folds which follows a quick inspiration due to sudden descent of the diaphragm. Air pressure is then built up below the adducted cords as the diaphragm ascends spasmodically, aided by the abdominal muscles, until the cords separate explosively and mucus is expelled. During any form of strong exertion involving use of the arms, the folds are again firmly closed preventing expulsion of air and collapse of the lungs so that a fixed origin for the arm and shoulder muscles is provided.

When the larynx is at rest and respiration quiet, the vocal cords remain abducted and move up and down slightly in sympathy with outflow and inflow of respiratory air. Ardran and Kemp (1966) on radiographic evidence emphasise that the cords

Full abduction   Gentle abduction   Gentle whisper

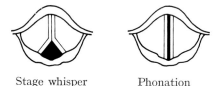

Stage whisper   Phonation

FIG. 17   Positions of vocal cords in action
Laryngoscopic view of vocal cords in phonation (open phases)
Coronal view of vocal cords in phonation, closed phase (from tomographs),
showing changes in bulk of cords

do not move in and out and obstruct the air passage but on the contrary are folded upwards into the ventricles and obliterate most of their cavities, the width of the glottis being only slightly less than the diameter of the cricoid. It is, however, common experience to see the folds moving gently up and down in a direct laryngoscopic view of the anaesthetised patient, while the airway remains widely open.

The cords are drawn wide apart to a position of full abduction in forceful inspiration. In quiet whispering the folds are slightly separated along the anterior two-thirds and a triangular aperture remains posteriorly. In a strong whisper the folds are adducted firmly along the anterior two-thirds and air is forced through the posterior triangle with considerable friction. (Luchsinger, 1965a, page 119.)

The anterior two-thirds of the vocal cords is known as the muscular portion or 'pars vocalis', and the posterior third is the cartilaginous or arytenoid portion and sometimes described as the 'pars respiratus'. In phonation the folds are adducted together in the mid-line or median position (Fig. 17).

PHONATION

In phonation the vocal cords are adducted by the interarytenoideus muscle and offer resistance to expired air in their closed phase until the pressure builds up and blows them asunder. Then the pressure immediately drops below the cords which are sucked back to their original position in the mid-line. This is known as the Bernouilli effect of air pressure in the larynx. Air thus escapes through the glottis in pulses on the siren principle which is economical of air. The alternating pressure working back and forth creates the sound waves which determine the fundamental pitch of the voice. Perfect phonation on any pitch depends upon the exact adjustment and balance of tension between the intrinsic muscles of the larynx and subglottic breath pressure.

For all pitches the mobile edges of the cords just make contact and brush together in the closed excursion of each phase. The glottal plosive, however, proves an exception; here the cords make abrupt contact for an instant, the breath stream being interrupted and then released explosively. The glottal plosive is used in dialect and precedes vowels in educated speech as a means of emphasis. It is also the normal mode of articulation for German vowels at the beginning of words. When its use is a phonemic aspect of language it is innocuous but when it is a physiological symptom of laryngeal tension and incorrect methods of voice production it can be harmful. Luchsinger and Arnold (1965) note that the soft attack denotes pleasant emotions of joy and pleasure while hard attack denotes moods of fear, anger and impatience. Hard attack is a symptom of laryngeal tension and if present in excess the sensitive membrane covering the folds may be damaged and the delicate laryngeal musculature strained. Koike, Hirano and Von Leden (1967) investigated soft attack, hard attack and breathy attack. Soft initiation of phonation was characterised by a long rise time from period of onset of sound to its maximum amplitude, and a small amount of air consumption. Hard attack was characterised by short rise time and considerable amount of air consumption.

Breathy attack showed a different pattern and a basic physio-logical difference, as would be anticipated.

The easy rhythmic excursions of the vocal cords in normal, healthy voice production can be heard in the normal vibrato or pulses of sound. This is not heard in breathy, strained or harsh voices and is therefore of diagnostic significance giving both physical and physiological clues.

The human voice is capable of a wide range of pitch; the un-trained singer can cover one and a half octaves and a trained

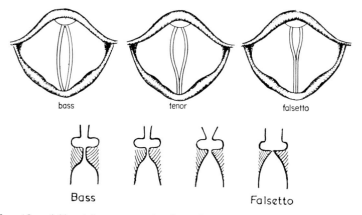

Fig. 18   (*Above*) laryngoscopic view of vocal cords in phonation, open phase; (*below*) coronal view of vocal cords in phonation, closed phase (from tomographs)

singer two and a half. It is impossible for the vocal cords to cover this range with the same manner of vibration throughout, and a different mechanism must accordingly be used for different parts of the compass. The tension, length and thickness of the vocal cords determine the pitch of the voice: considerable variations in the shape of the thyroarytenoid muscles being possible.

In cross-section the fold is wedge-shaped being flat on top and shelving away obliquely below but it retains this shape only for the middle notes of the voice. The vocalis muscle through its action on the conus elasticus is responsible for what are known as the thick and thin registers, or more usually the 'head' and 'chest' registers. Negus (1957) prefers the terms thick and thin since 'these describe actual facts' and have long been used in singing (Dawson, 1902). On *high* notes when many or all of the thyroarytenoid muscle fibres are in contraction, the vocalis muscle pulls the conus elasticus outwards, thus reducing the opposing areas of the vocal folds. This is clearly shown in X-ray tomographs (Fig. 18). On *low* notes, when elasticity of the glottic margins is at its maximum, excursions of large amplitude are possible. The conus is not pulled outward and medially for production of low notes. The thyroarytenoid and cricothyroid are relaxed, action of the vocalis deepens the opposing surfaces of the vocal folds to an extent of 3–5 mm. in depth. The large mass of muscle recoils relatively slowly when blown apart by lung air. In the high-speed motion photography of the Bell Laboratories Film (1937) the slow rolling apart of the opposing surfaces of the folds is clearly demonstrated, starting below and finishing above in a sort of figure-of-eight.

The alterations in the shape and tension of the vocal folds to the needs of vocal pitch require fine and exact regulation. The greatest skill in singing is necessary in effecting the transition from the middle to the falsetto or head register without a break, which cannot be avoided in untrained or strained voices. The thyroarytenoid and vocalis muscles working in concert have to be balanced delicately against the antagonistic action of the cricothyroid and posterior cricoarytenoid and the subglottic air pressure.

Added to the changes in length, tension and thickness of the vocal cords notable changes in the size of the laryngeal ventricles take place in sympathy with movement of the intrinsic laryngeal muscles and cartilages. Modification in resonance is produced by altering positions of the epiglottis and aryepiglottic folds which in the chest register may be drawn far back towards the posterior pharyngeal wall allowing only a very small aperture above the larynx. This constriction produces an acoustic filter which amplifies the lower harmonics and stops the higher partials. It is an important feature in producing the balanced tone of bass notes.

The famous Bell film mentioned above has been followed by others, such as those by Luchsinger, Vallancien, Timcke, Leden and Moore and others (Van den Berg, 1962) which contribute further insight into the function of the larynx in phonation. Van den Berg (1958 and 1964) has examined excised human larynges under air pressure by high-speed cine photography. Smith (1947) has contributed his experimental research with membrane cushion models. Luchsinger and Arnold (1965) having specialised in voice physiology and the physiology of singing for many years have given perhaps the most comprehensive account of the facts based on their own research and summarising that of others.

Rubin and Hirt (1960) have made a high-speed cinematographic film of the larynx at 6,000–8,000 frames per second, compared with the 4,000 frames per second of the Bell film. Voices were recorded simultaneously with the film by using a contact microphone applied to the thyroid cartilage. They studied in particular the transition from the middle to higher register because a break in the voice is particularly difficult to avoid in singing and a large part of a singer's training is devoted to obtaining a smooth transition. Considerable lengthening of the vocal cords takes place as pitch rises from the low to high fundamental but no lengthening of the vocal cords takes place in falsetto. In the transition period the taut and stretched vocal cords have to relax suddenly and in the untrained singer the vocal cords are described by these authors as 'wobbling loosely without touching each other, resembling banners waving in the breeze'. The true falsetto is achieved by an astonishingly complex series of intra-laryngeal adjustments. There are two methods by which falsetto is achieved. In the first there is an 'open chink mechanism' in which the vocal cords present a wave-like or rolling motion with the anterior section closing as the anterior opens in the same vibratory phase. Changes in pitch are achieved by changes of breath pressure. The second common vibratory pattern is one in which the margins of the vocal cords strike each other as in the fundamental register with the main mass of the thyroarytenoid less active and some activity in the medial fibres. In skilled singers the transition from head to falsetto registers cannot be detected by ear and both open and closed chink mechanisms may be used on the same note. A third type of mechanism is a stop-closure or clamping in the very highest range of falsetto when the two other mechanisms do not allow increase in pitch and is accompanied by progressive closure of the glottis from posterior to anterior commissure. When a pin-point opening remains there is a squeak or whistle. This is difficult to film because the epiglottis closes down over the larynx and the resonating chamber assumes its smallest dimensions. Sonninen (1968) has attacked the problems involved in another way as already described (page 37) and stresses the important function of the extrinsic laryngeal muscles in singing especially in the technique of 'covered voice' discussed more fully under singing (page 28).

RESEARCH IN VOICE PHYSIOLOGY

The physiological basis of phonation holds a persistent fascination for research workers, especially in the United States where many important research projects have been financed and research fellowships awarded to distinguished scientists from other countries to enable team collaboration. The result has been a wealth of valuable articles in scientific journals some of which must be mentioned for the benefit of the post-graduate student. It is often stated that such research is of little value to the ordinary clinician but this is not so, since frequently the discoveries made are relevant to diagnosis and treatment of the patient and it is the task of the clinical therapist to understand the value, see the relevance and apply new knowledge in practical ways.

Voice physiology research is aimed at discovering how this most remarkable human vocal instrument works. Although the scientist is the first to concede that the ear is still the best assessor of an individual's voice because psychological elements enter into the process as well as physiological, there are always different avenues to explore in an endeavour to explain the perfection of co-ordination and the infinite variety of delicate muscular adjustments which go into the production of voiced and voiceless sounds, oral and nasal sounds, rising and falling inflection, changes in volume and stress, and the reflection of feeling in vocal timbre, all happening simultaneously—flickering over utterance in a way it is difficult to explain in ordinary terms of cortical control of voluntary muscle.

HUSSON'S THEORY OF VOCAL CORD VIBRATION

It was Raoul Husson who first questioned the traditionally accepted view of vocal cord vibration. It had always been accepted without any reason to doubt that action of the vocal folds was regulated by the laryngeal muscles, and voice was produced by the rhythmic separation and recoil of the vocal folds under the influence of the subglottic air pressure as described in previous pages. This is known as the myoelastic, aerodynamic or tonic theory. In 1950 Raoul Husson put forward his neuromuscular, neurochronaxic or clonic theory of vocal fold vibration, in his famous address to the Paris Faculté des Sciences. His theory was later supported and ably defended by Portman, Robin and Laget (1956). Husson and his supporters maintained that the larynx was not *the* vocal organ but only one of the elements in the voice mechanism. They contended that every single vibration of the vocal folds was due to an impulse from the recurrent laryngeal nerves and that the acoustic centre in the brain regulated the speed of vocal fold vibration *'coup par coup'*. These vocal fold vibrations, which were the direct result of nervous impulses, set in motion the air column and it was not the air column which set in vibration the vocal folds.

The case of Husson was so well documented that those who immediately leapt into the battle and energetically opposed the neurochronaxic theory as utter nonsense had, none the less, to produce a considerable amount of counter-research to disprove it. No other research project, let it be said, produced a shred of evidence to support Husson's theory, and the excitement and stimulation the controversy engendered in the fifties is now old history. Nevertheless, a wealth of enormously valuable information was produced as a result of the research it stimulated and we learned more about the physiology of the voice in that decade than in any other, thanks to Husson's erroneously but sincerely conceived challenge. The fact that he was proved wrong does not matter any more. He must be respected for the fact that he had the courage to question accepted dogma and by questioning made others think.

For the postgraduate student the following excellent reports are available and are none the less instructive for the fact that they produce negative evidence of the validity of Husson's theory. Negus, Neil and Floyd (1957), Rubin (1960), Van den Berg (1958), Von Leden (1961) who devoted five years of systematic study to the problem, Weiss (1959) and Froeschels (1957) have all made valuable contributions to the subject.

PRESENT TRENDS IN LARYNGEAL RESEARCH

New instrumental methods for examining movements of the vocal cords, the change of shape of the laryngeal cavity in phonation, and action of individual muscles contribute further knowledge every year. Exploration of the problems involved is by no means exhausted because of the fascination which stimulates research projects.

A great advance in techniques for visual observation of the larynx virtually adds a third dimension to the image by amplifying its intensity when thrown on the fluorescent screen by electronic means. The image-intensifier opens up new vistas for inspection of sagittal and transverse X-ray tomographic studies of the laryngeal, oral and pharyngeal structures in action. The X-ray image-intensifier is an indispensable instrument in diagnosis of pathological conditions, for example in cleft palate, cancer of the larynx, and laryngeal palsy. Already many films have been made employing this method, and that of Vallancien is particularly clear. The work of Ardran and Kemp (1966, 1967) has already been described.

Another avenue of research into the complex problems of function of the intrinsic laryngeal muscles is presented by the possibilities of inserting electrode needles into individual muscles and obtaining electromyographs of muscle activity, a technique which has been extensively explored by Faaborg-Anderson (1964) but 'causes some discomfort to the subject which he does not always recognise as necessary'. Another snag is that needles are liable to jump out of muscles when there is too much activity in them.

The Laryngostroboscope: Stroboscopy is the procedure of illuminating a vibrating or rotating object with an intermittent flash of light instead of a continuous beam. By adjusting the frequency of the flash to that of the frequency of vibration of the object, the object can appear to stand still in any phase of its vibration. If the frequency of flash is raised slightly above or below that of the vibrating object it will appear to move in slow motion. A throat microphone is used to synchronise the strobo-scopic flash with that of the vocal pitch in electro-laryngo-stroboscopy. The application of electrostroboscopic illumination in indirect laryngoscopy is a great advantage in observing vibra-tion of the vocal cords and detecting abnormal movement, such as the cords being out of phase with each other or sectionally, which occurs both in strained voices and early malignancy. Luchsinger and Arnold (1965) say 'It may be stated that electron stroboscopy is indispensable for comprehensive laryngological diagnosis'. The equipment is expensive and it takes time and perseverance to grow so accustomed to it that it can be used routinely by the laryngologist as a diagnostic method. It is little used in England and in fact Mr Simpson of the Victoria Infirmary, Glasgow, is probably the only laryngologist using an electro-stroboscope in the British Isles. High-speed films which can be shown in slow motion serve the same purpose and again the equipment is expensive, a technical operator is necessary and time and space must be available. For practical reasons, therefore, filming of the vocal cords is confined to research projects.

Van Michel (1967) describes an apparatus called an électro-glottographe designed by Philippe Fabre in 1957. It consists of a generator of high-frequency waves which are passed through the larynx by two electrodes placed on either side of the thyroid cartilage. The modulations in frequency brought about by variations in impedance resulting from movements of the vocal cords are amplified and thrown on an oscilloscope screen or magnetic meter. This method of examination he claims to be useful in a wide range of disorders and with singers and has the great advantage of causing no discomfort to the subject.

To the average clinician, with none of these marvels of scientific research at his disposal, it is comforting to learn that the experienced voice therapist can compete successfully with electromyography and judge by ear the site of excess tension in the laryngeal muscles. Brewer, Briess and Faaborg-Anderson (1960) compared the electromyographic records of muscle imbalance in strained voices with the objective clinical assessment of voice and laryngeal function by Briess and found them to be substantially in agreement.

Animal experiments are also used in investigation of laryngeal function. The cat appears to be particularly suitable. Kirikae, *et al.* (1962) carried out an extensive and valuable study of the central motor innervation of laryngeal muscles in the cat under anaesthesia. Stimulation of the cortex of the cat was achieved by a stereotaxic instrument, movement of the laryngeal muscles being recorded electromyographically.

Zenker (1964) describes dissection of excised human larynges with staining of the thyroarytenoid muscle fibres and motor end plates which reveals an extremely complex system of fibre arrangements. Many fibres do not run all the way from arytenoid to thyroid but end in the interior muscle and can be linked to tendons within the muscle. Fibres thus connect different sections and layers of muscle and as they run in different directions they must be able to alter the pull within the muscle and influence different sections of the vocal cord. Zenker remarks: 'Our latest findings indicate how much more complicated the system is than it has so far been shown to be and how much greater is its plasticity. We have before us a keyboard upon which we are capable of playing in an enormous variety of different ways.'

While Zenker concentrated upon the motor fibres of the vocal cords, Kirchener and Wyke (1965) investigated the sensory mechanisms of the laryngeal joint capsules in cats. They found that the joint capsules are supplied with mechanoreceptors which are sensitive to mechanical stress and discharges from these mechanoreceptors into the nerves are capable of producing reflex changes in the tone of the intrinsic laryngeal muscles.

English and Blevins (1967) and Wyke (1967, 1969) further studied the laryngeal myotactic reflexes of the intrinsic muscles of the larynx in cats. The laryngeal muscles like skeletal muscles, are supplied with receptor nerve endings; these are very numerous, spiral in shape and like spring-coils encircle the individual muscle fibres. Discharges from these receptor nerve endings are capable of reflexly facilitating or inhibiting tone of the muscle-fibre groups with great rapidity in different sections of the laryngeal muscles at one and the same time. This mechanism, similar but doubtless more complex in the human, makes possible the rapid and precise moment-to-moment adjustments necessary in the tuning process of phonation and especially in singing. The mechanoreceptor reflexes originating in the laryngeal joints are involved in phonic co-ordination of the vocal cords and are complementary to the tonic myotactic reflex mechanoreceptors located within the laryngeal muscles.

The research findings of neuro-physiologists explain the extraordinary versatility of the human voice and the rapidity of movements observable in high-speed cine films which were previously quite inadequately explained in terms of the function of individual laryngeal muscles. Husson was aware of the need for a better explanation but unfortunately found one which could not be supported by scientific investigation.

It has been known for thirty years or more that the laryngeal mucosa is provided with a considerable number and variety of sensory nerve endings and that the corpuscular nerve endings are stimulated by mechanical stress and also changes in the intralaryngeal air pressure (Wyke, 1967). Stimulation of the mucosal system gives rise to the sphincteric reflex closure of the larynx which Negus (1949) described as a primitive and protective mechanism. The extreme sensitivity of the laryngeal mucosa which sparks off sphincteric closure of the larynx is of considerable significance in treatment of disorders of phonation. The irritability of the larynx arising out of even slight inflammation can be a self-perpetuating factor (a reflex servo system) in vocal strain and habitual hyperkinetic dysphonia which makes re-education difficult and accounts for the persistence of bad habits of phonation, in many cases grossly in excess of that anticipated at the outset of treatment.

4   Articulation
and resonance

The organs of articulation are the organs of mastication and deglutition adapted to the special purposes of speech. The lips, teeth, gums, jaws, tongue and hard and soft palates all co-operate in the articulation of consonants and vowels. Alterations in the size and shape of the oral cavity, which are brought about by alterations in the relative positions of these structures, produce sounds consisting of complex sound waves which are clearly distinguishable from one another and compose the vowel and consonant phonemes of spoken language. 'Frequency differences are the essential characteristics of the physical nature of speech sounds' (Ewing, 1930). These frequency characteristics are entirely dependent upon the placing of the organs of articulation in relation to compressed air in voiceless sounds and vibrating air in voiced sounds.

The Lips

The lips are mobile structures forming the orifice of the mouth and comprise the sphincteric muscle fibres of the orbicularis oris muscle. The risorius muscle retracts the angle of the mouth and 'produces an unpleasant grinning expression', Gray (1949) rather surprisingly informs us, overlooking its more pleasing risible function. The buccinator compresses and protrudes the lips (buccina-trumpet). The lips are used in the articulation of bilabial and labiodental sounds and also alter the shape of the oral cavity by varying degrees of rounding and spreading which contribute in part to vowel quality, as in the case of [u:] and [i:] and [ɔ:] and [a:].

The Tongue

The tongue is the most important organ of articulation as well as of swallowing. It is a highly mobile and active member entirely composed of muscle, capable not only of an infinite variety of movements, but also appreciable alterations in shape, thickening and thinning, bunching and humping, as it dances its way through speech. Alterations in shape are effected by the intrinsic muscles. These consist of an intricate network of superior and inferior longitudinal fibres and transverse and vertical ones. It is divided down its centre by a fibrous septum and is attached to the floor of the mouth by the frenum. The floor is formed by the mylohyoid muscle which arises along the inner edge of the mandible and is attached to the hyoid (Figs. 11, 12 and 19).

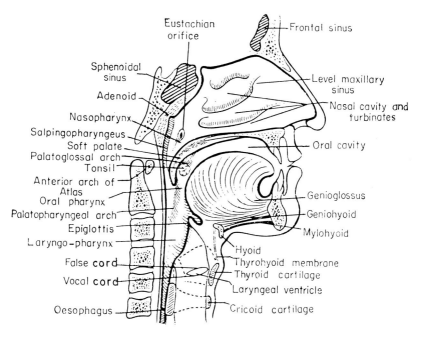

Fig. 19   Sagittal section through nose, mouth, pharynx and larynx to show relative positions of organs of articulation, resonance and phonation

The extrinsic muscles of the tongue are responsible for alterations in its position. The mylohyoid not only supports the tongue but assists in its elevation in swallowing and articulation of [k], [g] and [ŋ] and generally contributes to mobility. The genioglossus which forms the bulk of the tongue, protrudes it, and the lowest fibres are attached to the hyoid. The hyoglossus which draws the sides of the tongue downwards, arises from the horn of the hyoid and is inserted into the sides of the tongue. These movements of the tongue are closely associated with movements of the larynx through the common attachment to the hyoid bone.

The palatoglossus, another extrinsic muscle, is described in connection with the soft palate (page 58).

The tongue is responsible for altering the size and shape of the oral and pharyngeal cavities which act as coupled resonators to produce the characteristic quality of vowels and dipthongs. The majority of consonants are made by tongue movements against the teeth, gums and palate in such a manner as to cause plosion

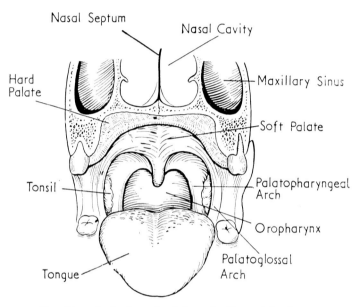

FIG. 20   Oral view of palate and pillars of the fauces

or friction. The only consonants in which the tongue plays a passive part are [p], [b], [m], [f], [v] and [h].

The vital contribution of the tongue in speech has always been recognised. Thus in the Bible we have a description of the 'confusion of tongues' and Moses telling the Lord that he is 'slow of tongue'. In Shakespeare's works there are many such references, for example Hamlet's injunction to the players to speak 'trippingly on the tongue', not to 'mouth', and Celia's 'Cry holla to thy tongue, I prithee; it curvets unseasonably'.

The word 'tongue' is no longer synonymous with 'language', as it is in French, except in the case of 'mother tongue', but the old usage persists in many idioms. We speak of one who is tongue-tied, of losing the tongue or finding it. We may caution a fellow to hold

his tongue or to keep a civil tongue in his head, while to put out
the tongue is symbolic of all the child would like to say but has no
time for in the need to make a speedy get-away.

The Soft Palate

The soft palate or velum when elevated divides the nasal cavity
from the oropharyngeal cavity. This is of primary importance in

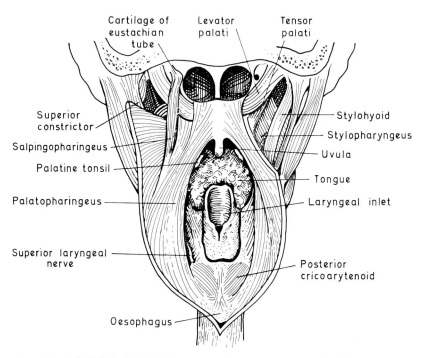

Fig. 21   Dissection of the pharynx, showing muscles of soft palate in
relation to tongue and larynx

swallowing and prevents the regurgitation of food down the nose.
Elevation of the palate is also of vital importance to the production
of good speech. The prevention of nasal escape of air is of great
importance in the articulation of consonants. Slight escape of
air down the nose (i.e. 'nasal escape' or 'nasal emission') does not
necessarily mean vowel nasality, but the ability to compress air
in the oral cavity is very necessary for the articulation of fricatives
and plosives. Massengil and Bryson (1967) carried out a cine
fluorographic study of velopharyngeal function as related to

perceived nasality of vowels in normal subjects, judged by a speech class of students. Although nasality increased with increasing size of palato-pharyngeal aperture as expected, some subjects were judged nasal despite complete closure and others even with as much as an 8 mm. gap were judged as having normal tone.

The muscles involved in the velopharyngeal sphincter of such vital importance to speech are difficult to assess individually and there are conflicting reports in the scientific studies relating the anatomy and physiology of the palate to reconstructive surgical techniques. Fritzell (1969) in his comprehensive and excellent report on his electro-myographic and cine-radiographic research into the activity of the velopharyngeal muscles in speech has clarified many questions and in the following description we rely heavily upon this work.

The velum is an entirely muscular structure forming a mobile flap which is attached to the posterior edge of the hard palate in front and hangs free behind terminating in the uvula. It is composed of several paired muscles.

The Tensor Palati hooks round the hamulus of the sphenoid and spreads out fanwise to meet its fellow from the opposite side. Its fibres divide into two layers posteriorly to enclose the musculus uvulae which forms the uvula. The body of the tensor palati forms the palatal aponeurosis to which the other muscles of the palate are attached. It is based on the anterior wall of the cartilaginous Eustachian tube. It is of little importance in speech and therefore its efficiency can be sacrificed in cleft palate operations when the hamulus is fractured in order to produce longer backward reaching palatal flaps. Plastic reconstructive surgery for cleft palate: the Wardill V–Y procedure (Morley, 1966; Braithwaite and Morley, 1963). Contraction of the tensor palati assists passage of the food bolus in swallowing and also effects opening of the Eustachian tube. Hence the practice of swallowing in order to equalise the external air pressure with that within the tube, to relieve feelings of pressure and deafness in air or underground rail travel.

The Palatoglossus is a small muscle arising from the transverse fibres within the tongue and ascends in the anterior pillar of the fauces to the palate forming the palatoglossal arch. It is of considerable importance in speech as Fritzell (1969) has demonstrated that the palate does not descend by the fall of gravity but is pulled down with rapidity in order to assist the essential quick flickering movement of the palate which is characteristic in articulation. Its action is antagonistic to the levator palati, another important muscle of the palate in controlling the palato-pharyngeal sphincter.

The Levator Palati arises in the petrous portion of the temporal bone, descends along the posterior and inferior border of the Eustachian tube and is inserted in the middle third of the soft palate to meet the levator fibres of the opposite side and interlace with other palatal muscles especially the palatopharyngeus.

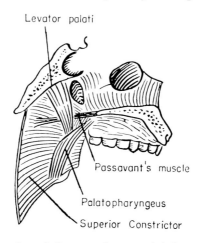

Fig. 22   The muscles of the nasopharyngeal isthmus and Passavant's
muscle (after Last)

It elevates the palate and its action is the most vital for competent palatopharyngeal closure.

The Palatopharyngeus muscle also arises in the palatal aponeu-rosis and enters the lateral walls of the pharynx. This muscle constitutes the posterior pillar of the fauces or *palatopharyngeal* arch. Specialised fibres of the palatopharyngeus muscle form a sphincter muscle at the level of the hard palate, running from its lateral and posterior border to encircle the pharynx inside the fibres of the superior constrictor of the pharynx. These fibres form Passavant's muscle which when contracted in swallowing raises a ridge, Passavant's ridge or cushion, at the level of the anterior arch of the atlas vertebra. Last (1960) states that it is incorrect to regard Passavant's muscle as part of the superior constrictor. Its fibres lie within the tube of the superior constrictor and are in continuity with the palatopharyngeus of which it is a part

(Fig. 22). Fritzell (1969) points out that there is considerable confusion in the literature concerning the anatomy and physiology of this muscle. At rest the soft palate hangs almost vertically. The nasopharynx varies very considerably in width and depth in different individuals, but on an average it is about 3 cm. in transverse diameter and 1 cm. in antero-posterior dimension, and is therefore not a very sizeable aperture. Lateral cine X-ray photography enables the accurate observation of movements of the soft palate and pharynx in speech. Calnan (1953) reported that there was very little observable difference in the articulatory mechanism of the velum for most of the vowels, nasals and

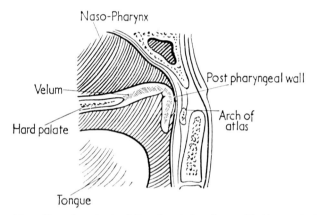

Fig. 23   Site of contact of the elevated velum with the posterior
pharyngeal wall in speech (after Calnan)

plosives. The velum is elevated and held at the ready before speech commences and then moves much less than is generally believed. Contraction of the salpingopharyngeus muscle which runs from the Eustachian tube to the thyroid cartilage also plays a part in closure of the pharynx by causing bunching of the lateral pharyngeal mucosa, and diminishing the transverse diameter of the pharynx by one third. The soft palate is raised highest of all for the vowel [i:], being lifted well above the level of the hard palate. The plosive consonants produce good elevation of the palate, but for [f] and [v] there is little elevation and little contraction of the lateral walls of the pharynx. Complete occlusion of the palatopharyngeal sphincter is not always present in non-nasal sounds, an observation also made by Russell (1931). In swallowing, complete nasopharyngeal closure takes place; a water-tight valve is formed by elevation of the palate, contraction of the lateral pharyngeal walls and forward movement of the pharynx as Passavant's muscle contracts.

It had long been accepted that Passavant's ridge played a vital part in nasopharyngeal closure in speech. Calnan (1954) in his article 'The error of Gustav Passavant' challenged the accepted view with the statement that Passavant's ridge appears at the level of the atlas vertebra which is *below* the elevation of the velum for speech. In the majority of people, the point at which the middle third of the soft palate kneels on the pharyngeal wall is appreciably above Passavant's ridge (Fig. 23). Sphincteric closure of the nasopharynx by Passavant's muscle and the levators of the palate occurs at the level of the atlas in swallowing only in these individuals. A minority of individuals, however, with perfectly normal speech obtain sphincteric closure through contact of the velum with Passavant's ridge. Nasal escape in these people is detectable, when a cold mirror is held beneath the nostrils (Greene, 1960). This may be associated with removal of adenoids in childhood.

It is now generally accepted that Passavant's muscle does not play a part in the speech of the majority of normal individuals. However, within the normal range there must occur differences in the relative dimensions of the palate and pharynx. In those individuals in whom the palate is rather short in relation to the posterior pharyngeal wall or in whom the pharynx is particularly deep and wide, compensation for the gap in closure may be obtained by raising Passavant's ridge. This modification takes place frequently in children after removal of adenoids. In cleft-palate individuals contraction of Passavant's muscle is more common and it is on this population that Gustav Passavant made his celebrated observations in 1873.

The superior constrictor was found to be consistently active in conjunction with the levator palati, by Fritzell (1969) but during connected speech it showed a great deal of variation. Activity related mostly to oral sounds and especially there was a burst of potential on 's', while nasal sounds were usually preceded by decrease of activity. Involvement of the palatopharyngeus was however not so consistent and clear in speech as the levator in speech. It does, or can, make a considerable contribution to lateral pharyngeal movement mesially and this is the basis of the rationale for pharyngeal flap reconstructive surgery in cleft palate which is discussed further in Chapter 13.

In conclusion we can say the levator palati is consistently active in production of oral speech sounds and is the most important of all the velopharyngeal muscles. The degree of activity varies with individuals and also in production of different vowel sounds. The palate rises in progressing from low to high vowels; from [aː] to [iː] and [uː]. The superior constrictor is also active throughout speech but less so than the levator.

THE RESONATORS

The resonators of the human voice are those air-filled cavities situated above and below the vocal folds to which the sound waves have access and from which they receive sympathetic reinforcement in their passage to the external air. The tracheal and thoracic cavities form the subglottic resonators. The ventricle and vestibule of the larynx, the pharynx, oral and nasal chambers compose the supraglottic resonators.

The subglottic resonators provide air spaces capable of vibration in unison with the vocal folds and so take part in the composition of vocal tone. The chest is especially sympathetic to notes of low frequency and resonates male voices of low pitch rather than the 'small pipe of the maiden's organ'. The size and shape of the chest can be altered by posture; stooping shoulders and a pigeon chest will not assist good vocal tone, while an upright carriage will certainly favour chest notes besides good respiratory habits. Alterations in the size of the thoracic cavity are, however, not very considerable and at best the chest acts as a universal, not a selective, resonator (Negus, 1949). Some deny the function of the chest as a resonator altogether, but this would seem to be an unreasonable view since vibrations can be felt by placing the finger-tips on the clavicles of male speakers, and can also be distinctly heard. The doctor's time-honoured practice of asking the patient to 'say 99' when listening to the reverberations of the voice in the chest through his stethoscope is undoubtedly established upon sensible and practical grounds.

The Supraglottic Resonators

The resonators above the glottis are capable of very considerable alterations in size and shape. The laryngeal ventricle is influenced by the action of the vocal folds (Pepinsky, 1942). Important variations in its shape and size take place in different vowels (Van den Berg, 1955). The forward and backward movement of the epiglottis and the contraction and relaxation of the aryepiglottic folds, extending from the arytenoids to the sides of the epiglottis, further alter the size of the laryngeal ventricle. Constrictions in this supraglottic cavity may impart nasal resonance to the voice.

The pharynx is of considerably more importance as a resonator than most textbooks on voice production acknowledge. It is tubular in shape and extends from the level of the lower border of the cricoid cartilage to the under surface of the skull. It is 13–14 cm. in length. Above, it is continuous with the nasal cavity, and below with the laryngeal inlet anteriorly and the oesophagus posteriorly (Fig. 19). It consists of the nasal, oral and

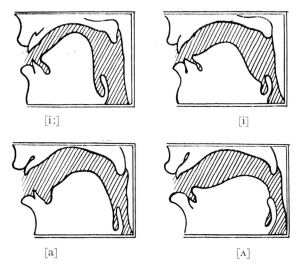

[i:]

[i]

[a]

[ʌ]

Fig. 24   Changes in oral and pharyngeal cavities as seen in lateral X-ray photographs, in articulation of vowels [i:], [i], [a] and [ʌ]

laryngeal parts formed respectively by the superior, middle and inferior constrictor muscles. These decrease the calibre of the pharynx upon contraction. The stylopharyngeus and salpingopharyngeus muscles reinforce the lateral pharyngeal walls and upon contraction raise and shorten them, decreasing the transverse and longitudinal measurements of the pharynx. At the same time, by reason of their attachment to the larynx, they assist in elevation of the larynx. This takes place in deglutition and to a lesser extent in speech.

The palatoglossus and palatopharyngeus muscles may also be considered in relation to the pharyngeal resonator. Their muscular arches form a flexible and variable arch of communication between the oropharynx and oral cavity and if over-tensed are capable of materially decreasing the dimensions of the oropharyngeal outlet and creating a 'cul-de-sac resonator' as West (1957) calls it.

The size and shape of the pharynx is further altered by the forward and backward displacement of the root of the tongue in relation to the posterior pharyngeal wall which occurs in articulation of vowel sounds (Figs. 24 and 25).

Lateral X-ray cine films of movements of the tongue and soft palate in articulation of certain vowel sounds, such as produced by the Haskins Laboratories, New York (Movements of the speech organs) show this changing shape of the pharyngeal resonator most dramatically, if the viewer concentrates upon observation of the pharyngeal cavity rather than of the oral cavity.

The Oral Resonator

The oral cavity, generally described as the chief resonator, has already been described fully in connection with the organs of articulation above. Its shape and contribution to resonance are dependent upon the position of the lips, the tongue, the soft palate and, of course, the degree to which the jaws are separated.

The Nasal Resonator

The nose's original and vital function in animals was that of olfaction, but in man this is no longer so, though it is a convenience and a pleasure to be able to smell. The tongue distinguishes between sweet, bitter, sour and salt, but we mainly 'taste' with our noses by savouring the aroma. Another important function of the nose is the warming, filtering and moistening of air before it enters the lungs. Nasal breathing, except in eating and speaking, is therefore highly desirable.

The nasal cavity is divided into two chambers by the nasal septum centrally and communicates with the nasopharynx posteriorly. It is divided into recesses or meati laterally by the turbinates (Fig. 19), which provide a fairly extensive area of mucous membrane for the necessary 'air conditioning', as Negus (1957a) puts it.

The nasal cavity is of considerable importance in resonation of the voice. Nasal obstruction reduces nasal resonance. Palatopharyngeal sphincteric incompetence and tension in the nasopharynx increases nasality. Both conditions contribute an imbalance of overtones in the voice which are recognisably

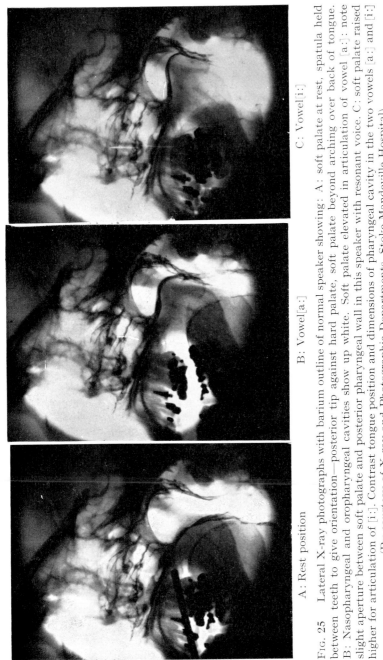

A: Rest position   B: Vowel[a:]   C: Vowel[i:]

FIG. 25 Lateral X-ray photographs with barium outline of normal speaker showing: A: soft palate at rest, spatula held between teeth to give orientation—posterior tip against hard palate, soft palate beyond arching over back of tongue. B: Nasopharyngeal and oropharyngeal cavities show up white. Soft palate elevated in articulation of vowel [a:]: note slight aperture between soft palate and posterior pharyngeal wall in this speaker with resonant voice. C: soft palate raised higher for articulation of [i:]. Contrast tongue position and dimensions of pharyngeal cavity in the two vowels [a:] and [i:]

(By courtesy of X-ray and Photographic Departments, Stoke Mandeville Hospital) abnormal. (The question of disorders of nasal resonance is discussed fully in Chapter 13.)

The character of the nasal consonants [m], [n] and [ŋ] is due in part to nasal resonance, but chiefly, it would seem, to the nasality of tone imparted to the voice by the bottling of the sound waves in the oral and nasal pharynx when the velum is slightly raised and the oral outlet is blocked by the lips as in [m] or contact of the tongue with hard or soft palate as with [n] and [ŋ]. Nasality may in fact be achieved by elevation of the dorsum of the tongue and constriction of the pillars of the fauces even when velopharyngeal closure is complete. This takes place in the speech of

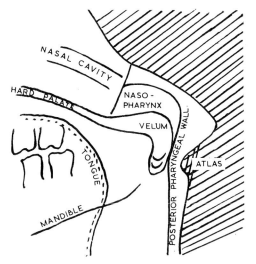

Fig. 26   Labelled X-ray tracing of normal individual articulating [i]

some English people but is more conspicuous in American dialects when the cul-de-sac resonator imparts a nasal 'twang' to the voice.

The nasal resonator's chief function is to act as a constant and universal resonator to the voice and it is responsible for clarity and beauty of tone. Skilful use of nasal resonance is an essential quality of artistic voice production. A relaxed oral and pharyngeal musculature, including the velum, though elevated, favours the vibration of air in the nasal cavity. Nasal resonance is utilised in some individuals by slight opening of the palatopharyngeal sphincter to provide a rich harmonic structure to the voice. This is the physiological basis of what is known as 'head resonance' and is especially heard or perceived in the 'head register', but

deep and resonant voices of men may also contain nasal overtones
due to a slight nasopharyngeal aperture.

Fig. 25 shows lateral X-ray photographs with barium outline,
a method actually first suggested by Mme. Borrel-Maisonny, the
French speech therapist who worked with the cleft-palate surgeon
Victor Veau. This is a nice example (among many others) of the

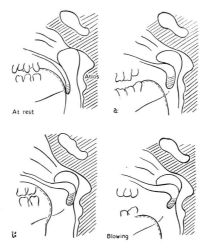

Fig. 27   Diagrams made from tracing over lateral X-ray photographs of
normal speaker showing position of palate at rest, articulating [a:] and [i:],
and blowing a carnival blower

contribution the speech pathologist can make to the work of a
highly specialised medical team.

The diagram in Fig. 26 shows the lateral X-ray photographic
tracing of a normal speaker articulating the vowel [i:] and is
labelled for guidance in reading the lateral X-ray prints in
Fig. 25.

Fig. 27 shows diagrams made from tracing over the lateral
X-ray photographs with Indian ink, after which the X-ray photographic print is bleached out leaving the diagram (Calnan, 1955).
Note the difficulty in defining the exact position of the soft
palate and uvula in relation to the posterior pharyngeal wall on
account of concentrations of barium which show up as black
streaks in Fig. 25. This interference does not occur when viewing
through an image intensifier which gives a much clearer picture
of the total configuration of soft tissues and bony structures
(page 51).

The Paranasal Sinuses

The maxillary frontal sinuses are traditionally included in the supraglottic resonator system and this belief is incorporated in teaching methods for 'forward tone placement'. It has even given birth to a method of teaching based on the erroneous belief that voice originates in the sinuses which still has a certain following (page 75). Latterly the part played by the sinuses in voice production has been relegated to the realms of voice mythology by modern techniques of vocal analysis. It is generally accepted that the sinuses play *no* part in resonance of the voice. Tarneaud (1961), also Hahn and her co-authors (1952) express this view in their appraisal of the resonating process. Negus (1957) in discussing the purpose and function of the paranasal sinuses in beasts and man, is in no doubt about the matter. He notes that the domestic cat has a loud voice of wide range and only a small volume of air-filled sinuses and that the giraffe with enormous frontal air spaces is unusually silent.

RELATIONSHIP BETWEEN ARTICULATION OF VOWELS
AND VOCAL RESONANCE

A resonant voice is desirable not only for aesthetic but for practical reasons. Quality, apart from rendering the voice pleasing, has the great advantage of giving it richness and carrying power without, however, making any extra demands upon the physical or nervous energy of the speaker. The fundamental laryngeal note is by itself of a thin and reedy quality but when transmitted to the resonating chambers above the larynx these, acting as acoustic filters, considerably enhance the sounds as already described (page 12). Luchsinger (1965e) emphasises that projection of the voice is dependent upon maximum resonance.

THE DEVELOPMENT OF VOCAL QUALITY

In order to develop its full strength and beauty the following factors which influence vocal quality must be correctly utilised:

1. Before the voice can be developed, the fundamental laryngeal note must be steady, clear and strong and this will only be achieved in the first place by adequate attention to breathing technique and laryngeal tension in maintenance of steady subglottic pressure.

2. The range of vocal pitch or register is also of great importance and must be attuned to the resonance pitch of the individual's

total resonator system; a voice pitched too high or too low cannot benefit to full advantage from its resonator.

3. The supraglottic resonators being in the main muscular and moveable structures must be voluntarily controlled to produce conditions of optimal resonance either by varying degrees of tension in their walls, or by alterations in the size of their orifices and cavities during the articulatory movements.

The texture of the walls of resonators affects the quality of tone very noticeably. Paget (1930), whose distinguished work on the artificial production of vowel sounds is of great interest, found that quality varied according to the materials of which his vowel resonators were constructed. Plasticine, glass, rubber, cardboard and wood all produced different tones, but as long as the characteristic resonance pitches of the vowel sounds (formants) remained constant the vowels were recognisable. The relaxed muscular walls of the vocal resonators tend to 'damp', stop or absorb high frequencies and produce mellow tone, whereas hard or taut muscular walls act as reflectors and produce harsh tone. If the walls of resonators are sufficiently thin and flexible, more-over, sound waves can cause these to pulsate and thus awaken sympathetic vibration of the air space on the other side. It is this factor which probably makes possible the use of nasal or head resonance even when the nasopharyngeal isthmus is closed, sound waves passing through the roof of the oral cavity and especially the soft palate or velum.

The resonance pitch of a cavity depends not only upon its size and shape but also upon the size of its orifice. In this connection Paget (1930) says, 'The musical pitch of a resonating cavity can be varied in three different ways, viz.: by enlarging the resonator which lowers the pitch, by enlarging the orifice which raises the pitch, or by lengthening the neck which lowers the pitch of the note produced by the resonating cavity. It follows from this that we can obtain the same resonant pitch from resonators of different sizes, provided we adjust the size of the orifice and length of the neck so as to compensate for the difference of volume of the resonator'. Van den Berg's (1964) work (page 25) is also relevant here.

These considerations explain how the small resonators of children can be adjusted to produce the same vowel sounds as adults, while parrots and budgerigars can imitate human speech despite gross differences in the structure, shape and size of their organs of articulation.

During speech the oral and pharyngeal cavities undergo an infinite variety of changes in shape and elasticity, each variation contributing a change in tone colour (resonance). Consonants and vowels succeed each other in rapid succession, as pitch and volume of the fundamental vocal pitch fluctuates, and infinitesimal alterations in muscular tension reflect the psychological and emotional state, throwing an ever-changing kaleidoscope of light and shade over the linguistic and phonemic characteristics of utterance.

THE VOWELS

It is usual to consider resonance chiefly in connection with vowel articulation because, although the voiced consonants are resonated, their vocal quality is partly obliterated by their characteristic dissonances.

The characteristic quality of the vowel sounds is produced, it is thought, by the coupling of the predominant resonance pitches of the oral and pharyngeal cavities. Although scientific methods of acoustic analysis have failed to prove whether it is the mouth or the pharynx which contributes the high and low frequency band-widths or formants respectively, the fact remains that the vowels are distinguished by two characteristic formants, one high and one low, provided by these linked resonators. The resonances of the vocal cavities are not too clearly defined according to Van den Berg (1958) and actually the formants of the vowels are damped to a certain extent and energy is lost so that they never compete with the predominance of the fundamental vocal note imparted by vocal fold vibrations.

Manuel Garcia (1805–1906), the celebrated teacher of singing to whom invention of the laryngoscopic mirror is attributed, was the first to recognise that the vocal folds affect quality as well as pitch. Russell (1931) more recently contributed to knowledge of the action of the larynx, pharynx, tongue and soft palate in speech and song. He used a laryngoperiskop for direct observation and photography of the laryngeal cavity, and lateral X-ray photography for observing movements of tongue and palate. He found that the laryngeal cavity undergoes radical changes not only when notes of different pitch are produced, as is well known, but also when different vowel sounds are formed. The vocal folds, for instance, become comparatively bunched and blunt-edged in the case if [i] but elongate and sharpen for [i:]. The ventricle of the larynx is also modified by the action of the false folds which follow the movements of the true folds. When relaxed they act as soft surface filters but when constricted they press down upon the folds and obliterate the ventricle. The tension favours high partials and produces the 'compressed' tone described by Aikin (1951). The epiglottis further influences vowel quality. It is pulled well out of the way for [i:] hence the invariable instruction to say [i:] to the patient subjected to an indirect laryngoscopic examination. The epiglottis, however, is pulled well back towards the cartilages of Wrisberg and shuts in the laryngeal cavity for the vowel [a] which undoubtedly accounts for that vowel's peculiar hard quality which has been likened to the bleat of a sheep. Negus (1949) has summarised the influence of the laryngeal cavity upon the tone of voice as follows: 'The larynx produces not only a fundamental tone but many overtones. It is by the relative amplification or damping of the overtones that sounds of different character and quality are produced, while others may be added in the resonating cavities themselves'.

THE PHARYNGEAL RESONATOR

The pharynx, the back resonator on which 'nobility of tone' would seem to depend (Paget, 1930), alters in depth constantly during speech as the larynx rises and falls in sympathy with the movements of the root of the tongue, and in singing with the rise and fall of pitch. The considerable changes in the size and shape of the pharyngeal resonator during the utterance of vowels, and backward, forward and up and down movements of the base of the tongue, are clearly seen in Figs. 24 and 25. These alterations in the resonator appear to be of as great, or even greater, significance in the determination of vowel quality as the alterations taking place in the oral cavity at the same time. Phoneticians, however, have concentrated almost exclusively upon the tongue positions in the oral cavity in an endeavour to describe the articulation of vowels. The charting of these tongue positions upon a vowel triangle (Jones, 1947) appears to be of limited, if indeed any value to the voice specialist. It is obvious that in speech the tongue position for any vowel is largely determined by the tongue position of adjacent consonants. The vowel is said, in fact, to 'resemble' the consonant, this being the nature of vowel similitude. This fact is confirmed by spectrographic analysis as Gimson (1962) stresses. The tongue, for instance, assumes very different positions for the vowel [i] in the following words: shilling, pithy, list, tit, kick. The pharyngeal and laryngeal articulation or resonation of vowels is less sensitive to movements of the blade and body of the tongue in the shaping of consonants. It is not intended here to underestimate the importance of the oral cavity as a resonator but to give the back resonator its proper due. Possibly the most important function of the front resonator is the provision of a funnel for the projection of sound, like a speaking trumpet or megaphone. The more open this funnel can be kept by the relaxed position of the jaws and tongue and the lips the better projection the voice will have. For this reason a bone prop is used to separate the teeth during articulation practice in some drama schools, believe it or not.

Finally, it is necessary to draw attention to the fact that the dimensions of the pharynx and the size of its nasal and oral orifices are also altered by varying degrees of tension in the pillars of the fauces and the soft palate. It is instructive to watch in a mirror the movement of these structures when speaking the vowel series: [a:], [a], [ɛ], [i:]; also to watch the play in tension, the rise and fall of the soft palate when [a:] is sung upon an ascending scale. Clear, bright ringing tones (voix blanche) are dependent upon lifting and tensing of the velum. Low mellow tones are achieved with the faucial arches well relaxed and the soft palate almost pendant and in this the observations of Paget (1930) are confirmed by those of Russell (1931) and Calnan (1953). Baritones and speakers with sonorous voices are often found to speak with a slight nasopharyngeal aperture. Van den Berg (1962) states that his investigations in conjunction with Albronda and Metz demonstrated 'that the closure of the nasal cavities by the soft palate during production of normal non-nasal vowel sounds is mostly incomplete'. A mirror below the nostrils may not be clouded in production of these vowels but the nasal clues are rather prominent in the spectrograph.

SOME CLASSICAL CONCEPTS OF ELOCUTION

Thinking the Voice Forward

Teachers of elocution insist upon the absolute necessity for 'thinking the voice forward' in the development of good vocal tone. A resonant voice is greatly a matter of thinking where to direct the air. The speaker should be taught to think upwards towards the mask of the face, and then outwards through the mouth and forwards. The injunction merely to speak out does not result in that necessary upward drive through the resonators, and as often as not produces strain, according to Birch (1948).

The exercise of humming to develop forward resonance and 'pure tone' by feeling the air waves vibrating in the mask of the face and on lightly closed lips is generally found to be very beneficial. The value of an instruction to 'think the voice' into the top of the head is presumably that it focuses attention upon the resonated voice rather than on what is going on in the larynx, and produces the necessary muscular adjustments in the throat and mouth. The hearing training which accompanies such teaching methods is probably of far greater value in eliciting the correct muscular responses than any verbal cues that may be given. The muscles of the throat, the root of the tongue and the larynx cannot be deliberately and directly controlled, but by listening to good patterns of voice and endeavouring to imitate them the desired results are eventually achieved, chiefly by means of the individual's auditory control or 'feed-back'. Taking place synchronously is of course the kinaesthetic proprioceptive and tactile feed-back which are less obvious but equally important factors in the learning process.

The Vowel Resonator Scale

Another popular method of teaching voice production, which can be used separately or in conjunction with the forward direction principle, is that of whispering the vowels when arranged in order of pitch resonance to compose a vowel resonator scale.

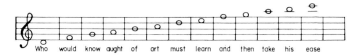

This method was invented by Aiken (1951) and has been adopted by most schools of speech training since (Thurburn, 1939). Shakespeare (1924) advocates its use in the teaching of singing and the well-known mnemonic for remembrance of the scale is his 'Who would know aught of art must learn and then take his ease'.

Practice in whispering vowels develops kinaesthetic feed-back as well as auditory sensitivity, and emphasises the necessity for an open and relaxed throat to produce good tone. The practice of vowels singly or in any combinations will probably be just as beneficial. The delicate adjustment of the resonators to produce the resonator scale cannot possibly be maintained in speech and it can be considered wasteful of effort to insist upon precise drill in the scale. As a precursory exercise for singing it is of more doubtful value. In order to gain conditions of maximal resonance in song, considerable liberties must be taken with articulation in order to 'hunt out' the positions of the muscular organs which will provide optimal resonance for the fundamental laryngeal note being sung at any time (Paget, 1931). The most excellent results obtained by the old Italian teachers of singing were achieved without recourse to the vowel resonator scale. Most teachers of the old school advocate practice of vowel sounds with flattened tongue, wide mouth and open throat, and emphasise most wisely the need for perfect respiratory control (Mills, 1906).

Efficient teaching in the forward production and vowel resonator scale methods undoubtedly produce excellent results. There is always a danger, however, that oral articulation may receive too great emphasis and other factors of greater importance be neglected. These factors are *relaxation of muscular organs, and a good vocal note evenly sustained by adequate breath pressure*. Unless due attention is paid to these aspects of voice production then perfect articulation will not achieve adequate results, at any rate with individuals suffering with strained voices. A certain school-mistress known to us, for instance, has such perfect articulation and such strong breath force that her whisper penetrates the far corners of a hall in the most embarrassing way, yet she invariably loses her voice with a cold, and is quite unable to sleep at night without cough lozenges to ease the irritating tickle in her throat— the symptom of daily vocal abuse. Besides which with every cold she develops laryngitis.

Sinus Tone Production

Yet another school of voice production that had a considerable vogue among the ignorant and gullible, advocates the development of 'sinus tone production' and maintains that the vocal folds are not essential to the production of voice because 'sound is absolutely *made* in the head' (White, 1938). This contention need not be refuted here, but the limitations of so distorted a view of voice are obvious. We treated a young man who had received a course in sinus tone production to 'strengthen' his voice; singing on a nasalised note pitched on G was a pronounced feature of his training. His 'vocal weakness' was, however, due to failure of his voice to break satisfactorily. Given speech therapy, he responded well to relaxation, correction of tense and shallow breathing habits, and to lowering of the voice to a suitable male register.

The part played by sinus tone in head resonance has already been discussed (page 69). The nasal resonator alone plays a major part in 'head' resonance and undue emphasis upon acquisition of resonance of imaginary origin in the air-filled spaces of the head may lead to an unpleasant thin and tinny quality to the voice and of course neglects the important principles of satisfactory voice production.

THE IDEAL OF BALANCED TONE

The aesthetically perfect vocal tone depends upon the perfect blending of overtones and this can only be achieved by the proper management of the whole resonator system, the larynx, laryngeal ventricle, pharynx, oral and nasal cavities, each of which plays an essential part in the production of 'balanced tone'. If the contribution of one resonator is excessive then there results an imbalance in tone. Excessive pharyngeal tone is achieved by constriction of the palatal arches, and raising of the back of the tongue, typical of the 'plummy' voice. Excessive tension in the nasopharynx and constriction of the oral outlet by the palatal arches and formation of a cul-de-sac resonator can cause nasality. Exaggerated lip rounding and compression of the lips imparts a 'cotton wool' or muffled quality to speech.

The harsh (grating or metallic) qualities of voices are all due to excess tension in muscular walls thus contributing dissonant components to vocal tone. 'How sour sweet music is when tone is broke and no proportion kept' and how infinitely pleasing is a musical voice such as that of Herrick's Julia:

> So smooth, so sweet, so silv'ry is thy voice,
> As could they hear, the damn'd would make no noise
> But listen to thee—walking in thy chamber,
> Melting melodious word to lute of amber.

It is small wonder that the Greeks considered a beautiful voice to be one of the indispensable attractions of a siren.

THE SINGING VOICE

Reference to the singing voice has been made here and there, but a comparison of speaking and singing technique at this juncture will provide a useful basis for a summary of the foregoing discussion.

Singing requires all that speaking does but far greater skill in all spheres. Breath capacity must be greatly increased and control of expiration and pressure finely opposed to vocal cord tension so that greater vocal volume and longer phrasing and wide variance in pitch is achieved.

In speech, pitch slides up and down a restricted scale of semi-tones covering a range of six or eight notes, three or four notes above and below the middle note. In singing, however, pitch covers one-and-a-half octaves in untrained voices and two to two-and-a-half in trained voices, an eighth or tenth above and below the middle note. The highly sensitive self-regulating auditory mechanism of trained singers has been analysed and recorded by Winckel (1952). Singers in an anacoustic chamber, where their voices did not resonate, automatically increased the volume and overtones of voice. In a highly resonant room they automatically reduced volume and damped their vocal overtones. Normally, singing pitch is of course tied to the chromatic scale and a fixed melody; absolute accuracy in pitching the singing voice and perfect control of the laryngeal musculature to prevent the voice from going off key is therefore essential, especially in changes from the thick to thin registers as explained by Van den Berg (1962).

The investigations of Rubin and Hirt (1960) have already been described (page 49), and the fundamental changes in the mechanics of laryngeal adjustment which takes place in transition from the head to falsetto register. A large part of training is devoted to overcoming the breaks or cracks in the voice during this transition and untrained singers are unable to conceal the transition. Within the falsetto range less breath is used but changes in tension of the vocal cords and increased resistance to the vibratory air force are responsible for rise in pitch.

The mastery of special singing techniques is necessary. The Italian school advocates the open singing technique, with open mouth and smiling lips, a wide open and relaxed throat being apparently the chief aim. For dramatic singing the 'covered voice' is advocated mainly by the German School because it gives added power and emotional tension to the voice. The technique necessitates descent of the larynx, simultaneous widening of the pharyngeal cavity and increased air pressure. Luchsinger (1965e) says by covering the voice is meant a slight darkening of the vowels on higher pitch levels to avoid excessively bright timbre in singing. Covering is used to facilitate changes from one register to another. It is suitable to Wagnerian opera. Brodnitz (1962) warns against the dangers of excessive use of 'covered voice' on account of the tension involved. It should be used by pop singers to obtain the necessary vocal volume to overcome the enormous volume of the band accompaniment but it is difficult to master and most of these performers are amateurs with no training so that they frequently damage their vocal cords. Schilling (1952) was of the opinion that open singing was more harmful than covered singing and that the latter method is only harmful when incorrectly practised and improperly mastered.

Sonninen (1968) examined the changing position of the larynx and movements of the laryngeal cartilages and trachea in covered voice in healthy professional singers. The larynx is pulled down low and forward to such an extent that the trachea is bent forward. This appears to be the correct and necessary technique in efficient covered singing and is not utilised by untrained singers. In open forte singing the vocal ligaments are longer, more tense and thicker than they are in covered singing; the vocal cords are subject, therefore, to more stress from air flow through the glottis.

Luchsinger (1965e) comments upon the cultural differences in singing style. The Italian and German styles have been mentioned. The Spanish 'flamenco' singing has a harsh, bright loudness to it which is much admired, so has also Greek singing, which has a certain nasal tone. These are types of traditional folk singing and in great contrast to the lilting sweetness of Welsh or Hebridean singing and the rich warmth of negro spirituals.

The management of vibrato in singing is a necessary skill. Luchsinger (1965) says that the ear can distinguish three acoustical parameters in the vibrato. These are firstly frequency per second of the oscillations which vary between 3 to 6 periods per second, followed by variations in intensity, and fluctuations in pitch. Opera and concert singers can utilise the vibrato and throbbing voice as a means of conveying emotion and dramatic intensity. Vibrato occurring with a higher periodicity is described as a tremolo and is considered a fault in singing. The well-known actor Sir John Gielgud has a characteristic vibrato which is unusual and assumes greater prominence on the stage than in his conversational speech.

A trill is considered a good measure of technical voice training and resonance potential. Vennard and Von Leden (1967) submitted the trills of four outstanding sopranos to spectrographic analysis. They concluded that the rate of pitch fluctuation in a trill is very little faster than that of a vibrato, but the extent of the pitch variation is increased so that the ear can detect the two pitches involved. At the same time an intensity modulation at double the rate of the pitch vibrato appears. Rhythmic contractions of the whole laryngeal structure also accompany a trill and the larynx can actually be seen to wobble in the throat.

Yodelling is a particular style of singing peculiar to the Swiss alps. It is thought to have originated in imitation of the Alpenhorn and the Shawm, an ancient wind instrument similar to the clarinet and common to all pastoral people (Luchsinger, 1965). The yodel consists of sudden jumps in pitch from chest register to head register on vowel sounds only, not words. Good air support is necessary and this is provided by activity of the diaphragm. The yodel has great carrying power and is an effective means of calling the attention of a neighbour on another mountain top, and is not as might be expected for rounding up lost sheep and goats.

The need for choosing the correct natural range of the voice is of great importance in singing since the outer ends of the singing range need very careful production and should not be over-worked, even in trained voices. Singing outside the natural vocal range imposes a serious strain upon the voice.

The quality or natural resonance pitch is also important in choosing the natural singing range. Quality, rather than range of pitch, may decide whether a voice is mezzo-soprano or soprano, but should not be allowed to count too much (Scholes, 1950). An exact definition of the ranges of singing voices is not possible since individuals vary greatly according to nature and the excellence or otherwise of their teaching. The middle notes of the various male and female voices given below are only approximately correct for average voices.

Tarneaud (1961) recommends that the length of the vocal cords as well as resonance should be taken into account when the proper register is in doubt, and quotes the investigations of Zwimmermann and Nadoleczny who measured the vocal cords of 4 basses, 6 baritones, 4 contraltos, 3 mezzo-sopranos and 21 sopranos with the Trendelenburg apparatus. In general the increase in length of the cords was closely correlated with drop in register. However, the length of vocal cord cannot be absolutely relied upon in females as the sole indication of appropriate register. One at least of the mezzo-sopranos in the above series had larger vocal cords than the contraltos. In the diagnostic laboratory of the future, vocal cord length and bulk may well be measured by the technique of using lateral X-ray photographs employed by Hollien (1960), supplemented by a spectrographic analysis of the overtones produced on a range of several notes which Winckel (1952) has shown is closely correlated to the efficiency of the voice in a particular register. Until such time as these diagnostic facilities are readily available to speech pathologists they will have to continue to rely upon a trained ear and tactile cues in assessment of optimum vocal pitch, as recommended by Zaliouk (1963) (page 171), and upon the use of pitch pipe, piano or other available instrument.

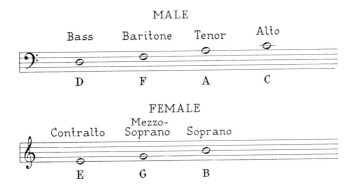

Articulation of the consonants in singing must be somewhat exaggerated, while vowel articulation and resonance must be adapted to the pitch of the laryngeal note and often has little resemblance to speech articulation. The vowel [i:] if it has to be sung on high C, for instance, will become metallic and nasalised if the speech articulation and raised tongue position is not modified in order to approach the neutral vowel [a:]. Diphthongs cannot be sustained but must be blended into pure vowels which strike a compromise between the two vowel elements.

Singing requires a more exacting performance in every department than does speech. The good singer must put his whole soul into the interpretation of a passage if it is not to appear wooden and stilted. This facility is dependent upon a complete mastery of technique; the control, not merely of the mechanics of singing but of fine shades of tone colour which defy analysis but convey the emotional message of a passage. No such extraordinary physical demands are made upon the speaker and even the art of the actor is not so exacting, although it approaches more nearly the performance of the singer. It was the great teacher Pacchiarotti who said 'He who knows how to speak and breathe knows how to sing' (Chi sa parlare e respirare sa cantare), but Hiller's less well known assertion 'well spoken is half sung' is a more accurate assessment of the relationship between good speaking and good singing. A good speaking voice is only an indication of naturally favourable anatomical structures and of singing possibilities.

Arnold (1962) has described the signs of favourable 'local constitution' which immediately indicate to the laryngologist when a person is endowed with a naturally good voice. These consist of roomy resonating chambers, symmetrical configuration of the larynx, a wide opening to the laryngeal vestibule with an erect and flat epiglottis. The larynx looks attractive and is easily inspected. The larynx, on the other hand, may look queer and constricted and cannot be easily inspected in those having inferior talents in phonic performance. In this connection we are reminded of the reference by Henderson (1954) in his description of Kathleen Ferrier's pharyngeal cavity which would easily have accommodated a fair-sized apple. However a short neck appears also to be an advantage and the long swan neck so much admired in medieval times presumably contributes to a weak voice. Yanaghira and Koike (1967) point out that the air volume available for maximally sustained phonation is not only dependent upon taking a deep breath in the correct way but is directly related to the vital capacity of the individual. This is dependent upon sex, height, age and weight, and a good deep chest. A big constitution favours production of a bass and a slight constitution is found in sopranos and counter-tenors.

Training in correct methods of voice production is a great aid to those speakers not favourably endowed anatomically. For the singer, good anatomical endowment is essential though this is not in itself enough. A good ear and musical talent are necessary, and dedication. Beautiful singing needs seven or more years of arduous practice in the acquisition of the requisite techniques before the art emerges and a sensitivity capable of interpreting human emotion imaginatively is liberated from the bonds of conscious striving.

5   Vocal synthesis

Voice is the product of the most finely co-ordinated, delicately balanced and harmonious movements of which the body is capable. An appreciation of the physiological characteristics of articulation and phonation cannot, therefore, be complete without consideration of the fundamental principles which underlie muscular movements. Co-ordination is obviously the prime essential in the execution of any action but physical relaxation and intellectual awareness of rhythm form the true matrix of co-ordination—the culture or medium in which it best develops.

THE RELATION OF RELAXATION TO CO-ORDINATION

The value of relaxation in the integration of muscle movements can best be understood if the processes which take place in voluntary movements are analysed. Broadly speaking, three different muscle groups are involved. The prime movers (protagonists) initiate the movement required by tensing and contracting. At the same time the antagonists which are responsible for contrary movement in the opposite direction must relax and in no way resist the prime movers. The synergists or bracing muscles simultaneously fixate the joint involved and so provide a fixed origin from which the protagonists may operate with maximal efficiency. The clenching of the fist gives a clear example of the action of these three muscle groups and is a classic example given in *Gray's Anatomy* (1949). The flexors of the fingers are the protagonists, the extensors the antagonists, the wrist extensors the synergists. As the flexors contract and the fingers clench, their extensors relax and stretch, while the extensors of the wrist contract and fixate the joint and provide a brace for the flexors. Should the antagonistic flexors fail to relax, the clenching movement will be hampered and if the synergists do not co-operate, the hand hangs limp and even greater difficulty in clenching will be experienced. Another example can be taken from laryngeal movement. In phonation the adductors of the folds are the prime

82

movers, the abductors the relaxed antagonists, and the posterior cricoarytenoids act as bracing muscles fixating the arytenoid joint capsules.

The efficient performance of any movement depends upon the proper co-ordination of prime movers, antagonists, and fixating synergistic muscles, and this co-ordination is ensured by the manifold connections which exist within the central nervous system (Gray, 1949). It can be seen that perfect balance must be maintained between the opposing forces of contraction and relaxation; any excessive tension in synergists or antagonists or adjacent muscle groups will throw the delicate adjustment out of line and render movement stiff, jerky and clumsy. The insidious influence of tension is not so evident in large movements as in fine; more conspicuous in manipulation of the fingers, lips, tongue and vocal folds, than in that of the limbs.

The smooth ebb and flow of nervous energy to the appropriate muscle groups requires perfect timing, a nicety and speed of adjustment quite outside the bounds of conscious control, and is dependent upon the unconscious organisation by the nervous system of the sensorimotor reflexes concerned (Sherrington, 1947, and Wyke, 1967, 1969, 1970). Although an action is conceived intellectually and performed voluntarily it is conceived in con- sciousness only in the broadest outline; the actual details of motor performance remain entirely involuntary and unconscious. Co-ordination is in reality learned by the nervous system through constant practice until a particular motor skill is perfected. In this process of learning, a perfect balance between relaxation and tension is struck and, as movements become organised, only those muscle groups which are absolutely essential to efficiency are eventually retained, and many other earlier and unnecessary helpers are discharged from service.

All the broad principles of co-ordination are learned in infancy and we witness their gradual evolution from the amusing jerky uncontrolled arm, leg and head movements at birth to the perfected skill in grasping, walking, talking, running and jumping. As Wyke (1970) says, speaking of the child's vocal development, 'This increasing efficiency of voluntary control of the phonatory musculature is contingent upon a parallel degree of subconscious maturation in the operational efficiency of the phonatory reflex systems—just as the child's developing ability to walk voluntarily is contingent upon the subconscious maturation of its postural reflex systems'.

SYNKINESIS

The progressive refinement of movements from the mass reflex activity of the infant and the selection and isolation of particular muscle groups to perform special movements is entirely dependent upon maturation of the nervous system. It is some time before the 'mélodie kinétique', as De Ajuriaguerra and Stambak (1955) call it, emerges. A toddler achieves thumb and finger prehension as he learns to pronounce crudely the first words at a year, but may not be able to put out his tongue without extending his fingers until three years, nor isolate thumb movement from that of the clenched fist. Finger and tongue co-ordinations are closely correlated developmentally. A child masters plosives first and difficult consonant blends last, and it is some years before the intonation and vocal patterns are perfected also.

The failure to isolate muscle groups and confine voluntary movement to the necessary muscles is known as synkinesis. It is a normal phenomenon in infancy but if it persists throughout life it is evident in varying degrees of individual clumsiness. This is a handicap in sport and in manual and lingual skills. It may reveal itself in poor and indistinct articulation or hoarseness and voice breaks in childhood. The significance of synkinesis in the motor aspects of speech and voice has been stressed in the work of De Ajuriaguerra and Stambak (1955) mentioned above. In pathological conditions of neuro-muscular disorder synkinesis and inco-ordination give rise to dysarthria and dysphonia (Chapter 14).

The learning stage of every motor skill is characterised by excessive concentration upon the task in hand, and an overflow of nervous energy throughout the body with enlistment of mass reflexes and vastly more muscle groups than are strictly necessary. The exaggerated high steps, the widely planted feet and the flexed arms of the toddler freshly launched in locomotion, as unsteady on his pins as a landlubber at sea, is as typical of this stage as is his lalling speech. With the infant, as already explained, immature motor maturation accounts for this inco-ordination, but the adult encounters much the same difficulties when learning to type, to play golf, to skate or to produce his voice in a different way. Generalised tension with inability voluntarily to relax unnecessary muscles delays the acquisition of the new motor skill.

NECESSITY FOR CONTROLLED RELAXATION

Relaxation is most necessary for co-ordination but partial or controlled relaxation is all that it is possible to achieve. Living muscle is never completely relaxed and is always in a condition of slight contraction which maintains it 'at the ready' for action. At any time there are varying degrees of muscle tone in the muscular systems of the body; thus there will be a considerable degree of tonus in those muscles maintaining posture, while the arms resting with hands in the lap and the crossed legs may appear completely relaxed if tested—if lifted and dropped. Complete relaxation is impossible in living muscle and extensive relaxation is only possible when the individual is lying down; at other times it would result in bodily collapse as complete as that of a puppet when the activating strings are released. Controlled relaxation is, however, a sensible aim. Relaxation of those muscles which are not engaged in maintaining posture or performing a voluntary movement results in improvement of that performance and, inadvertently, in the general efficiency of the whole organism. Excess tension throughout the body, even when resting as an accompaniment to anxiety, is a perpetual drain upon nervous energy, tiring the individual throughout the day and adding to his burden quite unconsciously. For this reason, controlled relaxation is always an important aspect of speech therapy, although it is by no means a panacea for all evils as its most ardent supporters believed in the past. Physical tension may be the result of excessive concentration upon the physical task in hand as already described and often interferes with the learning stage of the new skills demanded in voice production. More frequently, and especially in functional speech disorders, it is the reflection of the mental state of the individual, of his general anxiety and nervousness. Sherrington (1947) drew attention to 'the bodily resonance of emotion'. Relaxation will ease the somatic concomitants of fear, but it will not remove the fear itself. It is comparatively easy to conceal stage fright, but impossible not to feel it, if this is a situation which frightens the individual.

The great advantage of relaxation, therefore, is that by eliminating or reducing unnecessary tensions, it allows better control of voluntary movements and the development of the natural rhythm of the nervous system. Co-ordination may be considered as the unconscious and automatic neuromuscular organisation taking place in circumstances of relaxation, while rhythm is its psychological and conscious counterpart in mental experience.

THE NATURE OF RHYTHM

The rhythmic sense, the ability to apprehend and appreciate

rhythm, is in man both a remarkable phenomenon and a great intellectual asset. It is responsible not only for his athletic prowess, his feats in juggling and acrobatics, and the manipulation of tools, but also his ability, unique among animals, to sing, to compose melodies and to speak. The exact nature and basis of his delicate rhythmic sense or instinct is difficult to describe. Throughout the ages it has been recognised but has always defied exact definition. The universe and all living things are organised on a rhythmic basis but man more than any other creature appears to be most susceptible and responsive to its appeal.

Rhythm is most easily recognised in music, but is apparent in all man's artistic creations as a certain quality of symmetry and balance. As described by Thurburn (1939) it consists of pulsations of force or stress at sufficiently regular intervals to create a pattern, yet with sufficient irregularity to prevent monotony. It is connected with timing of movement, or expenditure of energy; it gives order to what might be a series of disconnected events; and it provides a design, a feeling of purpose and fulfilment. In its absence, energy unleashed creates chaos; the cacophony of an orchestra without a conductor provides an example. On the other hand an entirely regular pattern of rhythmic stress leads to stereotyped performance and monotony, lacking vital inspiration. Rhythm in music or speech allows considerable latitude but must keep within acknowledged limits. Sudden quickening of tempo to convey urgency and excitement or slowing down to convey solemnity are possible. Like the course of a river flowing down to the sea which is held up here or pours headlong there, is pitted by rain and rippled by the wind, its ultimate purpose is always known and felt. That which marks the great actor or soloist is not his technique but his emotional interpretation of a masterpiece through his fine sense of rhythm (Scholes, 1950).

SPEECH AND MELODY

Primitive man's awareness and enjoyment of rhythm must have developed with his growing intelligence, and song developed concurrently with speech or may even have preceded it. The most primitive races in existence today, the Australian aborigines for instance, may have no musical instruments yet all have well-developed traditional songs. The majority of primitive peoples, however, have both songs and primitive percussion instruments. The first musical instruments undoubtedly evolved from the rhythmic bangings which accompanied labour, such as the chipping of flints for tool making. The percussion which man enjoyed as he laboured was probably accompanied by song, all nations having their own labour songs to facilitate rhythmic movement and promote co-ordination and ease in strenuous muscular activity. Many young people, be it noted, can dance with frantic zest all night but can scarcely walk half a mile.

The simple African possesses an extraordinarily highly developed rhythmic sense, as the analysis of African music by Jones (1949) in his fascinating monograph has demonstrated. Tribal dances combine singing, clapping, feet and shoulder movements, and also drumming to an ever-changing rhythmic kaleidoscope of such complexity that a Westerner finds it hard to appreciate the various themes, and quite impossible to imitate them. By skilful flicking of the fingers, positioning of the hands and thudding of the palms it is only possible to produce a pitch range of eleven notes on the drum. African drumming is essentially harmonic, but it is a harmony composed chiefly of rhythms not pitch, and the main beats of the different rhythms do not coincide. African melody and drumming have grown up in close association with words. Many African languages are tonal, every word has its own pitch in a sentence and pitch largely determines meaning. The Africans do not conceive of melody in the form of abstract music but in the concrete form of word melody. Nonsense syllables, such as [pʌ-kʌ-vi-ti-ku], are composed to indicate the pitch and rhythm of drum music, the traditional pitch of the syllables in the language corresponding to the rise and fall of the drum music. The choice of words for lyrics is influenced as much by their pitch as by their meaning. This close connection between speech and rhythm provides a perfect and living example of the profound influence rhythm has exerted upon the evolution of language, especially in its more primitive stages. One of the many theories concerning the origin of language in Man is based on the belief that song preceded speech phylogenetically. Evidence is brought forward in support of this view from the ontogenetic development of musical vocalisation in the infant and the apparent recapitulation of syllabic utterance as it developed in the race and became genetically fixed (Stein, 1942).

RHYTHM AN INNATE ATTRIBUTE

Infant behaviour gives many instances of the instinctive nature of the rhythmic sense which indicates that it is a sense inborn and not acquired. The first vocalisation, other than crying, consists of gurgles, coos and trills which precede babbling and are nearer to song than speech, having the elements of time, inflexion and rhythm which are characteristic of melody and to the mother every bit as delightful. The toddler takes to chanting his own babble songs with complete spontaneity. The recognition of melody through the recognition of pitch rather than stress does not develop until later, and the ability to imitate a melody does not come until the age of $2\frac{1}{2}$ or 3 years according to Shinn (1909). However, an infant as young as 6 months may imitate three or four notes or inflectional shifts.

When speaking in chorus all school children develop a sing-song rendering of arithmetical tables or jingles, and this, being entirely self-imposed and developing without any external prompting, denotes the instinctive desire to provide what is auditorily satisfying and orderly and to avoid that which is disorderly, ragged and uncomfortable. Yet if an attempt is made to teach these same chant-addicted children to conform to an imposed rhythm and to march in time to music and a beat, however simple, it will be found to be impossible before the age of 6 years.

THE APPRECIATION OF RHYTHM

Since the rhythmic sense appears to be an instinctive urge in man it needs outlets and satisfaction. Rhythmic activity is always enjoyable, and arhythmic activity a cause of uneasiness and unrest. Successful motor performance brings an instantaneous feeling of ease and fitness. The laryngectomised patient who suddenly falls into the rhythm of fluent oesophageal speech when respiration, articulation, and phonation are co-ordinated feels a sense of achievement and fulfilment which is by no means entirely due to improved powers of communication.

Rhythm is appreciated through visual and auditory kinaesthetic and proprioceptive sensations. It is experienced in every fibre of our bodies even when we are not taking part in a rhythmic activity ourselves. There are few listeners to a Beethoven symphony, if the truth be known, who do not feel the urge to hum, tap, or nod through a favourite theme. There are many who actually succumb, and very annoying it is to witness the pale reflection of our own aesthetic appreciation in a fellow member of an audience.

RHYTHMIC STRESS, INFLEXION AND PACE IN SPEECH

The human brain, Walter (1953) has said, has a natural affinity to rhythm. 'Listen to the ticking of a clock, and note how long it takes for the unaccented sequence to resolve itself into groups, of two, three or four ticks'. Auditory stimuli are more easily retained, understood and reproduced if organised in patterns or rhythms. It is for this reason that verbal language has to be essentially rhythmic and melodic, composed of subtle variations in stress, inflexion and pace which follow the course of meaning and assist the understanding of the audience.

Fry (1963) has emphasised that in the comprehension of speech we depend on many cues besides the discrimination of consonants. Important cues are the stress and inflectional patterns of a language, the melody of heard patterns which we match against the established fixed patterns we have learned in infancy and early childhood. We have only to listen to the speech of foreigners speaking English to realise the importance of this aspect of intelligibility. Foreigners, when they have mastered vocabulary and syntax and are 'word perfect', may still be almost unintelligible because they retain the stress and intonation of their native language. Their foreign accent stamps them in fact as foreigners and the slightest trace betrays their foreign origin to the native. In *Learning to Talk* (Greene, 1960a) the comment of a weary English linguist (Joan van Thal) during an international congress of logopedics and phoniatrics is quoted. 'It is so much easier to understand French French and German German than French English and German English!' For real mastery of a language, to speak it like a native, the second language must be learned in early childhood, though the modern teaching method of the language laboratories promises a solution to the difficulties of acquiring a perfect accent later in life.

Winckel (1952) has shown that stress in speech is dependent upon increase in breath force and a fuller use of resonance. Inflexion is accomplished by minute adjustments in the length and tension of the folds which produce expressive pitch glides. Pace is varied by the slackening and quickening of the vocal and articulatory movements which regulate the speed of utterance. The meaning of speech is utterly dependent upon the factors of stress, pitch and pace, which are conceived intellectually as a rhythmic sequence of events and give coherence to what would otherwise be the utterance of a disconnected series of vowels and consonants (Thurburn, 1939). In linguistics these features are referred to as non-segmental characteristics of speech in contrast to the segmental features of vowels and consonants.

Fairbanks (1960) defining intonation and stress in the light of knowledge gained in the acoustic laboratory, states that intonation is an inclusive term referring to pitch as a function of time and may be applied to a simple inflexion or to long-term variation in phrases over numerous inflexional shifts. Stress refers to relative vocal prominence and is the combined effect of duration, pitch and intensity. Thus words appear to be compounded of increased duration, higher or lower pitch or greater intensity than neighbouring words. Stress and intonation have therefore subtly blended qualities of time, pitch and rhythm. Fairbanks in defining rhythm in speech as 'a pattern of vocal change' says that 'it is inherent in speech to be rhythmic' and draws attention to the need for regular lung ventilation and breathing patterns which underlie pause, stress, unstress, rate, pitch and intensity. Jerkiness refers to irregularity in this display or to spasmodic interruptions to inherent rhythmic patterns. Stammering is essentially a disturbance in this vital rhythm of speech.

Accent refers to the relative stress of a syllable in a word. If the traditional accent of a word is altered it becomes almost unrecognisable, as for example if the middle syllable of 'camera' is stressed and the first and third left unaccented. Totally deaf children, therefore, must be given kinaesthetic and tactile training in rhythm before they can integrate speech sounds and words in sentences and speak with sufficiently correct rhythmic stress to make themselves intelligible (Ling, 1963). Good articulation is not in itself sufficient to provide intelligibility. The 'scanning' speech of dysarthric patients is almost incomprehensible because it lacks traditionally accepted linguistic patterns of stress and intonation. Each syllable is uttered singly without pitch or stress variation (page 280). Rhythmic training is necessary in neurological voice disorders (Chapter 14).

Although little variety in word stress is possible, an infinite variety of rhythmic stress in sentences is permissible, meaning now being conveyed also by subtle changes in pitch and volume. By change in the melody of a sentence its meaning can be radically altered, though the phonetic structure remains unchanged. Thus the simple phrase 'Shut the door' may be command, question, wheedling request, tactful suggestion or the exasperated and hundredth reiteration that day. Practice in speaking the same single phrase in the greatest variety of ways helps those whose voices are colourless and monotonous on account of lack of variety in melodic cadence and stress.

Poetry which has marked stress or metre, the melody of which can be easily appreciated by ear and remembered, greatly assists co-ordination. The strength of the rhythmic concept in obtaining fluent and integrated speech is demonstrated by the speech of many clutterers who, quite unable to read or recite prose without a pronounced 'hitch or hobble' (Stanhope, 1932), have no difficulty with poetry having a pronounced rhythm.

The performance of rhythmic movements while speaking is another aid to co-ordination. Thurburn (1939) recommends the smooth tracing of a figure-of-eight with the hand in time to the rhythm of the metre. The humming of the melody of a phrase before speaking it is also an excellent method of developing the melodic appreciation of speech. The reading of good prose, of passages chosen for their vivid meaning and balanced phrases, also aids the rhythmic utterance and expression and is emphasised in training techniques by McAllister (1952). Although rhythm in prose is less conspicuous than in poetry by reason of the absence of repetitive metre, variations in stress and tempo are equally important in the artistic interpretation of a passage, ensuring the proper integration of all those aspects essential to good delivery. Pitch changes, moreover, keep the laryngeal muscles supple, as it were, and avoid overuse of muscle sets in maintenance of a monotonous and uninflected drone.

If relaxation and rhythmic training are made the basis of training in speech and voice production, the automatic co-ordination of respiration, phonation and articulation and melody is assured. This training also facilitates the use of only those muscle groups which contribute to efficiency. The technique thus acquired will faithfully serve both speaker and singer and amply repay the time spent in learning. Ease in performance will accompany any form of communication, be it oratory, drama, song, teaching, preaching or simple conversation. The degree of artistry achieved in the field of communication is largely a matter of individual ability, of course, but the degree of technique acquired is a matter of individual application.

6 Normal voice mutation: infancy to senescence

The voices of children in infancy and early childhood, under the age of seven years, have attracted little scientific interest in the past and there were few studies of the vocal characteristics of normal children to be found in the literature until quite recently Wasz-Höckert and colleagues made a unique study of the infant cry (1968). This is a field of voice research which would contribute valuable information to the fuller understanding of the psychopathology of childhood vocal nodules and also childhood speech and language disorders. It is noticeable that many children with articulatory faults due to poor co-ordination of the organs of articulation also have disturbed breathing patterns, hoarseness and monotonous vocal pitch. The inflexional patterns of normal children with retarded language development also have deficient vocal melody and monotonous inflexional patterns and rhythmic disturbances if one listens for these, although the average speech pathologist fails to do so in concentrating upon the phonemic confusions and articulatory defects of speech. Such deficiencies may be due to delays in neuromuscular maturation as well as intellectual cortical delays in the complex function of discriminating, storing, organising and recalling the melodic elements of language as described in Chapter 5. Monrad-Krohn (1947) has described these features of speech as the 'prosodic' quality which he defines as 'that faculty of speech which conveys different shades of meaning by means of variations in stress and pitch—irrespective of the words and the grammatical construction'. He has analysed the altered melody of language, the 'broken accent', or dysprosody of a dysphasic Norwegian patient who developed a German accent.

In collecting recordings of infants crying and babbling from 2 weeks onwards for a study in sound of *Learning to Talk* (Greene, 1963), Conway obtained recordings of an infant who later suffered from considerable delay in language development. This child's early vocalisation lacked the usual melodic inflexion and was limited to upward glides within a range of C_3–G_3 with no falling glides. The vocalisation, cooing and babbling melody and rhythm of infants undoubtedly contain important diagnostic clues for future speech proficiency. In its simplest aspect some infants vocalise earlier and far more prolifically than others. Profuse or negligible conversational and well inflected jargon occurs in different children (Greene, 1960).

At birth the larynx is very small. There is some difference of opinion as to the actual length of the vocal folds. Negus (1949) reports that they are 3 mm long at 14 days; 5·5 mm at 1 year; 7·5 mm at 5 years; 8 mm at $6\frac{1}{2}$ years and 9·5 mm at 15 years. There is a great increase in the size of the larynx between $2\frac{1}{2}$ and 5 years. The voice of the child of 5 years loses the piping pitch of the first years and this is an indication that infancy is over. Moses (1954) maintains that between 4 and 5 years a sex difference in the vocal range develops although there is no difference in length of the vocal folds between the two sexes. 'The basis of the adaptation is psychic: the four-year-old child is conscious of his sex and of a broad range of its implications'. This view is not generally accepted but has quite probably been insufficiently explored and requires scientific investigation. The boy is more aggressive and noisy than the girl and the games he plays and the language he uses probably denote his sex more than vocal pitch and tone.

Terracol, Guerrier and Camps (1956) state that the dimensions of the glottis of the infant vary in the actions of respiration and phonation and the function is essentially sphincteric. The hypopharynx is a hypersensitive zone which ensures that the slightest excitation produces a reflex spasm and closes the larynx. This can be detected clearly in the crying of the infant; the inspiratory wails and choking sounds when distressed are produced as a result of the safety mechanism of reflex sphincteric closure of the larynx, preventing inspiration of saliva into the trachea. The vocal folds Terracol *et al.* (1956) describe as being 7–9 mm at 8 days old and growing steadily until they attain a length of 15 mm at 3 years in the boy. They say no further growth takes place until 12 years or commencement of puberty.

The fibres of the vocalis muscle are incomplete at birth and develop alongside the more primitive thyroarytenoid muscle in which there is a sudden and considerable increase in size from the beginning of the ninth month. The increasing range of inflexion in the infant's voice from birth onwards is dependent upon the factors of growth and neuro-muscular maturation, which Von Leden (1961) states is not complete before 3 years.

Fairbanks (1942) reported an acoustical investigation of the pitch of experimentally produced hunger wails in his own male child at the 2 o'clock feeding at regular monthly intervals from 1–9 months. At one month the pitch varied from 153 to 888 cs; at 2 months from 63 to 947 cs; at 3 months from 89 to 2,120 cs; at 4 months from 214 to 1,495 cs and at 5 months from 229 to 2,387 cs[1]. The range then became more or less stabilised with range 207 to 2,631 cs recorded at 9 months. Fairbanks comments on the fact that very few coloratura sopranos can achieve a range in singing covering three octaves above middle C and equal to the vocal range of the 9-month-old child. He rightly attributes the regular and rapid rise in frequency up to 5 months to increased neuro-muscular development and not to increasing length of vocal folds. He attributed the plateau at 9 months to conditioning to the speech of the environment. This has been confirmed by Siegel (1969) with infants of 3 months of age, besides Osgood (1953) and Lennenberg *et al.* (1965) who studied vocalisation of infants in their first year.

Wasz-Höckert, Lind, Vuorenkoski, Partanen and Valanne (1968) carried out a spectrographic and auditory analysis of the infant cry. The subjects were 39 boys and 4 girls of age range 1 to 30 days, and 87 infants age range 1 to 7 months. They distinguished four characteristic signals produced by babies: birth, hunger, pain and pleasure cries. The birth cry is tense and raucous, 'voiceless' and short, about 1·5 sec. in duration or less. A cry is classified as the phonation produced in an expiration. The pain cry is tense, the longest signal, the best identified. Maximum mean pitch recorded was 740 c.p.s. and minimum pitch 460 c.p.s.: it has a mostly falling or flat melody. The hunger cry mean ranges from 500 to 320 c.p.s. and has a rising falling melody. The pleasure cry which does not appear till around 3 months has a rising, falling melody also with mean pitch ranges from 650 to 360 c.p.s.: it is never tense but lax: is often nasal and contains no glottal plosives, vocal fry or subharmonic breaks.

Wasz-Höckert *et al.* (1968) have also started studying infant cries in babies with pathological conditions which promise to be of great value in diagnostic pediatrics. For example, in babies with kinicterus it is well known that the level of serum bilirubin does not always reflect the presence or absence of neurological damage but acoustic analysis of the babies' cries does.

---

[1] C_1 is 64 c.p.s. and C_3 is 256 c.p.s.

This team played recordings of infant cries to parents, mid-wives and nurses. The most characteristic cries were the most easily identified and the less characteristic less well identified. The authors conclude that crying in the newborn is purposive. 'The baby is trying to communicate with the adult and it would be churlish not to respond'.

This fascinating study is accompanied by a disc of the cries which appear in the spectrograms in the book and includes the abnormal cries in Down's Syndrome, 'Crie-du-chat' and brain damage.

The same team (Valanne *et al.*, 1967) have examined the ability of human mothers to identify the hunger cry signals of their own new-born infants during the lying-in period and found that the mothers were successful in identifying their own babies on a tape recording including many others. Formby (1967) reported similar findings. The baby's cry has individual and personal characteristics as one would expect from the fact that they have different physiognomies.

Greene and Conway (1963) collected many recordings of crying babies in the first three months of life, some of which were used to illustrate the study in sound of how the infant learns to talk. We were impressed by the variation in the quantity, volume and quality of the cries of these infants. Fluctuations in volume, hard attack, tension and voice breaks, disruption of breathing, with breath catching, choking and hoarseness were apparent. Not all babies became hoarse after violent and prolonged crying. Volume was the greatest variable. Pitch changes were not so conspicuous, range being limited by the immaturity of the vocal folds. The happy babies' hunger cries were quite different from those of the unhappy babies, which expressed extreme distress. The whole gamut of human suffering could be heard in these primitive and reflex cries, from the pitiful complaint of discomfort or utter misery to the full blast of anger and aggression. Although I never met these babies, Conway confirmed the personality structure of the infants and their mothers from personal knowledge. The 'good' babies had calm mothers and the unhappy babies, anxious mothers.

Nurses and midwives are fully aware of the different vocal characteristics of the babies in their charge, which guide them in their assessment of how dire is the real need of a wailing infant. New mothers have to learn to interpret the cries of their offspring, and for the purpose of education such recordings as Wasz-

Höckert *et al.* (1968) have made are of course invaluable. They admit, however, that the spectrographic method has its limitations and it is not possible to rate quantitatively many characteristics, such as voice quality, tension, nasality, etc., and for these ratings they had to rely upon the evaluation by ear of the investigators. It is worthwhile describing, therefore the less exact scientific study carried out by Greene and Richardson (Greene, 1964) who studied recordings of infants in the first 9 months of life with a piano as a pitch guide, being interested in the earliest appearance of musical vowels as distinct from crying and scolding noises. The progressive development of inflectional glides in cooing and babbling was noted. The earliest appearance of an upward glide C_3–C$\sharp$ was in a girl 2 weeks old, and in the same child the range increased from C_3–E_3 at 7 weeks. A baby boy ranged from C$\sharp$ to F$\sharp$ in glides of a semitone on one breath at 5 weeks and achieved an inspiratory crow at $G_4\sharp$. This child had varied vowels and diphthongs and varied musical inflection at 16 weeks, rising and falling between $C_2\sharp$ and E_2. He produced these delightful musical glides up and down the scale within the range of $C_2\sharp$—E_2 and as a social response at 18 weeks when rhythmic syllables and babbling were developing rapidly. This child spoke early.

Upward glides appeared in these babies first, then rising and falling glides which increased in quantity and range progressively covering approximately an octave at 6–7 months. The influence of heard speech is obviously strong in this development and is present as what Piaget (1951) describes as 'contagion' as early as one month old. Vocal imitation is thought by Lewis (1951) to reach a peak at 3 months and then subside but my own experience is that there is a progressive increase along a continuum. Observers of the phenomenon have concentrated upon the aspects of articulation, the vowel and consonant imitation rather than vowel glides, inflection and rhythm, which we believe to be of great importance in the prognosis of speech development.

Authorities on child speech development maintain that genetically fixed babble patterns are similar in all children of all races and Wasz-Höckert *et al.* (1968) found no difference between Finnish and Swedish babies. Infant vocalisation, however, is individual and characteristic, also it varies in quality and quantity being dependent upon inherent personality and environmental stimulus.

The author's grandson, P., recorded at fortnightly intervals during the first year, could echo a rising vowel glide at 8 weeks, an ability which was soon lost. At 7 months he could imitate the syllable [gɔi] and once stimulated would play with this syllable spontaneously. On our gramophone record (Greene and Conway, 1960) Michael of 8 months imitates his mother's 'hullo' with better inflection than vowel definition. P. at 9 months imitated the rhythm of a simple melody but not inflection and had rocked to the rhythm of singing from 6 months. His babbling was not as varied nor so prolific as the children recorded by Conway nor were his inflexions so musical. He was very late in speaking and language development. He was anoxic at birth and there is a familial speech difficulty. The family gave much language stimulation, anticipating trouble, from the day he was born. It is interesting that this emphasis on training did not ameliorate the inborn traits. P.'s brother A. said [bu:] after feeding at least once a day after 7 days old. He gave inspiratory crows and responded to soft loving speech and smiling face with upward glides on [u:] and [ə:] at $4\frac{1}{2}$ weeks. This early promise was realised later in early speech development and high intelligence.

By 5 years the child's speaking voice settles under the influence of the environment at a median pitch in the region of middle C, or maybe two or three semitones higher. The child's singing range, which varies very little in boys and girls, covers the middle octave at the age of 7 years according to Tarneaud (1961). At 8 years the lower range is only slightly extended and the voice ranges from B_2 to B_3. At 9 years the range extends a little further in both directions from B_2 to D_4.

PITCH CHANGES IN CHILDHOOD AND ADOLESCENCE

The pitch breaks which occur in children's voices over the age of 7 years have received much attention on account of the need to understand and manage the voice mutation difficulties of adolescence in singing. Weiss (1950) in his comprehensive survey of the literature cites 334 sources. We are indebted to him also for his clarification of the problems involved.

Weiss defines 'break of voice' as a sudden and involuntary change in its pitch and *quality*. 'Voice break' therefore should properly be confined to the characteristic fluctuations in pitch *and* quality in adolescence during the period of voice mutation. The voice may rise or fall an octave and change register, rising to the falsetto or falling to the bass register. The voice 'breaks' analysed in the work of American workers described below either refer to the mutational period of voice break in adolescence or to 'shifts' in pitch during childhood. These shifts consist of abrupt and un-controlled rises and falls in vocal pitch due to poor co-ordination of the laryngeal musculature associated with general bodily growth. They do not have in boys the masculine quality which is so conspicuous and bizarre a feature of the real break of voice in adolescence. The young boy's resonator system naturally cannot produce the necessary resonance characteristics of adult male voice. This difference between real voice 'break' and vocal 'shifts' in pitch should be borne in mind when studying the important work of Curry (1940) and Fairbanks *et al.* (1949) which we are about to delineate.

Pitch breaks both up and down the scale were thought to occur only in adolescence until an oscillograph study by Curry into the pitch characteristics of adolescent male voices. He studied three groups of males: 6 10-year-olds, 6 14-year-olds and 6 8-year-olds. There was little difference in the mean pitch of the 10-year-old and 14-year-old boys which were 269·7 $C_3\sharp$ and 241·5 $C_3\sharp$ respectively. At 18 years the pitch dropped to 137·1 $C_2\sharp$ which confirmed the commonly accepted fact that the male voice drops an octave during pubertal mutation. The major drop in pitch occurring after 14 years was later than was anticipated. The voice breaks both up and down occurred within a 3-tone (6-semitones) range and were similar in both 10- and 14-year-olds, being only slightly lower for the 14-year-olds, and all occurring below the median pitch. These breaks were abrupt and quite different from the normal inflexional glides of speech and they were absent in the voices of the 18-year-old subjects.

Fairbanks, Wiley and Lassman (1949) studied the vocal pitch of 7- and 8-year-old boys and Fairbanks, Herbert and Hammond (1949) that of 7- and 8-year-old girls in order to discover whether the voice breaks in 10-year-olds reported by Curry (1940) were due to the beginning of adolescent voice mutation; the period of 'pubescence', the onset of adolescence and pubertal development, described by Weiss (1950). Fairbanks and his co-workers found that the voices of both 7- and 8-year-old boys and girls were pitched in the region of middle C and similar to those of adult females. The pitch of boys' voices at 7 and 8 years were similar to boys of 10 and 14 years. The pitch breaks, both up and down, in the 7- and 8-year-old boys were similar to the breaks in the voices of the 10- and 14-year-old boys and therefore could not be attributed to adolescence. Voice breaks were recorded in the 7- and 8-year-old girls as frequently as in the boys' voices. It seems therefore that this feature of pitch change of childhood voice is not sex-linked nor peculiar to adolescence or pubescence at 10 years. The vocal shifts would appear to be a perfectly normal physiological feature of juvenile laryngeal function. These shifts may also, we think, be aggravated by vocal strain imposed by vocal abuse in children who shout and scream at football matches and in the playground. Vocal shifts and subharmonic breaks were recorded in infants by Wasz-Höckert *et al.* (1968).

Luchsinger (1962) states that real voice breaks or 'stormy mutation' occur only in a minority of boys and are not the general rule. Weiss (1950) emphasises that the sudden drop or rise in the voice, changing momentarily from the childish treble to the adult male or vice versa is so conspicuous that it has accordingly been considered the main characteristic of the pubertal voice change, whereas the evidence is that it is actually uncharacteristic and unusual.

Dawson in his book *The Voice of the Boy* (1919) attributed pitch breaks to collapse of the voice due to misuse and vocal strain. None of his choirboys suffered from 'breaking' of the speaking voice or singing voice: their voices slid down the scale. He evaluated the pitch of their singing voices at frequent intervals and shifted them after $12\frac{1}{2}$ years from soprano to alto and gradually to tenor or baritone by 15 years as their voices dropped with growth of the larynx. He attributed failure to sing well in a boy to vocal abuse in childhood and advocated early training in breathing technique. The majority of experts stress the dangers for both boys and girls of singing during the mutational period and will not permit serious voice training to begin until 17 years with girls and 18–19 years with boys. Weiss (1950) points out that very few choirboys, possibly a mere 2 per cent, ever turn into good adult singers and this is attributed to the irreparable damage contracted in adolescence. Few singing teachers or choir masters instruct their pupils in the fundamentals of good voice production. Dawson (1919) stressed the need to cast off the antiquated shackles of bygone ages in teaching singing in schools. Moreover, the mutational period of the *singing* voice lasts very much longer than that of the *speaking* voice and this is often not understood and recognised by singing teachers.

Moses (1960), whose original contributions to vocal philosophy are of considerable interest, has discussed the modern trends in singing in relation to the history of opera and the castrati singers. He expresses the opinion that the appeal of vocal range in singing can be analysed from both musical and anthropological view-points. The latter incorporates the desire for unification of both sexes in vocal expression. He instances the admiration for the male tenor's production of high C in the soprano range and the popularity of the husky male notes of the female crooner. The singing range is largely determined by conditioning of the ear and muscular control to the conventional musical patterns. Wolfsohn (1956) was able to train his pupils to break away from convention and recover a range of 6 octaves similar to that of the untrained infant. Luchsinger and Dubois (1956) analysed the singing voice of Jennifer Johnson (a Wolfsohn pupil) whose range was found to be from low C (65 cs) to F_4 (2,960 cs). The highest notes consisted of sine waves (pure tones) and were apparently produced by compressing air through a narrow inflexible glottal chink in the same way as notes are produced on an ocarina (see page 49). The highest and lowest notes of this range, in my opinion, cannot be classified as singing but are freak noises having no musicality, despite the claim by Wolfsohn and his disciples that they are 'sung'. That the bat-like trills and animal grunts at the two extremes of vocal range are expressions of the racial unconscious related to the anthropological develop-ment of Man also seems to me highly questionable.

STORMY MUTATION IN BOYS

Those boys' voices which do undergo a prolonged and stormy mutation need not be considered pathological. The growth of the larynx which changes the childish treble to tenor presumably requires less time and is less demanding in adjustment than the larynx which changes the voice to bass. The deeper the voice drops the greater the difficulties in muscular adaptation, it would be logical to assume, also the greater the auditory awareness of change and self-consciousness engendered in the youth. Some adolescents may be proud of the vocal symptoms as a demonstra-tion of maturity and manhood, others may feel extreme em-barrassment. All depends on the personality. A stammering boy of 10 years responded well to speech therapy, for example, and stopped stammering for several months until his voice began to break at 12 years. This caused considerable self-consciousness and loss of confidence and return of the stammer. There was a pronounced increase in the number of breaks from falsetto to tenor and back when nervous, and very few when socially at ease and relaxed.

The breaking of the voice has always been attributed to rapid growth of the laryngeal cartilages and muscles and disturbance in fine co-ordination of the vocal mechanism. Nervousness and tension may aggravate inco-ordination. Difficulty in laryngeal management is only one aspect of the general difficulty in co-ordination arising out of the suddenly increased dimensions of the body at puberty. The clumsiness of the adolescent is well known; it is often attributed to self-consciousness, but the gawkishness of 'callow youth' is really the result of the dramatic elongation of the limbs which takes the boy unawares. He no longer knows his own length or strength, he knocks things over, slams doors, trips over carpets and spills from jugs and cups, seeming suddenly to be unaware that fluids shifted with too great impetus are propelled from their containers. The inco-ordination responsible for exaggerated and uncontrolled motor activity is amusingly similar to that of the toddler, and the boy leaves childhood with as much stagger and flourish as he entered it.

There is a considerable increase in the growth of the laryngeal cartilages at this time. The thyroid angle increases in boys and the 'Adam's apple' develops with a corresponding increase in length of the vocal folds. In girls the mean length is 15 mm before puberty and this may increase to 17 mm in a contralto. During the mutation period a boy's vocal folds may increase to a maximum of 23 mm in the bass voice. The minimum vocal fold length for the male is 17 mm so it can be seen that a tenor and a contralto may have much the same pitch range, but it is the larger resonators of larynx, pharynx and particularly chest which distinguish the male voice from the female.

Sometimes voice mutation is accompanied by chronic laryngitis in the male if strain is allowed to develop during the difficult period of growth. The voice is not only subject to pitch breaks but hoarseness. Curry (1949) investigated the question of hoarseness which is generally alleged to precede male voice mutation. He examined 40 boys aged 10 years and 40 boys aged 14. Three speech correctionists acting as judges agreed that 55 per cent of the ten-year-olds and 80 per cent of the 14-year-olds were 'hoarse husky', which confirms at least that hoarseness is more prevalent in the mutation period.

In some cases oedema of the larynx is such that the arytenoids fail to approximate and many writers speak of the 'mutational triangle' (Weiss, 1950) in this connection. This manifests itself in approximation of the vocal folds along the pars respiratus and separation in the cartilaginous portion. Such cases are few, however, and in the great majority of boys there is only a transient huskiness and fluctuations in pitch over 3–4 semitones as the voice gradually finds its mature level over a period of several months.

Voice mutation and vocal pitch are unquestionably tied to growth of the larynx and lengthening of the vocal cords. McGlone and Hollien (1963) found that the girls' vocal pitch is at its highest at 7–8 years and drops between 11–15 years 2·4 semitones and remains at much the same level throughout life.

Michel, Hollien and Moore (1966) recorded the speaking fundamental pitch of 15-, 16- and 17-year-old girls and found that the mean fundamental was 207·5, 207·3 and 207·8 c.p.s. respectively. This indicates that fundamental frequency is established at 15 years in girls and pubertal mutation is over.

Naidr, Zbořil and Ševčik (1965) carried out a five-year study of 100 boys at one school. They related changes in singing and speaking voice to anatomical changes in size of larynx, and height and weight of the boys. They noted changes in the voice occurring between 12 and 13 years with a striking loss of high notes. This corresponded with height of larynx of 30 mm and increase in body height. Between 13 and 14 years singing range became restricted with clearly prominent thyroid and considerable increase in body weight. The end of the mutational period occurred between 14 and 15 years. The voice reached its full depth with maximal growth of larynx, body weight and height attained.

This study by Naidr *et al.* (1965) indicates that there is little difference between the completion of puberty in males and females although onset of puberty is generally believed to be earlier in females.

There used apparently to be a difference in age of onset of puberty in females in hot and cold climates. In cold climates the average age was between 12 and 14 years but between 9 and 11 years in hot climates. Now there is less, if any difference, and puberty occurs earlier generally. This is attributed to improved diet and is an interesting change in socio-economic history.

The mutational changes in girls' voices are scarcely noticeable. The vocal folds do not increase so considerably in length, the minimum being 12·5 mm and the maximum 17 mm. The voice drops only 3 or 4 semitones below the original child's treble.

The girl's voice may be husky and this may be attributed to shyness or a cold but is generally due to hormonal changes. Amado (1953) believes hormonal imbalance leads to a lack of muscular tonicity and notes that some women's voices become husky before menstruation. Hildernisse (1956) reminds us that singers often have a clause in their contracts to exempt them from singing during the menstrual period. Tarneaud (1961) draws attention to voice change during menstruation and pregnancy.

Flach, Schwickardi and Simon (1969) examined 136 professional singers in order to find what influence menstruation and pregnancy had on their voices. There were menstrual voice changes for the worse in all of them. During pregnancy two-thirds of singers experienced voice changes which persisted after delivery in a quarter of this group. Perello (1962) attributes endocrine dysphonia to changes in the laryngeal mucosa and notes that the speaking voices of women frequently drop and show slight periodic changes of this nature, but it is only an inconvenience to singers and goes largely unnoticed in everyday life.

Lacina (1968) found 'premenstrualis laryngopathia' and vocal deterioration in quality of voice, not volume, due to congestion of the vocal cords of female singers. He found about one-third of female singers to be affected, and advocates a premenstrual drug but a period of 3 days' vocal rest during menstruation.

A husky voice may also be a symptom of sexual excitement. The soft husky tones of love-making probably have a psycho-endocrinological basis in that actual changes take place in the mucosal lining of the larynx. The husky voices of female crooners, film stars and actresses are much admired, envied and even simulated by women, and adored by men who are unconsciously excited by their sexual appeal. Eartha Kitt is popular with both male and female audiences.

The larynx of the adolescent girl may appear slightly reddened on inspection though there may be no vocal signs. Redness may be attributed erroneously to laryngitis or vocal strain whereas it may have a purely endocrinological basis. The voice should be rested and singing and acting avoided since it is just as possible to damage the female singing voice permanently as it is the boy's voice, though the speaking voice shows no impairment in most cases after strain in adolescence.

AGEING OF THE VOICE

Senescence describes the normal ageing process in man and senility the pathological condition. It is generally believed that the voice becomes weak and tremulous and high-pitched in old age, and it is obvious that the singing voice deteriorates much earlier than the speaking voice. There are great individual variations in age of onset and degree of vocal deterioration in old age. Much depends upon the quality of phonation earlier, a fine voice and especially a trained voice need not deteriorate at all in speech although the possibilities for singers naturally are reduced with age. Dame Sybil Thorndike, now 90 years of age, still has a fine acting voice but, of course, it has a mature and rich quality which is an indication of age. Martinelli, the Italian tenor, was still singing and recording at the age of 76 at the Metropolitan Opera House and sang the part of Terandotte at 82. Amado (1953) reminds us that several other male singers have preserved their voices at concert level over the age of 70. He names Malfia Battistini and Léon Melchissédec but no female singers of comparable age.

The cartilages of the larynx may begin to calcify and lose their elasticity after the age of 25 but this is not necessarily so. Zenker (1964a) says that the thyroid cartilage may still be elastic at the age of 70 years yet be rigid in much younger individuals. Pantoja (1968) examined the cartilages of 100 normal adults. He found that ossification in the thyroid cartilage begins in the inferior horns and progresses along the inferior and posterior borders and then along the anterior border and angle. He determined that calcification is not constant and may be absent even in the oldest patients. In singers and dramatic actors who preserve their voices into old age calcification presumably has not taken place.

Another aspect of ageing is the atrophy of the laryngeal muscles. Luchsinger (1962) describes the false cords as narrower and the vocal cords more visible in the laryngoscopic mirror so that the opening into the laryngeal ventricle appears very wide. The vocal folds are visibly less tense and may exhibit bowing. The mucous membrane can be reddish or show yellow or brownish pigmentation. The laryngologist sees the changes taking place in the larynx, and the laboratory phonetician records the acoustic changes and breaks in pitch by instruments. Long ago Shakespeare in *As You Like It* recorded from his own observations with masterly accuracy 'the sixth stage of man':

> The sixth stage shifts
> Into the lean and slipper'd pantaloon,
> With spectacles on nose and pouch on side,
> His youthful hose, well saved, a world too wide
> For his shrunk shank; and his big manly voice,
> Turning again toward childish treble, pipes
> And whistles in his sound.

It is only the untrained voices of men which rise in pitch, however. McGlone *et al.* (1963) investigated the vocal pitch characteristics of aged women, 10 women aged 65–79 and 10 aged 80–94 years. They found no evidence of a senile voice and rise in pitch nor drop in pitch. Saxman and Burk (1967) on the other hand examined a group of 9 women aged 30–40 years and 9 aged 40–50. They found the first group had an average pitch of 196·34 c.p.s. and the second group 188·58 c.p.s. from which they drew the rather sweeping conclusion that women's voices dropped in pitch with advancing age.

Mysak (1959) in a study of three groups of males of mean age 47·9, 73·3 and 85·0 years found there was a progressive upward trend in mean pitch levels although the males of the 47·9 year age group had lower levels (110 c.p.s.) than found in a student group of males studied by Snidecor (1943) whose mean pitch level was 129 c.p.s. The 85·0 year age group had significantly higher pitch levels than the 73·3 year age group. There was also an all-round slowing down in speech activity resulting in fewer words uttered per minute and with greater duration of pauses, which was thought to reflect a slowing down in mental processes of the aged groups.

Advances in medical science have resulted in the better management of the problems of the ageing body. Attention to diet and psychological health wards off many of the physical ills men and women were a prey to in the dangerous middle years. Ageing nowadays is less a question of years than of physiological age and retention of mental alertness, physical fitness and emotional equilibrium. Accordingly a healthy 80-year-old may be a youngster compared to an aged 60-year-old. Care and attention should be paid to preserving vocal efficiency in the active elderly since it preserves their social effectiveness and their youth. A hoarse and deteriorated voice greatly ages an individual in the ears of the listener and possibly of himself.

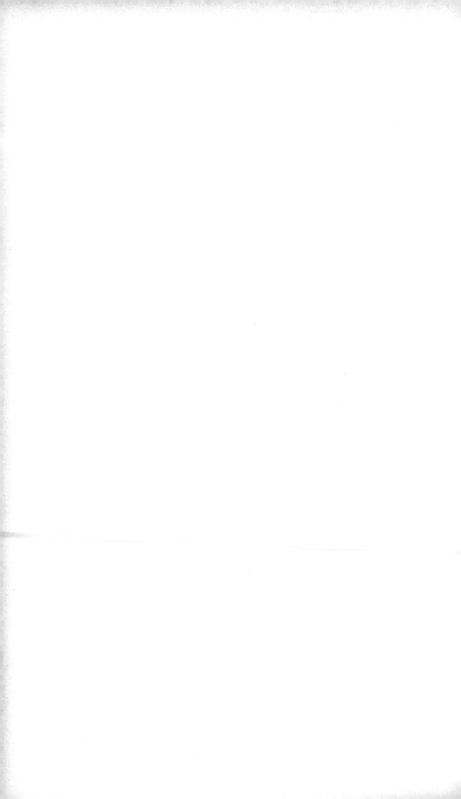

Part Two
Voice Disorders

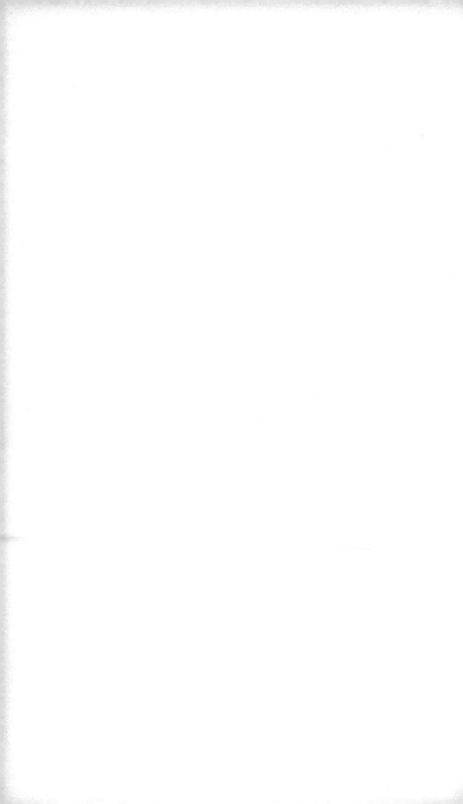

7 Hyperkinetic dysphonia: vocal strain

Aphonia means without voice. Dysphonia refers to impaired voice, that is, voice deviating in some way from the normal. This said, we have to admit that normal voice virtually defies definition and abnormal voice is even more difficult to describe since judgement depends so much upon the social and educational background of the listener. A speech therapist will have quite different criteria of normality to those of a manual labourer. In London and Southern England the melodious cultured voice is much admired and there is a far greater consciousness concerning good and bad voice and vocal deterioration, than in the north. On Teesside, for example, harsh voices are usual and this is reflected dramatically in the small load of patients referred to speech therapists from ear, nose and throat departments. In London there is a constant flow of every conceivable type of dysphonia and in Newcastle such patients are scarce. This is a reflection of social and economic conditions in the two areas, the difference between the affluent south and the poorer north where the struggle for existence is greater and the refinements of voice a low priority. The same observations are true for America and other parts of the world. It does not matter very much if a voice is beautiful or otherwise as long as it is adequate and suitable for that person's social and economic situation. What is important is any sudden change in the voice which makes it sound and feel different from what it has been in the past. A porter on the staff of a hospital had an excruciatingly harsh and grating dysphonia. I was often asked why I did not do anything about it. Eventually, when wishing to make the point I am making here in a lecture to a group of medical officers, I approached this gentleman tactfully and asked whether he would be so kind as to allow me to do a tape recording as his voice was so 'interesting'. Far from being upset, he was delighted, he said he had often been told he had an 'interesting accent'. The medical officers diagnosed by ear vocal nodules, laryngeal palsy and carcinoma and were impressed to learn that this was a constitutional dysphonia of long standing and the subject was not a patient at all.

We can say in general that the essential attributes of normal voice are basically audibility (appropriate volume), pleasing quality, and pitch appropriate to age and sex. Added to this, the voice must be suitably modulated and observe the linguistic melody as well as word and sentence stress. The voice must also be appropriately expressive. And here we come to the most intimate and subtle aspect of voice as an expression of personality. This aspect especially is of the greatest consequence in considering voice disorders due to mismanagement of the vocal mechanism, in which the inexperienced voice specialist may hear the mechanical faults and miss the emotional attitudes as an undercurrent in speech.

SCIENTIFIC DEFINITION AND ASSESSMENT OF DYSPHONIA

When the sound spectrogram was originally invented and produced commercially by the Kay instrument company there were great expectations of its possibilities in providing a scientific basis for classification of voice disorders. It was hoped that it would produce an exact method of description in place of the old method of subjective assessment by just listening and then describing with the adjectives a particular speech pathologist found most suitable. Such assessment cannot help being loaded with unscientific and personal bias as Renfrew, Mitchell and Wallace (1957) point out. No two speech therapists, let alone two lay persons, will mean the same thing by metallic, hoarse or nasal. Unfortunately the sound spectrogram has not lived up to expectations in practice. This is for various reasons. The fact that only 2·4 seconds of consecutive speech can be analysed at a time is a serious handicap. It does not allow a full assessment of temporal, pitch and stress aspects over an adequate stretch of connected speech. The segmentation of speech passages into 2·4 second periods even for a period of 30 seconds is a laborious business. Furthermore, the spectrograph confuses by the sheer wealth of frequencies it analyses so accurately, much of which is redundant to the human ear. It provides subliminal data which has no significance to the listener. For example, a spectrograph may give data indicating excessive nasality which can hardly be perceived by the ear (Van den Berg, 1962). When one realises that the spectrographs of normal speakers uttering the 'same' vowel are not only considerably different but that the *same* vowel uttered by the *same* speaker is never the *same* again but different each time, the complexity of the picture in regard to dysphonia can be estimated. An enormous number of spectrographs of different dysphonic patients uttering the same vowel would have to be fed into an electronic computer before deviations in a certain vowel could be determined, and then specialists might not agree on the classification in the light of what they *heard*, which is after all the thing that matters.

Johnson, Darley and Spriestersbach (1963) in their diagnostic methods in speech pathology, confine examination of voice quality deviations to nasality, breathiness and harshness. These three criteria are established by Fairbanks (1960) in judging the voice. He says hoarseness can combine both breathiness and harshness and most voice deviations can be placed in one of these three categories since they do not include so great a number of different qualities as most authors ascribe to voice disorder. Fairbanks stresses that pitch, intensity and voice quality are powerfully related to each other, as is to be expected from the involvement of the vocal folds in all three. Therefore prominence of one of these factors naturally influences the other and related variables.

Isshiki *et al.* (1969) also comment on the fact that electro-acoustic analysis reveals many features the human ear cannot detect and that the instruments now available are far inferior to the ear in making a comprehensive judgement of tone quality. They assess a four-factor method of rating dysphonia: rough (R), breathy (B), aesthenic (A), degree (D). Thus a vocal cord nodule may be rated (R) and a functional voice disorder with wide glottic chink (R.A.B.) This plan of assessment comes unstuck as soon as someone not a member of this team begins to wonder about what is meant by Aesthenic and Degree. Johnson *et al.* (1963) also recognise the psychological variable in vocal assessment but take the nonpsychiatric view. They say it is not possible to predict from a harsh and breathy voice that a certain speaker has personal adjustment problems but that we should be alert to the possibility of such a relationship.

SOME CAUSES OF DYSPHONIA

Dysphonia can be caused by:

(*a*) Misuse of the voice giving rise to vocal strain (laryngitis) or damage to the vocal cords

(*b*) Structural abnormalities such as congenital anomalies of the larynx affecting phonation, or benign and malignant neoplasms

(c) Abnormalities in the resonator system such as cleft palate (excessive nasality) and adenoids (insufficient nasality)

(d) Neuro-muscular lesions such as palsy or paralysis of the muscles of the vocal folds, pharynx, tongue and soft palate

(e) Physical disease such as hypothyroidism, myasthenia gravis and the endocrinological disorders

(f) Neurotic and psychogenic disorders

(g) Effects of drug therapy

VOCAL STRAIN (HYPERKINETIC OR HABITUAL DYSPHONIA)

In this section we are concerned with vocal strain which is the most common and perhaps the most easily reversible type of voice disorder. On account of the excessive muscular tension used it is often called hyperkinetic dysphonia.

Incorrect breathing, excessive tension in the larynx and an imbalance between glottic resistance and air pressure in individuals who use their voices considerably can cause a chronic laryngitis and weakness or tiredness of the muscles and laryngeal joints. This condition gives rise to varying degrees of hoarseness and discomfort. The voice may be harsh and strong at the beginning of the day and become weak and breathy by the evening. The throat is not sore and painful as it is with an acute infective laryngitis and no discomfort is felt on swallowing, but a certain tiredness and weakness of the throat may be found troublesome. Dowie (1965) discussing the nature of 'functional dysphonia' describes the disorder of muscle function and chronic mild laryngitis which so frequently sets in after an acute infective laryngitis and perhaps influenza. When an individual becomes run down and debilitated she, rather than he, becomes less able to cope with domestic stresses and things, as we say, get on top of one. The more harassing the environmental problems and the less adequate the basic personality the more the individual may focus on the vocal symptom and this may become the chief anxiety and cause of depression and inability to cope with life's difficulties effectively. It follows that vocal exercises alone will not cure the patient but the ear of a sympathetic, impartial and wise adviser is also most necessary.

It is common experience in laryngology to find little correlation between degree of laryngitis and redness of the vocal cords and tract and degree of dysphonia. Perello (1962a) in his comprehensive congress report on functional dysphonia comments on this discrepancy: an individual with a considerable laryngitis may present a perfectly normal voice while another with minimal symptoms may be severely hoarse. He therefore stresses the aspect of the patient's own complaints in diagnosis. 'Le laryngologue, le médecin général et le malade lui-même diagnostiquent' (the laryngologist, the medical practitioner and the patient himself make the diagnosis).

St. Clair Thompson and Negus (1955) whose preoccupation with organic and pathological features is predominant, comment in their section on laryngitis on the fact that hoarseness can exist with trivial or even imperceptible alteration in the vocal folds. 'On the other hand it is remarkable how men are able to talk, and basses and baritones sing, with inflammatory conditions of the vocal folds which would render women voiceless and tenors songless.'

Zilstorff (1968) says that there is nothing to prevent a singer performing with a moderate acute rhinitis, pharyngitis, tracheitis or mild laryngitis if his technique is right. If voice technique is poor then performance is impossible or produces long-lasting strain. Ordinary speakers with poorly produced voices, of course, have more trouble getting over colds and laryngitis, and teachers with vocal strain may lose their voices completely with every cold.

Moses (1954) in his interesting and valuable book on the voice of neurosis emphasises the need always to listen to the emotional content of the voice. He stresses the need to listen to the voice as the key to personality; that is to listen to the 'pathos', indicating the individual's estimate of himself in relation to others. He reminds us that the word personality is derived from Latin *persona* which was originally the name for the mouth-piece of the mask used by actors. In the course of time the meaning of the word shifted to the actor, a person in a drama, then to any person and finally to denote 'personality'. The symbolic connection with the voice was thus forgotten.

It is necessary to link the vocal characteristics with what the patient is feeling and which may be even unconscious at the time and repressed. Moses advocates objective and systematic listening and warns against the pitfalls of personal bias as to what constitutes 'good' and 'bad' voice and also against the dangers of intuitive assessment. 'In intuition one leaves the mental doors wide open to free association and one cannot prevent like or dislike from forcing itself on one's consciousness.' It is necessary to analyse the vocal symptoms systematically to be able to find a psychic explanation, avoiding interpretation of individual vocal

5

features. The speech pathologist is particularly prone to fall into the trap of dissecting and fact-finding when listening to dysphonia. In the preoccupation of doing so, he may fail to fit together the most important pieces of the puzzle. The characteristics of lack of energy and melodic change in depression may be missed, or the aggression and anxiety evidenced by hard attack and changes in variations in pitch, volume and stress. The shy withdrawn individual's voice may be weak, low and husky. It is, of course, impossible to relate voice qualities to emotions but over the course of time the speech therapist learns by experience to 'sum up' her patient—this includes a composite picture which includes facial expression, dress, hair-style, make-up, walk, posture and gestures besides voice. Then one is not deceived by the weak voice of the self-sacrificing saintly but selfish female who is only sorry for herself, nor the 'matey', familiar and boisterous manner of the bully with his aggressive and domineering voice. So, as we take the case history and listen to the complaints of the patient concerning his voice and the chapter of disasters which usually surrounds it, we must also listen to what he is unconsciously telling us through the pathos of his voice, his opinion of himself in relation to others which makes up his life and causes problems.

The average clinical laryngologist has, of course, none of the refined scientific techniques and equipment and unlimited time available to research workers and his examination may be considered relatively crude. Using a headlight, he places a warmed mirror behind the back of the tongue of the patient while pulling the tongue forward wrapped in a square of gauze in order to obtain an adequate purchase on this notoriously slippery organ. The patient is instructed to relax, not to gag and to say [iː]. This examination is called an indirect laryngoscopy and may be upsetting to the patient although a cocaine spray often helps relaxation. A direct laryngoscopy is one involving anaesthetising the patient and introducing a laryngoscope down the throat in order to obtain a direct view of the larynx. This provides a means of more thorough investigation for pathological signs but does not yield direct information concerning the movement of the cords on phonation and is only of indirect value to the speech therapist.

Crude as the indirect laryngoscopy may be, it provides the essential information for the therapist to work on and includes assessment of the health of the throat and vocal cords, the degree of laryngitis from the redness of the cords, and swelling and collection of mucus, also movements of the cords and position in phonation. There may be a glottic chink on phonation with incomplete approximation of the arytenoids or the cords may appear flabby and bowed which is a condition commonly called an 'internal tensor weakness' by laryngologists. If there is chronic laryngitis present it is probably due to vocal strain and if there is no sign of laryngitis the dysphonia most probably is a purely psychological manifestation. It is of very great help to the therapist if she can look over the shoulder of the laryngologist and see the larynx of all her patients for herself and discuss the diagnosis with him.

Sometimes the ventricular bands are seen to be pressing down on the vocal cords with obliteration of the ventricles in persons using excessive tension when phonating. The voice is harsh and sometimes there is a double note which has given rise to the use of the term 'ventricular band voice' based on the belief that the false cords are producing phonation independently or in conjunction with the vocal cords. Patients with so called ventricular band voice were found by Ardran and Kemp (1967) to exhibit obliteration of the ventricles and no vibration of the ventricular band. Van den Berg (1955) describes the harsh metallic voice produced when the ventricles are obliterated and the higher harmonics not filtered. Ellis (1952) emphasised that the extrinsic muscles of the larynx assist in adduction of the ventricular bands and the extreme tension evoked in this movement. Perello (1954) advocates a relaxant lotion, such as Parapint, which allows natural movement of the muscles to reassert itself.

Vocal strain occurs chiefly in those whose occupations make severe demands upon the voice, such as teachers, lecturers, preachers, singers, actors and salesmen. People who have to speak in noisy surroundings may also strain the voice working in shops and factories. Professional use of the voice is not the only cause of trauma, and shouting at football matches or parties, shouting at a child or a dog or a deaf relative, even abnormal laughing or giggling habits (Briess, 1964) can cause strain.

Irritants can aggravate the mild chronic inflammation in the larynx due to vocal strain or may, of course, be the original cause of laryngitis contributing to vocal strain. A smoky, dusty or over dry atmosphere with non-humidified central heating or air conditioning can be harmful. The sensitive mucus membrane of the larynx becomes dry and irritants provoke coughing. Excessive smoking and neat spirits act as irritants but the "beery bass' may be due to hours spent in the smoky, hot atmosphere of saloon bars rather than to alcoholic consumption. A hoarse voice and a red face are not necessarily the marks of the boozer but often go with red hair and blue eyes and a sensitive skin (Munro-Black *et al.*, 1964). Such individuals are prone to laryngitis and are particularly sensitive to atmospheric irritants.

The following case history is very typical of vocal strain:

Mr Brown. Aged 47, was the headmaster of a primary school, a dynamic, enthusiastic teacher and organiser and enjoyed his work. At 43 years he had taken a two-year part-time University course and at 45 a year's full-time course in child development. He was working on a thesis concerning the difficulties of teachers in the first three years of their professional career. Three months before being referred for speech therapy he had an attack of flu and sore throat but was too busy to take sick leave. Since then he had become increasingly aware of discomfort in the throat and presented at the ear, nose and throat department at the end of the winter term. His larynx was red and there appeared to be an 'early leukoplakia'. It was decided to try speech therapy and if no improvement was gained, to review the patient for possible biopsy plus stripping of the vocal cords at Easter.

Mr Brown had given up smoking fifteen years before and he had also given up class teaching recently and confined himself to administration, telephoning, interviewing parents, staff and pupils. He loved teaching and missed the four daily lessons he habitually gave and felt he was not doing his job properly and that the children were suffering. He had been depressed and anxious before seeing the laryngologist and became convinced he had cancer of the throat.

He was tense, an inveterate and entertaining talker, breath intake was good but he inclined to talk in long phrases, running out of breath towards the end and forcing the voice out with extreme laryngeal tension on residual air. He was treated in the classic fashion with relaxation, breath control, phonation exercises and vocal projection, besides phrasing. He was an apt pupil and his technique improved rapidly during the Christmas holidays. When school reopened he was persuaded to start teaching again, since it appeared that this might be even less abusive to the larynx than his administrative work. As the term progressed his throat still felt terrible, he said, although he was quite sure he was not straining it in school any more. However, the moment he crossed the threshold in the morning he noticed the discomfort returning. Perhaps this was purely psychological? In the morning when he woke, his throat was comfortable now and his voice sounded good. Careful questioning revealed the information that Mr Brown always travelled up to London in the company of local friends, commuters like himself in a smoking compartment which was noisy and crowded. He admitted that during the 40-minutes journey he never read his paper but talked most of the time. He enjoyed immensely these discussions about world affairs, politics, etc., which got him out of 'the educational straight jacket'. He was persuaded that this activity constituted the further vocal abuse responsible for an aching throat by the time he arrived at school. Once he explained to his companions why he must sit in a corner or even another compartment and read, his cure was rapid. At Easter when his larynx was examined it was found to be normal in appearance and no surgery or further treatment was necessary.

Moore (1962) and Dunker and Schlosshauer (1964) have filmed the vocal cord vibrations of normal and hoarse individuals and analysed the abnormalities of movement which can be seen quite clearly. Irregularities occur in the duration of consecutivce cycles; the closed phase may be tighter and longer than normal or not be achieved at all; the vocal cords may vibrate at different speeds and the cord on one side execute two or three excursions to one excursion from the opposite cord. Sections of the vocal cords may approximate at different moments, not presenting a clean and regular edge on account of failure in sections of the thyroarytenoid to contract. This can be understood in terms of disturbance of the myotactic reflexes described by Wyke (1969), just as the cords being out of phase can be ascribed to greater congestion and oedema in one cord than the other, increasing its weight and reducing its elasticity.

These defects in movement due to laryngitis can be heard as pitch breaks, hard attack, grating, breathiness, etc. Phoneticians have invented new terms of reference recently to denote some aspects of dysphonia with which a speech therapist needs to be familiar. Vocal fry, creak and glottal roll are now popular. These symptoms are described as an unperiodic phonation of the vocal folds in a lower frequency range than the normal pitch register. It appears in infant cries and adult speech and can be seen in spectrograms as trembling, narrow harmonics of lower intensity (Wasz-Höckert *et al.*, 1968).

As the individual tries to overcome his vocal weakness, he puts more force into his efforts and tension increases in the larynx. The muscles contract and air pressure below builds up before it is forced through the glottis and a vicious circle is created. The vocal cords are bathed in mucus which is nature's method of protecting and lubricating them and in the circumstances of excessive friction in vocal strain there is often an excess of mucus on the vocal cords. The patient complains of a 'frog in the throat' and keeps clearing his throat which necessitates compressing the cords together and forcing air through them to blow away the beads of mucus. This causes further trauma to the delicate membrane and mechanism. All sorts of anxieties may develop concerning cancer, loss of job and financial difficulties.

HOARSENESS IN CHILDREN

Constant shouting obviously imposes a strain upon the voice. The trained speaker or singer can produce a considerably louder voice when performing in a theatre than the average person when shouting, but the trained voice suffers no injury because it is properly produced. Children who yell at the tops of their voices in the playground often suffer from chronic hoarseness. This is particularly common between the ages of 5 and 10 years (Ellis, 1952). When one hears the vocal pandemonium that breaks loose from children pouring forth from the confines of school buildings, it is a matter for astonishment that more children do not suffer from vocal strain. It is reported that in Germany 40 per cent of school children have hoarse voices (Seth and Guthrie, 1953). Boys are more commonly afflicted than girls, and the incidence is high below the age of ten and diminishes considerably as children grow older (Curry, 1949). A state of mild chronic laryngitis generally accompanies the dysphonia and the folds may be swollen and show incomplete adduction in the arytenoid region. Baynes (1969), found 7·1 per cent of children suffering from chronic hoarseness with the highest incidence in children in the first grade at school.

The voices of children are difficult to re-educate because it is almost impossible to persuade them to rest their voices or to produce them correctly. Speech therapy is, therefore, best left till the age of 11 years if dysphonia still persists. As a result of shouting less as he grows up the child's voice generally becomes normal of its own accord.

In all cases of vocal strain the condition undoubtedly depends upon the native constitution of the individual, general health and resistance to colds, and the reaction to stress (Sedláčkova, 1960). Some babies are noticeably hoarse after an excessive bout of crying and these may be the children who develop dysphonia later or are chronically hoarse throughout childhood. Flatau and Gutzmann (1907) describe such cases of congenital hoarseness and the variations in the type of voice and voice production in children and a predisposition to vocal disorder. A mild laryngitis may persist in many cases and is aggravated by colds and is often associated with enlarged adenoids and tonsils which are a 'culture bed of infection' (St. Clair-Thomson, 1955). The hoarse, muffled, denasalised voices of these children are characteristic and quite diagnostic of the condition (Greene, 1957; Pfau, 1954; Makuen, 1911). Medical and surgical treatment alleviate the laryngitis.

As a rule no treatment is prescribed for mild chronic hoarseness in childhood and it is considered best not to develop speech consciousness in these children. Hoarseness which becomes progressively more severe, also loss of voice, needs further investigation as this is frequently associated with vocal nodules.

The voice changes and dysphonias which occur in adolescence present somewhat different problems and are considered under voice mutation (Chapters 6 and 11).

HOARSENESS IN ASTHMATIC PATIENTS

Asthmatic individuals are sometimes referred for speech therapy for breathing exercises and treatment of hoarseness and there may be some doubts as to the value of speech therapy. The aetiology of asthma is very difficult to determine and there is almost equal evidence of its being a familial and allergic disorder as of its being a purely psychosomatic symptom. It seems to depend upon the personal bias in training of the investigator. Although the purely psychogenic cases occur many cases are due to allergy. It is hard to explain infantile eczema, for instance, leading to bronchial asthma in childhood on any other basis, also specific allergy to food or pollen.

Bastiaans and Groen (1955) give a clear and simple review of the aetiology and treatment of asthma. They are of the opinion that asthma is of psychogenic orgin and that the disorder originates in the unsatisfactory relationship with a domineering yet devoted mother. The child's reactions are inhibited either by discipline or by his own pattern of self-control and an inner conflict develops, the main feeling of which is that of oppression. The oppressed sensation is somatised in the form of difficulty in breathing and asthma which becomes an unconscious and reflex reaction to emotional stress. Bastiaans and Groen (1955) list ten characteristic features which form the 'core' of the asthmatic personality. Perhaps the most interesting to the speech therapist and relevant to treatment is the difficulty in solving personal problems by 'talking it over' or 'giving and taking'. They comment 'none of our asthmatic patients could be considered as capable of adequate communication in personal contact'. Medical treatment, drugs, inhalations, desensitisation and psychotherapy are all prescribed and a combination of these different modes of dealing with the problem may be necessary.

The voice of the asthmatic is generally breathy and wheezy, there being both laryngeal and respiratory symptoms. The laryngeal mucosa may be slightly congested as a reaction to allergy or continual coughing up of bronchial mucus. A real vocal strain may be present in patients who use their voices considerably. Breathing is always wheezy in chronic cases even between real attacks of asthma. Breathing is clavicular and the over-development of the upper chest with permanent changes in circumference of the thoracic cage may be evident.

We have found that relaxation and reassurance and treatment along the general lines for vocal strain are beneficial with asthmatics. Instruction in correct breathing technique, with emphasis upon abdominal patterns to counteract the clavicular, is very helpful. By learning to relax and practise abdominal breathing when an asthmatic attack threatens the patient may often ward off the attack. Having faith in something to do which will help, immediately allays anxiety and the very real fear of the attack itself which is exceedingly uncomfortable and frightening, especially for children, on account of the feelings of asphyxiation. Whether these are psychologically determined or not does not minimise the actual experience of asthma.

'MYASTHENIA LARYNGIS'

If the vocal folds are insufficiently tensed by the action of the thyroarytenoid muscle on account of muscular strain and vocal abuse, the slackness produced accounts for slight 'bowing' of the folds under subglottic air pressure in phonation. This allows a certain amount of unvibrated air to escape through the glottis. The voice thus produced lacks volume and resonance and is described sometimes as 'asthenic', breathy or husky. It is also sometimes called 'paretic', which is not a very suitable term since the muscles are not affected by paresis (slight paralysis). If the breathy voice is the result of vocal abuse then it is a symptom of strain. For this reason it is sometimes referred to as hyperkinetic phonasthenia, which means literally excessive muscular tension vocal weakness. A film star celebrated for her deep husky voice is reputed to have deliberately acquired such a voice by screaming and this would appear to be a good example of hyperkinetic phonasthenia. However, the vocal change was probably due to damage to the vocal cords and permanent thickening of the mucous membrane. We have seen many such cases in pop singers. A careful laryngological inspection and diagnosis of the actual appearance of the cords is necessary.

Chevalier Jackson (1940) gave the condition of vocal weakness the confusing name of 'myasthenia laryngis', which gets confused with 'myasthenia gravis', a neurological myopathic disease (page 254), manifesting itself in weakness of laryngeal and all other muscles. Jackson described his myasthenia laryngis as associated with vocal strain and found it commonly occurred with singers and actors and that it often developed immediately after a performance. It may occur before a performance if the performer is under stress or anxious over a difficult new part which he has been practising assiduously. Local application of a mild astringent lotion is beneficial and produces an immediate clearing of the vocal tone. The effect may be in part psychological, but the local irritation of the mucus membrane sets off a reflex tensor action in the laryngeal muscles and tendency to bowing of the cords is dispelled. Most laryngologists specialising in voice have their own pet prescriptions (Zilstorff, 1968; Punt, 1968). The moment the voice is heard to be right and feels right the singer or actor is reassured and once the effect has worn off he no longer remembers the vocal weakness.

When, of course, the condition of vocal weakness is due to vocal abuse speech therapy will be necessary or referral to the performer's singing professor.

8 Hyperkinetic dysphonia: vocal abuse

The vocal cords are not only remarkably resistant to vocal trauma in the vast majority of people but possess remarkable powers of recovery when traumatised. Vocal abuse has to be persistent to produce lasting changes in the mucous membrane covering the vocal cords. Shouting at a football match, a scream

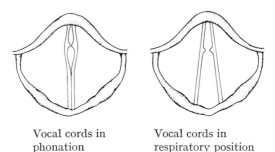

Vocal cords in
phonation

Vocal cords in
respiratory position

FIG. 28   Vocal nodules

of fright, an exacting operatic performance may produce a tiny localised sub-mucous haemorrhage in a capillary but this is absorbed and disappears in the course of a few days if the voice is used normally. Continuous vocal abuse, however, may perpetuate and aggravate the condition and lead to formation of established vocal nodules. Singer's or screamer's nodes as they are often called, are non-malignant neoplasms due entirely to vocal trauma. Starting initially with local haemorrhage and oedema they appear as soft red swellings on the edges of the vocal cords where the amplitude of the excursions and friction between the opposing lips of the cords is greatest in phonation. This is approximately at the middle of the anterior two-thirds of the cords, since the posterior thirds of the cords do not vibrate in the middle and head register (Fig. 28). The nodes which are at first red and soft gradually fibrose as connective tissue proliferates around the bleed and chronic nodules white in colour and conical or hemi-spherical in shape are formed. The diameter seldom exceeds

122

1·5 mm. In children they are usually larger, flatter and softer than in adults (Kleinsasser, 1968).

Vocal nodules occur most frequently in children according to Sedláčkova (1960) and Kleinsasser (1968). Heaver (1958) found nodules to be more common in boys than girls under the age of 20 years, then incidence decreased in males with advancing age and increased in women especially during the middle years. Vocal nodules in men are extremely rare, in fact.

Seeman (1959) reports that many deaf children suffer from vocal nodes as a result of vocal abuse.

Sopranos singing above their natural range may develop vocal nodes since many are mezzo-sopranos but the fashion today is for soprano singers. However, Zilstorff (1968) stresses the fact that if the singer is properly trained and has acquired the correct singing technique damage does not develop. We have, in fact, only encountered vocal nodules in untrained singers such as music teachers teaching singing in school, men and women taking part in amateur operatics, choirs, madrigal and folk groups, etc. (Greene, 1968).

PERSONALITY FACTORS

There is a constitutional and personality factor common to individuals who develop vocal nodes. They are mostly energetic, active, hard-working and anxious besides being talkative. Arnold (1962) and Luchsinger and Arnold (1965f.) state that vocal nodules present the reaction of local tissue to mental strain imposed by difficulties in adjusting to the demands made by society in persons of a certain personality structure. Arnold (1962) notes that the disorder is common in pyknic and athletic types and rare in asthenics. They develop in vociferous and aggressive individuals rather than in soft-spoken and gentle-mannered people.

There is such a strong anxiety component in the personality structure of these individuals who suffer from vocal abuse producing organic lesions in the larynx of vocal nodules, polyps and contact ulcers that one is led to believe that they are akin to psychosomatic disorders such as stomach ulcers or migraine. The reflex sensory and motor neural mechanism of the larynx is presumably governed by parasympathetic pathways. Dowie (1965) has commented on the frequency of vaso-motor rhinitis and menstrual and gynaecological troubles associated with dysphonia.

Psychosomatic patients as described by Linford Rees (1967a)

are not necessarily neurotic but may be well adjusted and successful people. They are anxious, tense, ambitious and self-driving, always competing with their fellows and trying to excel them. The business executive, the singer and actor have this tension, ambition and drive besides many housewives and committee women on a smaller stage. They may be perfectionist and find it hard to delegate responsibility and resent offers of help which they may regard as interference and it is not surprising that they develop fatigue and exhaustion. They are, of course, productive, responsible and reliable. The old saying 'if you want something done ask your busiest friend' takes advantage of the psychosomatic personality which cannot refuse to undertake an interesting job and enjoy social commitment. Therapy for vocal abuse needs always to take into account the anxieties of the individual and must attempt to bring them out into the open so that the patient can recognise stress and take steps to protect himself from strain and overwork. From the study of identical twins brought up in separate environments it is calculated that 80 per cent of personality and neuroticism is genetically determined and only 20 per cent is due to the influence of the environment so that the psychiatrist and the speech therapist have a problem on their hands when dealing with the over-anxious. Nevertheless better adaptation to everyday life at home and at work can be achieved by dealing with the voice problem and discussing personal difficulties on a sensible and practical level.

EXTRANEOUS IRRITANTS

Besides the personality, degree of vocal use and bad habits of voice production, it is generally agreed that aggravating factors can contribute to development of nodules. Allergic tendencies and a vasomotor rhinitis are often associated and may be psychosomatic symptoms of anxiety. Chronic laryngitis is a symptom of vocal strain and generally precedes formation of nodules but sometimes an acute respiratory infection, laryngitis and cough may precipitate formation of nodes if the patient has to use his voice considerably. Constantly coughing and clearing the throat is harmful to the vocal folds on account of the sphincteric spasm engendered against strong air pressure in order to dislodge mucus with what can only be described as a scraping activity. Catarrhal conditions are very difficult to cure and particularly common in middle age. Brodnitz (1953) gives advice on this subject. Medical treatment is not effective e⸱   ⸱⸱ ⸱ is a stress symptom or mucosal reaction to air pollution. The patient is often unaware of the habit he has formed and must be advised to desist as far as possible.

Cigarettes in quantity are a proved irritant; the great majority of these anxious patients are addicted to smoking. They should be encouraged in every way to stop or drastically cut down smoking. The connection with lung cancer is generally known but it should be pointed out to the patient that excessive smoking and chronic laryngitis can eventually produce malignancy.

Atmospheric irritants, air pollution, such as fumes in industry, diesel engine fumes, cement dust in building, or carbon from printer's ink contribute to laryngitis and cough. However, using the voice incorrectly and continuously against background noise is undoubtedly the basic and most damaging factor in formation of vocal nodes.

In the first stages, prior to actual formation of the nodes, beads of mucus may be seen collecting on the folds at the predestined site in an indirect laryngoscopy. This, to the laryngologist is a clear sign of vocal abuse. At this stage the voice may be slightly husky and hoarse or the patient in an effort to compensate for lack of volume may continue to produce a harsh and strident voice. As the nodes become established and increase in size, the cords have increasing difficulty in approximation, air wastage occurs and the voice may be lost, but more commonly it is harsh and hoarse, maintained by excessive laryngeal tension. The throat may ache and the throat feel sore after talking for any length of time, and especially by the end of the day.

Treatment depends on the size and structure of the nodes. Soft and recently formed nodes will disappear with voice rest and not recur if a course of voice therapy is followed. Long-standing and fibrous nodes need to be removed surgically under general anaesthetic. The patient generally spends a night in hospital and is discharged the following day. Ideally he should be referred for voice assessment and voice recording by the speech therapist before operation and the plan of speech rehabilitation explained. After surgery complete vocal rest and written communication should be observed for 4 or 5 days until the vocal membrane has healed. Whispering generally means varying degrees of approximation of the vocal cords and is not advisable. Voice rest should not exceed a week as it is now thought that it is not good for muscles and joints to be inactive for any length of time and this follows the current view in physical medicine that immobilisation of limbs should be for the shortest possible period (Zilstorff, 1968).

VOCAL NODES IN CHILDREN

There are few comprehensive studies reported in the literature concerning vocal nodes in childhood. Hoarseness in children often goes uninvestigated. If nodes are present surgical removal is not often undertaken on account of the size of the larynx, danger of trauma to the vocal cords, and also the probability of recurrence on account of failure to prevent the child abusing his voice. Nodes may be removed in special circumstances only if of long standing and with evidence of increasing voice impairment, or if a child wants to sing or act. Parental anxiety should not be a determining factor and parents are generally reassured when they learn that the condition will improve in adolescence as the child grows up and behaves in a more decorous fashion. Arnold (1962a) says that vocal nodes should never be removed in childhood on account of the mechanical difficulties involved in surgery and danger to the larynx mentioned above.

Voice therapy should be attempted in all cases although it is difficult to get young children to co-operate or agree that their voices need improvement. They are talkative, lively and noisy youngsters who enjoy yelling in the playground, playing cowboys and Indians or soldiers and enjoy shouting in support of their team at football matches. It is not easy to persuade them to remember methods of voice production and proper vocal volume at the height of their enjoyment and excitement and indeed one wonders whether it is right to do so when the fault is innocent, the damage slight and childhood so short. In all events, the teachers and parents of children will have to realise their responsibility in the matter and endeavour to exert control of the child in and out of school. Sometimes a lively child is not allowed to be noisy at home especially by a 'nervy' mother who cannot stand noise or if neighbours in adjoining apartments complain. Then the child needs to let off steam in the playground and in the gang. The home background of the child must be carefully assessed and taken into consideration when instituting any vocal rehabilitation programme. If anxiety and stress within the family or at school are manifestly the underlying cause of self-assertion and aggression being expressed overtly in vocal abuse, then of course there is need for speech therapy aimed at alleviation of the child's emotional difficulties. As with the treatment of adults, exercises alone are not enough, nor the prevention of shouting.

Not all laryngologists or speech therapists favour a permissive attitude to vocal nodules in children so I am particularly grateful to Miss Z. Harrod for permission to quote the following case history.

Peter, aged 8 years, was referred for speech therapy with a husky voice of one year's duration and recent diagnosis of minute vocal nodes. He was a noisy child who constantly shouted and talked loudly but had always had an exceptionally deep voice. His mother reported that his voice improved during the holidays when he did not shout at play-time in the playground. He was fond of taking his dog for walks in the fields and constantly shouted instructions to it to come back. He was not given any voice production exercises but cautioned about shouting and told to make a great effort and talk quietly for a week. His mother promised to co-operate and see that the therapist's instructions were carried out as far as possible. Peter was also told that if he did not try hard he would have to stay in during school play-time and stop taking the dog for walks. He was seen a month later by which time his voice was back to normal and when referred to the laryngologist it was discovered that the nodes had 'entirely disappeared'.

Boone (1966) describes the case of a 7-year-old girl who had been hoarse from infancy. Vocal nodules and thickening of the vocal membrane developed and the nodules were removed and cords stripped. After 10 days of vocal rest the voice failed to return. Boone attributes this to psychological factors but organic factors must have played a part. The period of vocal rest was too long especially as establishment of new muscular co-ordination and reflexes was necessary. Moreover, stripping of the cords (page 165) results in some delay in vocal recovery. The child responded immediately to vocal exercises and reassurance, obtaining voice in coughing, then vowels and later in words.

The question of hoarseness and vocal abuse in childhood and its psychological concomitants have not been widely studied in the past, as already noted. Eva Sedláčková (1960) filled in many gaps in our knowledge and made a valuable contribution to speech pathology in her extensive review of the literature and original observations. Not only has she examined the larynges of children suffering from chronic hoarseness but she has examined them periodically over the course of years as they grew up. She stresses that the hyperkinetic dysphonias of childhood and vocal nodules are different stages in mismanagement of the vocal organs and linked with personality in exactly the same way as they are in the adult. The personality of the child expressed in voice disorders is a symptom of anxiety as a reaction to social pressures. These children have an inherited familial temperamental disposition.

She draws a distinction between the chronic cases of childhood hoarseness and nodules due to vocal abuse and the nodules which develop in adolescence through singing. The nodes in children form on the middle section of the fold. In adolescents, they form at the classic junction of the anterior two-thirds of the vocal folds and the speaking voice is unimpaired. Sedláčkova's electro-laryngoscopic pictures show clearly the site of the swelling in cases of childhood hyperkinetic dysphonia. These children used rather deeper pitches than they should which accounted for the site of damage at the point of the vocal folds' widest excursion. She also studied the pneumographic records of her children and noted their numerous irregularities such as rapid drop in thoracic pressure at the end of phonation; exaggerated contraction of the abdominal muscles; the expiratory movement far exceeding that of the normal; arrests of expiration during speaking and inverse breathing patterns.

The course of the nodes and evolution depends upon the severity of temperamental factors and degree of vocal abuse. In the majority of cases the nodules disappear spontaneously during adolescence; especially dramatic changes may take place in boys during voice mutation as rapid growth of the folds is realised, the voice drops and the stress points of the cords shift.

Sedláčkova further reports that in some of the more pernicious cases of vocal abuse structural changes in the vocal folds take place. These changes may be irreversible and the voice be permanently impaired. In hypertrophic laryngitis, the swollen folds may begin to thin at the edges and separate on phonation which is a sign of hypotonia in the muscle. Later, atrophy of the edges may be apparent with insufficient glottal closure associated with permanent weakness of the vocalis muscle. In some cases the transition from the hypertrophic condition plus vocal nodules, to that of atrophy as the nodes disperse, is marked by a thinning at the edge of the fold. At the same time a longitudinal furrow develops lateral to the vocal ligament. The furrow deepens and finally this medial atrophied portion of the fold is seen lying at a lower level than the portion lateral to it and failing to vibrate. This is the 'sulcus glottides' which has been reported upon in adults and was thought to be of congenital origin, but appears to be the result of mechanical trauma in childhood. Such cases explain the probable aetiology of some of the patients with post-mutational hoarseness described by Arnold (1958) in his discussion of 'dysplastic dysphonia'. He refers to types of hereditary and congenital hoarseness in cases of hyperkinetic dysphonia and irregularities in the levels, width and bulk of the folds in cases of sulcus glottides.

VOCAL NODES IN POP SINGERS

Pop singers play an immensely important role in entertainment in the modern world appealing to a far greater audience than singers of lieder and opera. They follow in the train of the troubadours and singers of ballads, and in their turn add to our heritage of folk songs as jazz folk did. They are therefore not to be under-estimated, although professors of singing in the classical style do not recognise their vocalisation indeed as singing. The senior coach of the Covent Garden opera company has said he would not consider them seriously as candidates for the chorus (Miller, 1970). Their numbers are legion and they give pleasure to millions. They perform in pubs and workers' clubs, in night clubs, on television and radio. They are largely untrained, having musical sense and personality and pleasing voices but some, it must be admitted, have little natural vocal endowment. For many it is a short life but a lucrative one and when the voice is lost through vocal abuse they drop out of 'show biz', but this is not necessary if their voices are taken in hand and trained in time. For the world-famous stars of the Top Ten as well as the galaxy of lesser singers, it is a serious problem when they run into trouble with their voices, as many do.

The vocal gymnastics and tricks peculiar to each singer, the double notes, acute pitch changes, the scoops and swirls have to be executed against the deafening competition of amplified music from the band accompaniment. Despite the use of a hand micro-phone they must still 'belt it out' at the top of their voices, as one pop star explained. In disc recording, head-phones are worn so that the singer can hear his own voice and the technical acoustic engineers are responsible for the splicing in of sound effects and play an important part nowadays in making many hit records. The sound-pressure levels created by the bands and rock and roll groups are so great that they exceed the safety levels for avoidance of hearing impairment. Lebo and Oliphant (1968) in an investigation into music as a source of acoustic trauma found temporary threshold shifts in hearing among performers and in some individuals permanent cochlear damage.

Although a successful performer does not have to take part in long performances, 'on the way up' he has to do so and the vocal cords may suffer damage. The least crippling condition appears to be a permanent thickening and scarring, even a battered fringe-like edge to the vocal membranes. This may of course contribute to the peculiar husky or broken tones of the voice which causes the particular appeal and heart throb in the fans, but there can be only one acceptable Louis Armstrong. The speaking voice deteriorates long before the singing voice. These singers may consult a laryngologist on account of sore throats and increasing discomfort. The laryngologist, if wise, hesitates to operate for fear of damaging the voice by improving it un-recognisably—he generally gives reassurance and perhaps medical treatment (Greene, 1968). He may remove the tonsils if a source of infection, although this is not altogether free from hazards either, as resonance changes may be produced in the resonant character of the singing voice.

The common run of cabaret and pop-group singers perform for many hours on end starting at midnight and going on into the early hours. When not singing they are smoking and talking in a dry, hot and polluted atmosphere. It is not surprising that chronic laryngitis and vocal nodes are common.

Vocal nodes which go on increasing in size eventually deprive the singer of his voice and surgery cannot be avoided. Sometimes there is a sudden flare-up of a polypoid fringe (see under polyps below) along the edge of the vocal cord following laryngitis or a particularly severe bout of vocal abuse. In this case the vocal cord or cords must be stripped (the operation is called technically 'decortication'). It is advisable to tape-record the singing and speaking voice before operation as a precaution against possible law suits besides being essential to the vocal rehabilitation pro-gramme (Kleinsasser, 1968). After stripping of the vocal cords the voice takes sometimes as long as 3 months to recover fully and lose a husky, veiled tone. Although the cords heal very quickly lesions in the mechano-receptor reflex system must persist and this accounts for the disturbance in tuning of the laryngeal muscles in phonation. In all our patients the voice has suddenly become clear much later than was anticipated after operation. Singers become anxious during this interval and it is necessary to warn them that there will be a delay in full vocal recovery despite learning to produce the voice more satisfactorily.

Speech therapy which provides advice on how to spare and

conserve the voice despite the nigh impossible demands made upon it during performances, must be given, besides instruction in relaxation, breathing, and phonation. When the vocal cords have recovered and are healthy in appearance the singer must be referred to a competent teacher of singing so that he can learn techniques in how to produce a loud voice without strain. Although obvious difficulties and conflicts present themselves in acquisition of new techniques for improving an old and successful way of singing, the gifted artist generally succeeds in adapting breathing and vocalisation technique to his own particular needs. It must be remembered that sheer volume of voice in itself is not damaging. In Wagnerian opera a soloist has to sing against a hundred instruments which provides an even greater volume of sound than amplified pop, besides which the operatic star, of course, cannot have recourse to a microphone. The world's most famous singer, Caruso, developed vocal nodes because he was a baritone but forced his voice up to a tenor register (Sonninen, 1968). This produced much vocal strain and towards the end of his career his voice deteriorated and the huskiness can be detected in the phonographic recordings which have been preserved. It was on account of his great talent as an actor and interpreter that he retained his popularity.

Singers, even the most successful, are anxious before performances and the emotional volatility and temperament of artists is well known. Their imaginations aggravate their vocal symptoms and they need sympathy and understanding as Punt (1968) emphasises. A laryngologist is often present in the opera house when big performances are in progress, ready to administer medication and reassurance behind scenes. The pop singer or amateur performer must rely on comfort from visiting the busy hospital consultant and the speech therapist can achieve good results with speech therapy before passing the singer on to a singing teacher. Although trained singers can, in emergencies, sing with a cold and infective laryngitis (Zilstorff, 1968) the untrained or poorly trained singer with signs of vocal abuse and chronic laryngitis should never do so. The performance will be disastrous and this will not only aggravate the vocal condition but be psychologically traumatic. All singing should be forbidden until the larynx is perfectly healthy again and reported as such by the laryngologist. If in financial difficulties the singer must get some other quiet, temporary job, but must manage satisfactorily on sick benefit and savings.

Brodnitz (1953) in *Keep your Voice Healthy* and Punt (1967) in *The Singer's and Actor's Throat* have written with sufficient simplicity for the educated layman to benefit from reading up the subject of vocal strain and its avoidance, and are suitable for recommendation to patients as supplementary study to a course of voice therapy.

VOCAL CORD POLYPS (see Chapter 16)

Patients may be referred to the speech therapist for voice therapy following removal of a polyp which may have been a vocal node, but some laryngologists appear to refer to unilateral non-malignant neoplasms as polyps indiscriminately to distinguish, perhaps, from the bilateral and distinctive vocal nodules. An exact diagnosis is important to the speech therapist and the histological report gives the necessary information. For example, the following histological report on what was referred to as a 'polyp' clearly indicates a nodule due to vocal abuse: 'Section showed vascular and oedematous polyp. One dilated blood vessel in the connective tissue has undergone recent thrombosis'. In this case a vocal nodule had developed larger on one cord than the other where only a little swelling and inflammation was visible. Probably speech therapy alone would have cured the condition had surgery not been decided upon.

Scarring of the vocal cords as a result of surgery used to be not uncommon but should never occur now that the relatively new Kleinsasser (1968) technique is being used. An endolaryngeal surgical microscope is used which provides a three-dimensional magnified image of the vocal cords and their surfaces in great clarity and detail. This facilitates operating with less risk of removing chunks from the vocal cords since a minute irregularity of the surface looks like a mole hill. The technique necessitates the use of long-handled delicate instruments for stripping and nipping. Speech therapists are advised to request permission from a surgeon using the technique to watch in the operating theatre as one clinical session is more instructive than many hours of studying books can be.

CASE HISTORY ILLUSTRATIONS

Adult with Vocal Nodules

Mrs Q. aged 30 years. Vocal nodules situated bilaterally at the junction of the anterior two-thirds of the folds. Voice severely hoarse and breathy, breathing shallow, considerable pharyngeal tension. She was recognised by a hospital colleague as a girl who had served with her in the Forces ten years previously, and whom she remembered vividly because she shouted in a harsh, strident voice and was an inveterate talker. The patient had recently left work in an office in order to help in her father's shop and this gave an opportunity for talking all day to customers and travellers. She was nervous and talked to conceal her shyness. She was aware that she talked too much and far too loudly, but all members of her family behaved similarly and moreover they always talked against the wireless which they liked to have on at all times and at 'full blast'.

She responded slowly to treatment but was never placed on vocal rest. The pitch of her voice was not lowered appreciably; the reduction in pharyngeal and laryngeal tension and insistence upon normally quiet speech was sufficient to cure the nodules by reducing the friction between the vocal lips.

An interesting aspect of this case was the exhibition of mild hysterical symptoms. She rejected any suggestion that she was worried about her voice or that her throat caused discomfort or tickled, even though a paroxysm of coughing often occurred during her visits to the clinic. Her indifference during a laryngoscopic examination suggested hysterical anaesthesia. She also confessed to the conviction which she knew was 'silly' that the pimples in her throat came to a head before menstruation and broke away with a sharp prick at its onset. It was possible to persuade her that nothing of the sort happened and that concentration upon better voice production was the only cure for her vocal disorder.

The long discussions which formed a part of every treatment session were undoubtedly necessary and cathartic.

Pop Singer's Larynx

Johnnie, aged 23 years, was a gifted versatile variety artist—he sang with enormous verve and feeling, was able to vocalise in a range of 2 octaves, was an excellent tap dancer, drummer and impersonator. He had been singing in South America since the age of 15 and latterly had made a name in Europe. His fame was increasing and he had hopes of getting into the Top Ten with a hit record. He had recently acquired an excellent manager after years of battling alone working incredibly hard, fixing his own engagements. The future looked good. But his voice had begun to deteriorate and every performance became an anxiety. At first only his speaking voice became hoarse and with extra effort his voice was not too bad when singing and he was able to conceal the lack of control and make cracks and pitch breaks sound as if meant. He had a few lessons with a singing teacher in Chile some 9 years before but he had no singing technique to support his natural musical gifts. Although he used a hand microphone when singing, the noise of the band was such that he still needed to produce every decibel he could muster.

Eventually Johnnie could sing no more and in despair presented himself to a laryngologist who reported that his larynx was in a real mess, inflamed, with 'polypoid fringes' along the edges of the vocal cords. The cords were stripped (à la Kleinsasser) and he was instructed to sing no more for the time being and follow the instruction of the speech therapist to whom he was sent. He saw her once, then his laryngologist again, who pronounced the cords to be fine and healthy, and proceeded straight away to fulfil engagements in Sweden, France and Germany. In Germany the hoarseness returned and he went to the most famous laryngologist available who pronounced that he was suffering from vocal nodules which must be removed. At the same time Johnnie met a colleague who advised him to return to London and see the author. After sorting things out with his London surgeon who is a close collaborator in hospital, but not private practice, Johnnie, much frightened by now at the prospect of losing his voice altogether, agreed to obey orders and follow the speech therapy regimen. He gave up smoking and had never drunk much. Whispering for two weeks cured the newly formed polyps and laryngitis. Instruction in relaxation and breathing were given and later vocal exercises and singing exercises. No professional engagements were booked for three months. For the first time the patient had a real holiday, swam and played squash and enjoyed himself in a quiet way. Much time was devoted to discussion of the problems involved in Johnnie's way of life. It became apparent that he did more damage to his voice when leading a normal life and feeling on top of the world off the stage than on the stage. After performing all night, he would collect up a party and dance down the streets of Majorca or wherever, singing at the top of his voice, then repair to a bar for a meal during which he entertained everybody with jokes, songs and impersonations, being an individual of bubbling spirits and a born comedian. He slept little and enjoyed life in a perpetual state of excitement. Of course he had his moods and depressions like all 'hypermanic' personalities. Gradually he began to see that he must grow up and mature and that he could not abuse his system and his vocal cords at 23 in the same way as he had in his teens. This needed a great effort of adjustment but he was dedicated to his profession and determined not to retire from it early as most pop stars are forced to do, following a brief meteoric flight with great financial profit. Finally Johnnie went to a good singing teacher and then back to work. He has had no further laryngeal symptoms.

CONTACT ULCERS

The aetiology of ulceration of the folds in the arytenoid region was first related to vocal abuse by Jackson (1935). He gave the condition its now accepted name of 'contact ulcer' on account of

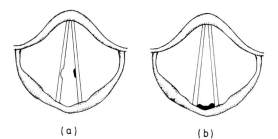

(a)   (b)

A: Contact ulcers over vocal processes of cords with hammer and anvil effect in phonation

B: Pachydermia of the posterior commissure

FIG. 29   Contact ulcers and pachydermia

'the trauma of hammer and anvil' with which the arytenoids strike each other in the forced type of phonation employed by these individuals (1945) (Fig. 29). This action causes inflammation, and eventually ulceration and granuloma or neoplasm on the mucous membrane covering the arytenoid region of the fold. Contact ulcers may be confined to one fold only or both may be involved. It is almost exclusively a male complaint. It will be remembered that the vibration of the arytenoids in the chest register was mentioned earlier (page 42). The ulcers develop in individuals having deep throaty voices. Women for the most part do not employ sufficiently deep voices to develop contact ulcers, and are more prone to the development of vocal nodules.

CONTACT ULCERS AND PACHYDERMIA

Kleinsasser (1968) states that contact ulcers are not actually ulcers or granulomas but consist of 'craters' with highly thickened squamous epithelium over connective tissue with some inflammation (oedema). The classical description of the visual appearance is a raised granuloma on one side and crater on the other which fit on contact of the cords like a ball and socket. In well-established cases of contact ulcers the epithelium of the anterior two-thirds of the cords may be thickened. In early stages of the condition, there may be only signs of oedematous swelling over the vocal processes and some hoarseness. In more severe abuse the voice is harsh, hoarse and deep and excruciating to listen to. It is almost exclusively a male complaint.

Newly formed contact ulcers should not be operated upon but treated with voice rest and speech therapy. With established contact ulcers surgery is necessary and perhaps stripping of the hyperplastic epithelium from the anterior sections of the cords. This thickening develops through the effort to approximate the vocal cords as the separation of the arytenoids increases with development of the ulcers. In an indirect laryngoscopic view, bowing of the vocal cords anteriorly is often observable. Absolute voice rest must be observed after surgery until the epithelium has grown over the mucosal defects after which voice therapy is essential, otherwise the contact ulcers will recur.

There has been and still is considerable confusion over the distinction between laryngeal pachydermia and contact ulcers, of which at this juncture it is necessary to give brief mention (see also under hyperplastic laryngitis, page 346). Virchow described contact ulcers exactly in 1860 in a patient who was a Prussian lieutenant commanding troops in a garrison, but called the condition 'pachydermia'. Jackson (1935) invented the name 'contact ulcer' because of the trauma of 'hammer and anvil' with which the arytenoids strike each other in phonation.

Negus (St. Clair Thomson and Negus, 1955) did not recognise any such thing as contact ulcers and stated: 'We have no experience as an entity but only of similar but variable appearance of hypertrophic laryngitis sometimes due to misuse of the voice, especially in foul air with excess of tobacco or alcohol, or syphilis, or early and especially senile tuberculosis and what is generally recognised as pachydermia'.

Arnold (1962) distinguishes between the contact ulcers and granuloma of the cartilaginous portions of the folds and the pachydermia of the posterior commissure, the area between the arytenoids, which is caused by chronic infections and irritations. Kleinsasser (1968) describes this condition and illustrates it under the term 'interarytenoid pachydermia'. He says it is an isolated lesion confined to a particular region. The development of a primary carcinoma in the interarytenoid region is extremely rare and it need not be considered as a precancerous condition. The thickening of the folded epithelium prevents closure of the glottis and the voice is harsh. Little can be done surgically or medically to alleviate the condition. The area may be resected but there is grave danger of post-operative scarring and even restriction of the movement of the arytenoid cartilages as a result.

Contact ulcers are, it seems, far more common in America than in Europe where the condition is very rare (Brodnitz, 1961). In the past 6 years in the busy ear, nose and throat department of the general hospital of St. Bartholomew's, London, I have only had three cases referred, all men. One with advanced lesions was operated upon and another cured by speech therapy only.

The third was caught early and had only oedema over the vocal processes. Two of these patients were referred with a diagnosis simply of vocal nodes. This indicates that more cases may occur but be given the wrong name and speech pathologists not having access to medical notes or indirect laryngoscopy may not be aware of the true condition. The high incidence of contact ulcers in the United States may be a social phenomenon related to a fashionable 'dark brown', deep voice which to my in-experienced ear is as characteristic of the cultured Harvard accent as it is of the 'Oxford' (or Oxbridge) accent of which Mr Edward Heath provides a very good example.

Bilateral ulceration of the folds in the arytenoid region can follow intratracheal intubation (Wattles, 1949) which is the usual method of administering general anaesthetic and given nowadays more frequently than formerly for minor operations. The folds of women suffer damage more often than men because their larynges are smaller. In any event ulceration as a result of anaesthetic intubation is very rare and should heal quickly if the patient does not abuse his voice subsequently. Complete vocal rest is advisable until the cords heal and speech therapy should not be necessary since the initial trauma has nothing to do with bad voice production.

Extraneous irritants are known to aggravate ulceration of the folds—a dusty atmosphere, chemical fumes, excessive smoking and drinking—but it is doubtful whether these things in themselves are ever the primary cause of ulceration. Removal of the specific irritant may result in immediate alleviation of the symptoms if the folds are still in a mildly oedematous stage, and heavy smokers are reported to have lost ulcers within twenty-four hours of ceasing to smoke (Myerson, 1952).

REVIEW OF THE LITERATURE

New and Devine (1949) have reported upon 53 cases of contact ulcer of whom 47 were men; in 41 the condition was unilateral and in 12 bilateral. The six women in this group had all developed contact ulcers following intratracheal anaesthesia, of the 47 men three cases only were the result of anaesthesia and the remaining 44 were of 'indeterminate aetiology'. From this group 39 patients were treated surgically, and 32 of these were eventually cured. In all, 73 operations were performed, some patients being subjected to one operation and others to as many as five. The authors comment upon the fact that the patients were all individuals such as salesmen and managers who used their voices a great deal and were living on a plane of high nervous tension. Speech therapy was not given.

Peacher and Hollinger (1947) reported the results of research into the value of vocal re-education in the treatment of sixteen cases of contact ulcer. An experimental group of six individuals who could receive weekly speech therapy were given instruction in vocal re-education. A control group of ten individuals were treated surgically or by vocal rest or both, but given no special speech instruction. The results of this experiment showed that the contact ulcers did not heal in either the control or experimental groups unless the patient changed his method of voice production. All those who received vocal re-education showed a cessation of symptoms with total or nearly complete disappearance of the ulcer. Ulcers in the experimental group took from one to four months to disappear and in the control group from seven months to three years.

The patients in the experimental group were not made to rest their voices at all, the contention being that if the individual uses his voice correctly talking will do no harm.

All the patients exhibited the vocal characteristics listed below and these faults had to be corrected in the vocal rehabilitation programme.

1. Extreme tension of the speech musculature coupled with generalised bodily tension

2. Forcing of the pitch far below the optimum
3. Glottal plosive attack
4. Explosive speech patterns

    (*a*) Predominant stress pattern
    (*b*) Rigid melody or confined pitch range
    (*c*) Considerable breath pressure
    (*d*) Loud intensity

5. Hoarse quality

Peacher (1961) followed up 70 patients over periods of one to twelve years following vocal therapy; five had a single recurrence of the condition and one of these developed malignancy. There was an operated and non-operated group: 34 patients had 80 operations before and during therapy, and 36 patients had no operations. The operated patients had an average healing time of 26·52 weeks and non-operated group 10·05 weeks. The operated patients were not a control group but had advanced pachydermia and required surgery before therapy. There were 62 men and 2 women and mostly engaged in speaking professions. Some had concentrated voice therapy and others extended over two to eight months. The average number of hours of treatment was 5·6–8·0 but no correlation was found between healing time and length or numbers of hours of treatment. There was no correlation between time of healing and other factors such as smoking, drinking, voice rest and ability to carry a tune or duration of hoarseness prior to treatment. They confirm that the two main factors contributing to the condition are vocal abuse and emotional tension. The vocal abuse includes glottal attack, too low a pitch, poor breath control and excessive coughing and throat clearing. A film made by Von Leden and Moore (1960) in the Voice Research Laboratory of Northwestern Medical School shows the action of the vocal cords in contact ulcers. The mechanism of the arytenoid joint was also examined by these workers (Von Leden and Moore, 1961). The cartilages perform a rocking movement in two planes making a wide excursion in low frequencies and in the deep throaty voice produced the prolonged approximation of the surfaces in the region of the vocal processes exposes them to greater stress.

Brodnitz (1961) reported on 26 cases and confirms the relation of contact ulcers with stress; four of his patients developed stomach ulcers and a fifth a duodenal ulcer after healing of a contact ulcer. He also found no correlation between incidence and smoking or drinking. A constant urge to clear the throat and also a characteristic pain which radiates to the ear were present. He comments on the difficulty in effecting a cure which is admitted by all therapists. He uses Froeschel's chewing therapy (see page 172) and in advanced stages of treatment advocates use of an amplifier so that the patient can monitor his speech and reduce the hyperfunction. Amplification is gradually reduced until the patient develops a soft voice. The patient with contact ulcers gives the impression of trying to shout all the time and the use of amplification certainly is a useful corrective procedure, far more effective than listening to recorded speech.

Cooper and Nahum (1967) reported on sixteen patients of whom 13 were cured and the rest were improving. They stress the need for early diagnosis and voice therapy and describe three stages or degrees of severity, it being far easier to treat a patient in the first stage and obtain a cure than in later stages when all reports agree that treatment is long and difficult and relapses occur. They describe the first stage as one characterised by vocal fatigue and hoarseness by the end of the day with an oedema developing on the arytenoid region which may improve with rest. The second stage exhibits continual hoarseness and fatigue with occasional pain in swallowing and severe inflammation over the arytenoids. The third stage exhibits constant severe hoarseness, fatigue and pain in swallowing and talking, and ulceration of the cords which may require surgery.

All therapists treating patients for contact ulcers emphasise the need to develop vocal flexibility and attack the monotonous pitch employed which is so characteristic in this type of dysphonia. Burkowsky (1968) explains that variation of fundamental frequency accompanies alterations in length, thickness and tilt of the vocal cords so that on adduction shifting parts of stress can occur and the glottal impact not always fall in the same region. In his interesting account of a 71-year-old preacher, Burkowsky describes how he was put on a month's vocal rest and his wife testified that he wrote everything down during this period. He presented after this with a visibly worsened laryngeal condition. It was found that during the month of rest he had spaded over an acre of land, cleared scrub, and played the clarinet which increased tension in the head and neck. The heavy physical labour necessitated fixation of the thoracic cage and sphincteric closure of the larynx which was not good for the existing contact ulcers.

Nahum (1967) directs voice therapy to raising the pitch level and developing 'optimum pitch' and mentions the need for reducing vocal volume.

Cherry and Margulies (1968) describe three patients suffering from contact ulcers which failed to heal when treated by conventional vocal rest and voice therapy. They were found to suffer from pharyngo-oesophagitis due to peptic acid reflux. They suggest that peptic reflux while the patient is asleep can seep into the posterior larynx and cause inflammation and ulceration. They treated gastric acidity with suitable medication and advised the patients to sleep on raised pillows. The ulcers were cured after a period of 3–6 months. They do not deny that vocal abuse may also be a contributory factor and that voice therapy is advisable, but stress the need for peptic reflux to be included as a factor assessment in diagnosis. Cherry and Delahunty (1968) experimentally painted the vocal cords of dogs with gastric juice and found this produced inflammation and then ulceration, which adds confirmation to their observations on contact ulcers in human beings.

Case Report

Mr E., aged 50. A decorator permanently employed in a newspaper printing firm, working day and night shifts. Happily married with two sons out at work. An F.O.C. (i.e. father of the chapel) of his trade union. He had always had a 'dark brown' voice since adolescence which was admired by his wife who adored him. A very impatient and rather aggressive man who did not suffer fools gladly, and an immense talker, but friendly and 'hail-fellow-well-met'. It was thought that he might be thyrotoxic but this was not proved. He had suffered increasingly with sore throats and laryngitis, then lost his voice suddenly with none of the usual symptoms of laryngitis. He was referred to the laryngologist and then for speech therapy with a request for treatment of 'vocal abuse and vocal nodes'. His voice was so painfully rough and deep that contact ulcers could be diagnosed by ear alone and when the medical notes were consulted there was illustrated the typical site of lesions over the vocal processes. This is mentioned specifically since it indicates that vocal nodes, even in a progressive ear, nose and throat department, can be diagnosed as vocal nodes in Britain. Of course they are, but of a particular type, which is of less significance as regards treatment for the laryngologist than for the speech pathologist.

Mr E. had been warned that the 'nodes' would have to be

removed surgically if they did not disperse with speech therapy and if he did not cut down smoking and shouting and apply himself with zeal to his speech course which he regarded with grave suspicion. He had come to hospital to have his tonsils out, not to fall into the clutches of a bunch of females. At his first interview, he proceeded to tell us quite frankly we were on probation and explained that in his opinion all women were absolutely senseless. For example, his wife was a marvellous woman but—she had been driving with him for 25 years and did not know how to put on the brake. He had parked the car on a slope and forgot to put on the brake—as he crossed the front of the car to the pavement he realised it was mowing him down. Moreover if nothing were done not only would he be damaged, but the bonnet of his new car and the boot of the car in front. He therefore stopped the car and held it with a mighty push and yelled to his wife sitting in the front seat to put on the brake. Instead she asked 'Where is it? How do you?' His shouts were heard by his son in their third floor flat and he came to the rescue. It was this incident which, it seems, produced the contact ulcers and loss of voice.

Mr E. besides his personality problem, worked in an atmosphere of printer's ink dust, smoked heavily, talked too much and vocalised in the wrong way. He was too self-conscious to perform any exercises and needed teasing to put him at his ease. He was physically fit and had no breathing problems, and apart from his job, cleaned the house and windows and even did the washing when his wife was at work. He was not even tense; he leaned back in his chair and enjoyed being tough with people and telling them what he thought, without being the least offensive, but on the contrary charming and entertaining. He promised to cut down smoking and did so; he relinquished his post of F.O.C., not that this stopped his active participation in trades union disputes and strikes of the printers. Although his union was a different one he could not possibly work for some reason which we were at a loss to understand. We never got to the bottom of this, but at least his voice was rested as he was at home decorating the flat from one end to the other, and with his wife out, had nobody to talk to and he was forbidden to sing. We suggested whistling and chewing gum if he felt lonely.

The chief feature of vocal abuse was endeavouring to produce volume (psychologically to shout all the soft-heads down) on a deep monotonous note devoid of inflection. Recordings were played back to him and he was given an amplifier to practise with at home. Imitation of phrases on a higher pitch and with exaggerated inflection were practised. At first he objected to a voice which sounded 'pansy' and said he could not possibly talk like this. The men at work waggled their hips at him and flicked back their hair and patted their curls. Recordings demonstrated that he was only changing from baritone to tenor and the pleasure expressed by charming students with beautiful voices at hearing his improved voice was very therapeutic.

After one month's treatment twice weekly and two months once weekly, Mr E.'s voice was sufficiently improved to request an indirect laryngoscopy. There was no sign now of contact ulcers, but the vocal processes were seen to 'toe-in' with too great contact while the anterior two-thirds of the vocal cords were rather slack (internal tensor weakness). A month later, after two week's summer holiday no abnormal signs could be observed in the larynx. Mr E. still lapses into his old bad phonatory habits in an argument and is in grave danger of suffering a relapse. He will therefore be followed up in the speech clinic, as he works nearby, for another three months or more.

GENERAL CONSIDERATIONS

In discussing the rehabilitation programme for patients suffering from vocal strain and vocal abuse with the concomitants of chronic laryngitis, vocal nodules or contact uclers, there is no need at the outset to make fine distinctions in treatment. We are dealing with a common aetiology, consisting of an admixture of mechanical and psychological stress manifesting itself in symptoms of varying degrees of severity of hyperkinetic function. Chronic laryngitis is the mildest symptom of trauma, contact ulcers the most severe. We can therefore lay down general principles or guide lines in treatment of the underlying causes of dysphonia and deal subsequently with problems involved in correction of specific faults. This then will be the plan for this chapter.

The Role of the Laryngologist

The laryngologist is responsible for the diagnosis and the medical and surgical treatment of the patient. No case of hoarseness should ever be accepted for treatment by a speech pathologist without first having obtained a report from a laryngologist. It is imperative that malignancy should be excluded besides other illnesses and there is grave danger to the patient in treating even the mildest case of hoarseness without obtaining a laryngological inspection and diagnosis first. Brodnitz (1953) insists that hoarseness should be properly investigated if it persists for more than two weeks after onset. Lederer (1948) describes hoarseness as 'the danger signal' of so many disorders and diseases that a very full investigation is needed. This may include all of the following: a case history; indirect or direct laryngoscopy; an examination with X-rays of the upper respiratory tract including nasal sinuses, chest and neck; examination of the ears and hearing test. Examinations of sputum and of the blood are also made if indicated. It may be some time before the patient is referred for speech therapy or these investigations may be proceeding concurrently with vocal training. A speech pathologist should be aware of this

144

and take an intelligent interest in results of tests as frequently they have some important bearing on treatment of vocal symptoms. The intricacies and possibilities in differential diagnosis of dysphonia will unfold more clearly in later chapters. An obvious example of the need for the speech pathologist to have knowledge of a patient's medical treatment is the possibility of drug therapy for illness unrelated to voice but producing a dysphonia. The relationship may not be immediately detected by the laryngologist and dysphonia thought to be a functional disorder.

When the ear, nose and throat investigations are complete and medical treatment for infection carried out and surgical treatment finished, and it is certain vocal abuse is the chief cause of dysphonia the patient is referred for speech therapy. It is seldom nowadays that patients are placed on vocal rest except immediately postoperatively, as this is considered old-fashioned. An important responsibility of the laryngologist is to reassure the patient that there is no malignancy and allay the cancer fears which may have developed either before or since attending hospital and the subsequent rather alarmingly thorough examinations, especially a direct laryngoscopy under anaesthesia. This often leaves the throat sore and the neck stiff and anxious patients focus on the discomfort felt, and when told there is nothing really wrong, may feel resentment and assert their throats are worse than before they came into hospital. If the patient is a heavy smoker the laryngologist will warn against the dangers of contracting cancer at a future date. If there seems to be considerable anxiety a short course of a tranquillising drug may be prescribed. The laryngologist also needs to explain the need for speech therapy and in every way support the authority of the speech therapist in taking over treatment. Voice therapy is sometimes considered unnecessary and too time-consuming by the patient, especially if the voice recovers completely after surgery.

If the speech therapist can arrange to hold her out-patient clinic in the ear, nose and throat department during the consultant's clinical sessions the team approach is cemented. The therapist can be introduced to the patient, have the laryngeal condition demonstrated by indirect laryngoscopy and have pathology explained. Any speech therapist who has worked under such ideal conditions recognises that close collaboration and teaching from the laryngologist is of immense help in increasing the effectiveness of therapy based upon a sound knowledge of the laryngeal pathology. This is an aspect of voice therapy sometimes overlooked in research projects which endeavour to assess phonation and vocal characteristics. These, voice scientists believe to be woefully misunderstood by clinical therapists because the latter's means of description of voice is conflicting and inadequate. When related to the laryngological report and visible condition of the larynx, adjectives such as hoarse, breathy, hard, are more easily understood and in any case are not vitally important, merely convenient.

THE ROLE OF THE SPEECH THERAPIST

The first need in the speech therapy programme is to ensure that the patient understands why he is referred for treatment and what is meant by vocal strain or abuse. A brief description of the plan of therapy should be given.

It is often necessary to reassure again that the condition is not related to cancer. Often a patient has not understood explanations fully. Professional people, speech pathologists and doctors, fail to realise that the specialised language and vocabulary they use, *is* specialised to lay people. The simple lay term 'vocal abuse' is not easily explained or understood. The patient should be allowed to talk and ask questions in the quiet surroundings of a speech clinic. His contacts with medical staff hitherto, unless attending a private office, will have been in the limited privacy of an ear, nose and throat examination bay, one of many in a large clinic. A general ward also offers no privacy. Patients are often too shy and overawed to ask questions and expose their ignorance. When they gain confidence with the therapist they frequently say 'I know it's silly, but does that mean . . .?' and the therapist is astonished that a most elementary point on which the whole of a reasoned and logical explanation hinges has just not been understood at all.

Brodnitz (1962) in this connection comments on the need in treatment to encourage individuals to ask questions and demand explanations and to avoid the authoritarian attitude in teaching. Singers and professional actors are, as he says, too often trained like seals to perform motions they do not understand, being rewarded or punished in their attempts by praise or scolding. They may as a result produce good voices but they have no idea of the rationale behind their training and no idea of how to preserve and care for their voices. Speech pathologists in dealing with professional voice users are constantly amazed at the ignorance of their patients over the most simple and obvious reasons for relaxing, breathing, pitching and resonating the voice. Voice therapy is distinct from voice training, it would appear, for just this reason and accounts for the fact that the speech therapist may successfully correct vocal abuse when the teacher of singing or dramatic art cannot.

Time must be devoted to explanation and discussion therefore, and it must not be taken for granted that the patient understands because he has been told once. Asking the patient to 'tell back' the instructions given or explain what he has been practising at home and why, often reveals utter confusion over the aims of treatment. This does not mean the patient is a fool but that our teaching has failed. Our own knowledge acquired during years of training and experience blinds us to the difficulties of our speciality, a fact that we constantly forget in our relations with not only the layman but also our medical colleagues. We must remember that the patient is a student in training and, as is well known, students need to be introduced gradually to new facts and told them an extraordinary number of times before they are assimilated.

THE CASE HISTORY

The patient's presence in the clinic being in fact due to being an inveterate talker renders it generally very easy to obtain a frank and full account. It is much simpler than when dealing with disturbed and depressed patients. The anxious talkative person confronted by a new or strange situation often has difficulty in curbing speech and exhibits an inability to stop talking which was aptly described by T. E. Lawrence (1941) in reference to the active archaeologist: 'with a voice that splits when excited and a constant feverish speed of speech . . . a man of ideas and systems'. Such people do not sit and read alone or rest but are only happy when busy and when in the company of others.

Information is required concerning the duration of the voice disorder and an attempt must be made to date its origin and the circumstances which precipitated hoarseness. The patient's working conditions need to be known, whether noisy and how much talking is necessary and when and to whom. Telephoning in an office full of typewriters or carrying out secretarial duties for a deaf employer in a quiet room may constitute the chief vocal abuse. Details of the home background and leisure activities are equally necessary. The working conditions may be quite innocuous as described in the case history of the head master (page 116) but the use of the voice in leisure hours may be at fault. A deaf relative is often a cause of vocal strain, there is a need to shout and there is also a great drain on the patience with consequent mental and laryngeal tensions arising. Domestic quarrels between husband and wife and much argument with 'difficult' teenagers and children when voices are raised can cause vocal strain—anger and aggression taking its toll of the vocal cords.

Investigation into the patient's pastimes in his leisure hours often reveals that these are limited but at the same time an inordinate amount of time and energy may be spent on quite unnecessary tasks. Men tend to become over-meticulous about their work and their gardens, but women are unquestionably the worst offenders with regard to domestic duties. The fact that a woman's work is never done is frequently her own fault. It may be due to lack of planning or the maintenance of a ridiculously high standard of cleanliness in the house, or insistence upon waiting hand and foot upon the rest of the household. A widow with chronic laryngitis, for instance, who worked long hours as a clerk maintained that it was essential to get up an hour earlier than seemed necessary in order to heat water for her adult son, clean his shoes, cook his breakfast and call him in good time. In fact she thought she strained her voice calling up the stairs to him every morning for he had considerable difficulty in rousing himself and in remaining awake. Were she not to care for him in this way, he would most certainly never get to work in time and would lose his job in the bank.

In such cases it is necessary to persuade the patient to behave rationally. This is generally not so difficult as would at first appear since beneath the apparent devotion there rankles a deep resentment; if the truth be known this is often accompanied by a critical and nagging attitude and strained relations within the family. Clarity of view is always lost in these mild anxiety states but can be reversed by sympathetic discussion, and this must naturally form an important aspect of treatment.

An interest in the patient's general health should be taken especially if run down after an attack of influenza. A long weekend, a few days' holiday and complete change can work wonders and relieve stress symptoms, such as loss of appetite or insomnia. Sometimes the individual's restless energy can be channelled into more satisfying and healthy pursuits. Hobbies and social activities may be encouraged to get a teacher or business executive away from work. Singers under contract in variety clubs and cabaret lead very debilitating lives and attention must be drawn to the need for getting adequate rest and considering health, diet and holidays—especially between engagements.

The heavy smoker of cigarettes must be helped to reduce the number smoked per day. The average number smoked needs to be ascertained—it is generally considerably more than the individual confesses to since it is a common human failing to admit to only the least of our faults. A definite target of the maximum per day to be smoked may be agreed between patient and therapist and the former then reports on his success on keeping to the limit. Some people can cut out smoking altogether by a superhuman effort of will, others find it easier to cut smoking down gradually. Some can afford to take a cure. It is a difficult task in any case to accomplish. Moral support and encouragement from the therapist is most helpful. It is difficult to resist self-indulgence such as food when put on a diet if unassisted and it is easier to succeed if reminded and praised for achievements. Deprived of cigarettes many resort to the consolation of sweets and then the middle-aged put on excessive weight. This may be only a temporary phase but if it helps to reduce smoking it is the lesser of two evils. Smoking of a pipe or cigars and cheroots can replace cigarettes. One of our patients found it easier to give up cigarettes when he had one or two cheroots a day to look forward to.

Sweet-sucking for relief of an irritating 'tickly' cough is another problem. Acid drops and many cough sweets are irritant. Glycerin and menthol are considered harmful, blackcurrant pastilles appear to be soothing and harmless. Chewing-gum is thought to be positively beneficial, keeping the jaws active and the throat relaxed. Chewing therapy as invented by Froeschels (Froeschels and Jellinek, 1941; Froeschels, 1948) is used in treatment by Brodnitz (1953) besides many continental therapists in voice therapy.

The question whether a patient should change his occupation often arises. Unless he is obviously unhappy in it or unsuited to it, and unless a more satisfactory one can be found without difficulty, the aim should be to cure the vocal disorder while keeping the patient at work. Dysphonia in itself is insufficient reason for change of occupation. It is a very serious step in most cases to assume that because of vocal strain teaching or salesmanship must be relinquished. When an individual is trained in a profession he cannot give it up without serious financial consequences. If vocal re-education is successful it is not necessary to make any

change in occupation. Once the technique of voice production
has been acquired the voice will be found to be adequate for all
purposes. Only if there is reason to believe that dust or fumes are
causing chronic irritation and laryngitis should the patient be
advised to find other employment. Wearing of a mask often provided by the management may have been neglected and may give
adequate protection if consistently worn during working hours.
Masks, however, are unpopular as they are hot and suffocating and,
of course, restrict talking which is another penalty for the patient.

The pernicious habit of clearing the throat to excess has to be
corrected. Von Leden and Isshiki (1966) have analysed 'cough at
the level of the larynx'. They describe the opening phase of the
glottis with deep inspiration, the closing phase with rapid and
firm closure of glottis and ventricular bands, followed by the
opening phase of expiratory explosion and dislodging of foreign
matter. Patients may complain that they *must* cough or choke.
Clearing of the throat can be effected in different ways varying
from hawking and acute glottal shock and scrape to a quiet and
breathy clearing operation. The latter is adequate and generally
employed in polite society and individuals do not asphyxiate.
The patient must be warned against the damaging effect of the
powerful clearing of the bronchial tubes and vocal tract first
thing in the morning. Habit is a potent factor in all this, the
patient often unaware of it and able to desist in large measure
when his attention is directed to the fault. Recording the patient,
especially with amplified play-back is a helpful deterrent.

VOCAL ASSESSMENT

The assessment of voice production needs to be related to the
foregoing description of vocal strain and abuse, and factors contributing to the condition must be carefully observed and noted.
This can be done perfectly adequately by the experienced speech
therapist while taking the case history and just listening to the
patient and watching him. There is no real need to give specific
tests although the patient, if a singer or instructor, for instance,
may be asked to demonstrate his singing or shouting and voice
production under certain circumstances. It is also always useful
to have the patient's own description of his voice before trouble
began. He may be able to produce an earlier recording of his
speech. Briess (1964) an expert in treatment of voice disorders
is able to identify the imbalance in muscular tension in the
laryngeal muscles by correlating the sound produced with the

history and laryngoscopic findings. His clinical findings correlated closely with the electromyographic recordings of patients in an experimental study which was carried out (Brewer, Briess and Faaborg Anderson, 1960). It is interesting to note that listening to the voice alone on tape recordings is useless to Mr Briess and he insists that he has to watch his patients as well (Briess, 1964). As would be expected, after treatment and improvement in voice production, electromyography showed a reduction in tension in the previously over-active adductors and tensors and a better balance or spread of activity to all the intrinsic laryngeal muscles.

The following list of headings under which observations can be classified will be useful to the student:

1. *General Deportment*

    At ease and relaxed or anxious and tense
    Posture of head and torso—good/stiff, erect/slouching
    Mannerisms: gestures, fidgeting, head movements, facial
          expression, throat clearing

2. *Breathing*

    Thoracic movement: control, abdominal, upper thoracic or none visible. Control of breath during speech: inspiratory whisper; breath holding with sphincteric glottal tension and air escape at end of phrase, speech continuing with insufficient breath support. Nasal inspiration not oral during speech

3. *Vocalisation*

    Throat relaxed or tense: balance between supra- and infra-
          hyoid musculature
    Pitch: too high or low for age, sex, build; inflected or monotonous
    Maintenance of vocal note: steady or with pitch breaks
    Quality: resonance balanced/excessive chest or head re-
          sonance/breathy/harsh/nasal emission/nasality
    Volume: Weak or loud; shouting glottal attack to overcome
          tensor weakness

4. *Articulation; open vowels or tense jaw and muttering through teeth*

An hour should be allowed for the first interview. Having obtained all the information required treatment should be commenced immediately. No time should be lost in starting the cure and no patient should be assessed and sent away without being given help in what to do about his voice 'until next attendance'. Students in their anxiety to assess often fail to give the patient some positive advice and exercises and may allow the patient to leave depressed and frustrated. After explaining what he is doing wrong it is essential to explain how it can be put right. Nothing impresses and reassures more than being given something to do about it. This provides concrete evidence that treatment will be structured and cure is in sight. The nice cosy chat has its uses always and the need to establish a reassuring and sympathetic atmosphere is recognised but this must not obscure the need for an active frontal attack on the bad habits of voice production.

A recording of the patient's speech should be made and played back to him and this should be kept for demonstrating the progress made later on in treatment.

If an improved vocal note is obtained at the first session it should be recorded and played back so that the patient can criticise his performance. This is the beginning of basic and essential hearing training. It is through the ears the individual has in the main to learn to control his voice. An imitation of the patients' voice production by the therapist, and a forced and easy vocal note demonstrated and contrasted by her is also valuable.

Advice should be given on how to conserve the voice while still impaired. Vocal rest will not be prescribed but the need to cut down speaking at least temporarily must be emphasised: to speak at work only when necessary, not to gossip and yarn in the pub, talk against TV at home, go to noisy parties, etc. Also the need to speak *quietly* and not shout must be stressed in some cases. Persistent shouters should undergo a hearing test since they may be raising their voices in order to hear themselves, not to shout the therapist down. Loan of a pocket amplifier (see instruments list, page 422) to patients suffering from vocal abuse to use at home can be of benefit. Hearing the voice thrown back instantaneously, automatically causes the patient to tone down the volume of his vocal output.

After speaking with amplification for a spell, the patient switches off with the instruction to go on speaking wtih just as little effort. If he raises his voice amplification is again introduced, and the process repeated until the voice remains quiet without amplification. Patients often enjoy using instruments at work and at home as they rest the voice and throat. There is no need, of course, to confine use of the instrument to practice periods.

A speech trainer, if available, can be used in the clinic and some recording machines such as the Uher 4000 Report L can be played back *while* recording with pause button depressed and serves the same purpose. But these cannot be carried around at home or at work.

The aim in treatment and the object of each exercise at every stage of treatment should be given so that exercises are understood and performed intelligently. Explanation must be suited to the educational level and intelligence of the individual. A simple-minded person or child will be satisfied with talk of balloons, voice box and echo, while an interested seeker after truth may require a lecture, with diagrams, on the anatomy and physiology of the vocal instrument and the physics of sound and a reading programme of suitable books.

Exercises in relaxation and respiration must, in most cases, be started at once and the foundation of good voice production thus laid. Slight inflammation often persists for several weeks and the folds are noticeably red but this chronic laryngeal condition due to strain does not need complete vocal rest. As speech habits improve it clears up as a natural result of the reduction in vocal abuse.

Treatment should follow a plan which embraces the introduction of carefully graded exercises and the logical and slow progression from the simple to the complex which is the fundamental basis of good teaching. Exercises should never lack variety. Even though devised to develop the same function, there are many ways in which methods may be varied and made interesting and stimulating. Exercises practised in the clinic can be written in a note-book. Adults as well as children can forget instructions and waste time between treatments in practising exercises wrongly or not at all. With aggressive types it saves some argument as to what was prescribed and prevents misunderstanding. Most patients, however, are conscientious about practice and application especially if their jobs are in jeopardy and some have to be cautioned against overdoing it. The best exercises are those which the patient consciously applies while he is speaking in everyday situations, that is by remembering to relax, to breathe adequately and phrase his speech into shorter word groups, reduce volume and increase inflexion.

Briess (1959 and 1964) as he describes his therapy, does not favour the division of voice therapy into work on separate aspects of voice production in treatment of the specific laryngeal muscle dysfunction mentioned on page 151. He teaches 'phrase design' with rising and falling intonation, working upon choice of vowel, pitch and subglottic compression simultaneously. He cautions against inspiring too much air and too often. This plan is most successful in less severe cases of vocal strain such as individuals who have recently produced symptoms of vocal strain and in whom the breathing and projection of voice are reasonably adequate. In our experience, when patients suffer from long-standing tension and vocal abuse, attention to detail is most necessary. Once vocal exercises are introduced, and this should be almost at once, all aspects of voice production are immediately brought into play in a co-ordinated action on the part of the whole vocal tract from the lungs to the articulators.

At the beginning of treatment intensive therapy is best if it can be arranged; fifteen-minute sessions daily or three times a week are better for breaking old habits and laying new ones than one long session per week.

10 Treatment
of hyperkinetic
dysphonia: exercises

It is advisable for the student to base the plan of treatment or vocal re-education on the following five basic steps:

1. Relaxation and reassurance
2. Breathing technique
3. Phonation
4. Vocal flexibility and interpretation
5. Self-expression

Naturally the above is an artificial demarcation of function and early in treatment all five aspects begin to be fused. A vocal note involves a balance between relaxation, tension and confidence besides breath control. Flexibility involves control of expiration and glottal tension besides self-expression. Emphasis in treatment depends upon the needs of the patient after careful assessment of his difficulties and faults in voice production. A sufferer from slight vocal strain will need different treatment from one with vocal nodes, or contact ulcers. One patient may need little instruction in breathing technique and much relief from laryngeal tensions, another may be found to have been relieved from laryngeal tension when breathing technique has improved.

The following description of treatment is an attempt only to teach the student a systematic plan and the concept of a logical progression from one stage to another based on sound principles of cause and effect. The student therapist who originally works to a plan works gradually away from it as experience grows and she evolves her own system and adjusts it to the particular needs of each patient. The treatment schedule recommended is for the learner and allows for imaginative interpretation and infinite variety; in fact if 'exercises' are to become real therapy, individual interpretation and inspiration is essential. For this reason very few exercises are given but sufficient, it is hoped, to indicate avenues of approach. There are numerous books describing better and more interesting exercises and the student is directed especially to study those of Birch (1948), Grant Fairbanks (1960), Johnnye Akin (1958), Elise Hahn *et al.* (1952) and McAllister (1952), besides others referred to in the text. Uris (1960) is recommended for entertainment and sound common sense. For advanced training in conversational techniques and public speaking we refer the reader to Oliver (1961) on the development and expression of personality and Soper (1963) on public speaking. Oliver, though concerned only with normal speech, also recognises the need for personality adjustment. He cautions against the danger of losing the wood for the trees, of finding the voice only to neglect the word and stresses the need to heal the personality as well as the voice. Other recommended reading is Hanley and Thurman (1967), and Barrett (1968), but there are many others, normal voice being far better covered than dysphonia in the literature.

RELAXATION THERAPY

Relaxation, which used to be regarded by early speech therapists as the panacea for most speech and voice disorders, has naturally fallen into some disrepute in modern times. I use methods for inducing relaxation far less than formerly and no longer use the couch and prone relaxation. The custom of otolaryngologists of prescribing tranquillising drugs to anxious patients referred for speech therapy has in large measure dispensed with the need for working intensively on physical relaxation before breathing exercises are introduced. Nevertheless, instruction in relaxation is still necessary so that when the patient comes off the drug, relaxation can be maintained. Dependence upon even the mildest and most innocuous drugs is to be discouraged.

Reviewing the literature we find that relaxation is not discarded but in use in modified forms and under the guise of different semantic terms of reference. For example, Willmore (1959) bases treatment on the concept of 'vocal homeostasis' and says 'an over-riding aim in all voice therapy is the reduction of misplaced effort and tension'. A new approach to old problems is always refreshing and homeostasis certainly gives relaxation a new look.

Although bodily relaxation may be easily achieved by the patient, it is not in itself enough for correction of faulty habits. The difficulty of obtaining canalisation, or 'carry-over' of technique learned in the clinic, into everyday life is well known. Vocal strain can be seen as a lack of balance with symptoms of hyper- and hypofunction in both bodily and mental spheres.

The organism must be restored to a healthy stage of equilibrium both mentally and physically, and a dynamic resting state (controlled relaxation) combined with optimal function in daily activity (co-ordination). The fine balance between the action of the lateral cricoarytenoid and posterior cricoarytenoid muscles in maintaining equilibrium of the criocarytenoid joint, as described by Stroud and Zwiefach (1956), is an example of vocal homeostasis (page 42). Brewer *et al.* (1960) gives many examples of imbalance. The adjustment of sub-glottic pressure to the bulk and tension of the vocal folds as described by Van den Berg (1964) is another.

Barlow (1959) in discussing anxiety and muscle tension notes that anxiety has been termed the 'mal du siècle'; he writes as follows: 'We know very little about Angst (anxiety) which may even proceed from the birth trauma or be a primitive version of original sin. Freudians consider anxiety to arise from the repression of anger or love. Theologians associate it with the Fall, Behaviourists with undigested food in the stomach, Kierkegaard with the vertigo that precedes sin. Buddha and many philosophers regarded it as concurrent with desire. Anxiety is inherent in the uncoiling of the ego; it lurks in old loves, in old letters, and in our despair at the complexity of modern life'. Barlow also quotes the work of Mitchell (1908) who drew attention to the fact that neurotic patients benefited from rest, relaxation and physical therapy, including a light stroking massage given over the entire body to induce relaxation. This, we opine, was the original source of inspiration for relaxation therapy as practised by speech therapists in England during the first quarter of this century, and later. Barlow (1952 and 1954) himself is an exponent of 'postural homeostasis' and stresses the need for releasing muscular tension by achieving correct posture and a balanced resting state between tension and relaxation. Better understanding of the relation between relaxation and posture may be gained by reading Barlow's publications. Treatment for patients with muscle-tension pain associated with poor posture necessitates referral to a doctor of physical medicine. Muscle tension alone due to anxiety can cause pain also in neck, head and back (Barlow, 1959; Linford-Rees, 1967) and the individual will benefit from relaxation. Relaxation is not in itself enough if it does not help resolve the underlying condition which revives the individual's ingrained habits of posture. The patient has eventually to learn to recognise the tensions which disturb homeostatic balance in everyday activity.

The relation between anxiety and physical muscular tension

has long been recognised. Psychiatrists use the couch in the analytic situation, recognising that relaxation is valuable if not essential. Jacobson's book on progressive relaxation (1929) is the classic source of reference to the subject. Wolpe (1958) used Jacobson's methods of relaxation when employing reciprocal inhibition of neurotic responses as an aspect of behaviour therapy (Eysenck, 1960). Rippon and Fletcher (1940) wrote much earlier on reassurance and relaxation and based therapy for relief of anxiety and fear on 'induced relaxation'. It is fashionable to discard relaxation therapy but it must be remembered that there is a wealth of well-documented evidence that reaction to stress is far less when a patient is relaxed and at ease than when tense and upset. For example, in a scientifically controlled experiment the reaction of patients suffering from allergic asthma and hay fever to artificially introduced pollen was found to be measurably greater when tense than when relaxed.

Since vocal strain is the result of both mental and physical tension, vocal re-education will fail unless it achieves physical and mental relaxation. Tension is the natural bodily accompaniment of fear and anxiety, the primitive and instinctive animal reaction to danger which throws the muscular system into a state of readiness for attack or flight. Modern man deals intellectually with the circumstances of life which alarm him, he attacks with words and is 'touchy' or else retreats into himself, avoiding uncomfortable situations. In either case his primitive defences are unconsciously thrown into action by the sympathetic nervous system; the bodily state then reacts upon consciousness (Fink, 1943), the original nervousness is aggravated by the somatic symptoms, and thus a vicious circle of fear and tension is created (Ladell, 1940). Physical relaxation, which can be cultivated deliberately, materially assists in slowing down the over-active nervous system and to a certain extent this allays anxiety. Relaxation will never entirely remove real anxiety, of course, but it eases panic and gives the mind time to take stock of the situation, and to approach personal problems rationally. When in a reasonable frame of mind we receive suggestions and act upon them more readily than when in an emotional ferment. A pebble thrown into a whirlpool is of little consequence but when cast into calm water it breaks the surface with ripples which, spreading in concentric rings, set off on a journey the limits of which are defined only by the imagination.

Relaxation can be of considerable therapeutic advantage from the purely mechanical and physical aspect; its great value as a means of attaining the rhythmic co-ordination of the muscular movements of speech has been described elsewhere (Chapter 5). The damaging effects of tension upon the laryngeal and pharyngeal musculature have also been detailed in connection with vocal strain. It is impossible in most cases, however, to achieve voluntary relaxation of those most vital parts of tongue, throat and larynx simply by drawing the patient's attention to the existence of tension. For this reason it is necessary to teach general relaxation of the whole body which will eventually overflow into the speech mechanism. It must not be forgotten that many patients really enjoy supine relaxation and find it remarkably beneficial. Others may object, in which case relaxation may be taught more effectively with the patient sitting in a comfortable chair. Children and adolescents frequently dislike supine relaxation and are embarrassed by it. They may enjoy movement exercises followed by an interval of relaxation while sitting quietly and engaged in discussion.

The following plan for relaxation therapy can be adapted to the needs of the individual patient and the preference of the therapist. Many therapists nowadays feel supine relaxation is absurd and unnecessary. As long as the patient learns to relax by some method in which he and the therapist have implicit faith, the particular method is not so very important.

Teaching Supine Relaxation

The easiest way in which to learn how to relax is undoubtedly while lying comfortably on a couch or hospital examination bed in a quiet room and with eyes shaded from direct light.

Before starting relaxation therapy the therapist should fully explain his reasons for thinking it desirable, and thus obtain the co-operation of the patient. Otherwise it is perfectly natural for embarrassment and astonishment, if not suspicion, to be felt at being asked to lie flat on the back when expecting nothing but vocal exercises.

The fundamental principle in teaching relaxation is the development of kinaesthetic and proprioceptive awareness by contrasting muscular tension with muscular relaxation. Feed-back and monitoring is as essential in re-education of the neuro-muscular system as in hearing training. Although muscular relaxation can be taught separately, the ultimate aim is to link auditory and muscular mechanisms in speech production as previously described (page 152).

In order to convey the idea of relaxation, which is very often a totally foreign experience, the therapist should ask the patient to flex the therapist's arm while he demonstrates to him the following three degrees of muscle tension:

1. A considerable degree of tension in which the arm is tensed to resist manipulation
2. A lesser degree of tension in which manipulation is not resisted but anticipated, which is the degree habitually exhibited by the patient
3. Full relaxation in which the muscles do not in any way support the arm which falls limply to the side when dropped

Now explain that it is impossible at first to obtain voluntary relaxation of the muscles of larynx, chest and throat but since the body works as a whole, tension or relaxation of any part tends to overflow into all parts of the body at the same time. If voluntary relaxation of the neck, arms and legs is achieved this will spread to the muscles of speech and voice and the desired result will automatically be achieved. Relaxation of the arms and legs can now be taught. Give instructions in a quiet slow voice and suggest relaxation through both manner and movement.

1. With the patient lying on his back, shoulders on couch and head supported by a pillow, instruct him to let his arm relax and become heavy while the therapist supports it by placing her hand just above the elbow. Gently manipulate elbow, shoulder and wrist joints. Tension is felt in the limb at first like a rod resisting manipulation as the patient tries to anticipate it. Attention must be drawn to this behaviour and tension brought into the focus of consciousness.

2. Teach relaxation of legs in same way. Support the thigh with a hand just above the knee. Lift and drop leg, rotate ankle.

3. Remove pillow and support back of head with interlocked fingers, gently lift, lower and rotate head, which should appear extraordinarily heavy when neck is properly relaxed. Draw attention to any tension in facial expression.

Should such exercises prove ineffective, stretching exercises are often helpful, contrasting tension in forceful purposive movements with the relaxation and relief which accompanies its abrupt cessation, as recommended by Jacobson (1929).

4. Instruct patient to stretch the arms stiffly down the sides, trying to touch the therapist's hands with the finger tips. Notice

the feel of strain in arms and shoulders. Relax and enjoy the ease of the resting period. Repeat three or four times.

5. Stretch the legs, pointing toes to touch therapist's hands, feeling tension in the backs of legs. Relax and then repeat.

6. Arch the back lifting small of back off couch. Relax and repeat. With the feeling of ease in mind, try to hold on to this sensation and to remain passive and helpless while the therapist flexes arms, legs and head as in exercises 1, 2 and 3.

Relaxation Through Suggestion

Some individuals respond less well to physical suggestion than to suggestion through mental imagery, while lying with eyes closed and listening to the description of a peaceful scene which creates an image of ease and peace. The patient then goes on to imagine or consciously develop his own peace of mind. This type of individual frequently claims to be perfectly relaxed until tested, when he tenses involuntarily. The irregular and shallow breathing which accompanies failure in relaxation, however, is generally perfectly evident if one watches the rise and fall of the chest which testifies to the persistence of tension in the supposed state of relaxation. Every patient should be able to relax voluntarily and especially when the limbs are flexed; if he cannot, it is perfectly certain that his mastery of the art is quite insufficient to stand up to the far greater demands made upon him in everyday life.

Instruction in relaxation should be followed by five minutes in which the patient lies undisturbed, resting peacefully with hands folded over the abdomen. If during this interval breathing becomes deep, easy, regular and rhythmic, the relaxation period should end by drawing attention to the change in breathing which has taken place, and to the movement beneath his hands. That this is the natural way to breathe and approximately the correct way when speaking should be explained; also, that it is intended to develop breathing in this way in place of the patient's customary breathing pattern. The patient who relaxes in the peace of the clinic is very open to suggestion, and this factor can be utilised to good effect when suggesting ways in which the patient may cope better with his difficulties at home and at work.

Relaxation When Active

Relaxation is not difficult to achieve when supine and concentrating upon nothing else, but when up and about it is far more difficult. The habitual tension of the individual generally returns as soon as he rises from the couch, but can be dissipated by further exercises directed at relaxation of head, neck, arms and torso when sitting or standing.

1. Sitting at ease, let the head hang forward and swing it gently from left to right feeling the head as heavy as a cannon ball swinging on a rope.

2. Standing with feet apart, lift the arms up from the sides to a horizontal position, imagining the fingers are attached to the floor by strong springs which resist stretching. Pull against this resistance as arms lift and feel the uncomfortable tension in the axillary musculature, then relax arms and let them drop heavily with the force of gravity alone. Do not '*bring*' them down to the sides.

3. Flex the patient's arms as they hang limp by his sides and flap them loosely. Now let him swing both arms together from one side to the other in an easy rhythmic motion. This is a soothing and very satisfying exercise.

4. Standing with feet apart, the patient drops the body forward from the waist allowing the arms to swing loose with fingers brushing the floor. Gently press the patient between the shoulders and his whole body including the head should swing loose from the waist, suspended from the vertebral column.

5. Sitting in a comfortable chair the patient stretches luxuriously, yawns and then settles down for a doze, shutting the eyes and breathing deeper and deeper, slower and slower until a deep easy respiratory rhythm is attained.

BREATHING AND BREATH CONTROL

The paramount importance of developing correct breathing technique—that is central breathing or the diaphragmatic intercostal method—is emphasised by all teachers of speech, drama and singing. It is generally recognised that development of vocal skills and improvement of impaired voice cannot be achieved without attention to breathing and breath control. Mills (1906) wrote: 'Singing and speaking may be resolved into the correct use of the respiratory system, *above all else*. For the voice user all breath that does not become sound is wasted. The sole purpose of breathing in speech is to cause the effective vibration of the vocal folds. Before the larynx can be effectively used the source of power, the bellows, must be effectively developed. A well-developed chest and complete control of expiration are necessary for the perfect use of the voice'.

We can in fact learn a great deal from the old textbooks on the subject and these make refreshing reading when under the impact of 'voice science' with its tendency to disregard the human element. Among the author's book treasures is the 8th edition of Mrs Emil Behnkes' work *The Speaking Voice* (1897). In her preface she says that 'long experience with every class of professional voice user has proved that nearly all vocal faults of speakers which result in failure of voice and in throat troubles commence in wrong methods of breathing as applied to voice use, while control of the breath is the foundation of all good voice production, and a good aid in its development'. Much attention is paid to strengthening those muscles which take part in the mobility and elasticity of the thorax, enlarging the vital capacity and improving the power of the voice. The recommended exercises are delightfully illustrated by photographs of a gentleman in singlet, long pants, white plimsolls and always a white handkerchief attached to a broad canvas belt, presumably for removing perspiration from the brow and from the mustachio of the upper lip. The lady wears a full black calf-length dress with long sleeves, high collar and a rather small waist, black stockings and *no shoes*, which appears to be the sole concession to physical exertion and is in contrast to the dress of the manly, athletic figure of the gentleman exponent of the art. In all, 18 exercises for developing the external chest muscles are given.

Following development of capacity of the chest fundamental training was given by Behnke in 'vocal methods' which underlie the acts of pronunciation, intonation, emphasis and modulation. Vocal methods consist of instruction in the best method of supplying the lungs with the motor power of voice-air (ordinarily called 'breath-taking'), by which means the vocal cords, the tone-producing element, are set in motion. It also teaches economy of expiration of air, so as to produce efficient and even voice without waste of breath.

Celebrated professors of singing in the past laid stress upon development of chest and abdominal muscles. Singers lay on the floor with weights upon their abdomens which they had to lift and lower. Just after the second world war, I treated a Hungarian-trained singer of Wagnerian opera of 55 years of age. She taught me a great deal about breathing technique in the process of my obtaining for her some vocal recovery from a vocal-cord palsy after thyroidectomy. Subsequently she was able to take up an appointment as a singing professor in a well-known private girls' school.

Although physical exercises for development of the chest may not be taught and practised today the need for the student to be physically fit and strong is recognised as essential (Punt, 1967). Open-air sports and improved diet have improved health and physique generally and so largely dispensed with the need for muscular exercises which were probably most necessary in the Victorian era.

Posture is obviously an important consideration in voice production which needs little emphasis but requires some mention in case it is overlooked. Rounded shoulders, pigeon chest, a sagging body which folds the chest at an angle upon the abdomen in a crease at waist level will not allow good expansion of the lungs or control of expiration, nor a good chest resonator. Posture is also allied to personality and confidence. The upright carriage, straight shoulders of the individual who looks you squarely in the eye as an equal has a good opinion of himself in contrast to the diffident, stooping and withdrawing personality. The latter, of course, is not often met in vocal abuse, which is correlated to the aggressive and assertive and often seemingly very confident individual, although this may be a compensating cover-up for anxiety and timidity.

Johnson, Darley and Spriestersbach (1963) discussing diagnostic methods in speech pathology, despite their determination to be nothing if not strictly scientific, have a few observations wrung from them which they have 'rather arbitrarily placed under the heading of "Posture" for want of a better term'. They confess as follows: 'In the absence of relevant research findings, clinical experience and current knowledge concerning the speech-producing mechanism suggest that articulators and resonators function most effectively when they are held in positions that are not markedly deviant in relation to the long axis of the body'(!).

Finally, it is necessary to mention that the paramount importance of teaching breathing technique to increase volume of air intake and control of expiration with an economy of breath expenditure to meet the requirements of phrasing and interpretation is now questioned by voice scientists. It is probably going out as relaxation comes in with the perpetual see-saw of change and denigration of time-honoured practices. To the conservative, the belief that breathing technique is not so important strikes as heresy, but specific attention to breath control is largely avoided by Briess (1964) and Brodnitz (1962) in their very different methods of phrase design and chewing therapy respectively. Nahum

(1967) makes no mention of relaxation or breathing techniques in treatment of contact ulcers. The swing away from breathing technique arises, it seems, out of the experimental research regarding air flow through the glottis and study of the aero-dynamics of phonation. Isshiki and Von Leden (1964); Isshiki (1965); Yanagihara and Koike (1967); Rubin *et al.* (1967); Isshiki *et al.* (1969).

The emphasis upon laryngeal tension, resistance to velocity of air flow and subglottic pressure have a direct relation to voice disorders due to hyperkinetic function. A patient, more probably a male, may be breathing adequately as regards volume of intake and region of lung expansion but flow rate is primarily at fault because of sphincteric closure of the glottis. It is often apparent that breath is held up by the larynx under extreme tension and forced through the vocal cords causing friction between their opposing surfaces. Vocal volume is obtained without rhythmic vibration of the vocal cords, such as takes place when they are adducted and tensed in a manner just right in relation to breath pressure. In such cases, particularly conspicuous in contact ulcers and vocal nodes, the release of laryngeal tension by the introduc-tion of exercises which produce a breathy attack and relaxation of laryngeal and external frame muscles, leading to a clear and well-sustained note, is a priority. Training in listening for a pleasing vocal note and awareness of kinaesthetic sensation of ease opposed to tension, of comfort and discomfort in phonation, are more important than general relaxation and breathing technique. On the other hand while training takes place, development of aware-ness of general relaxation and realisation that vocal power comes from the lungs not the voice box is unavoidable.

Wyke (1967 and 1969) speaks of the 'tuning' of the laryngeal muscles, a term peculiarly well suited to the vocal musical instrument. It is this tuning which is grossly disturbed in vocal abuse and takes time to re-educate. After stripping of the vocal cords there is an organic dysfunction and until full healing of the mucosal and myotactic reflex system has taken place the voice will not recover fully (page 130), despite improved technique.

Introduction to Breathing Exercises

First describe to the patient how it is difficult for the pear-shaped lungs to expand in the upper thoracic region which is encased in a bony cage, whereas it is easier to expand in the lower region where the lungs are larger and the ribs are free in front and

separated by a large area of elastic muscle. Give a demonstration
of the correct breathing action, how when the lungs fill the
abdomen wall comes forward and the ribs lift, and as the lungs
empty the abdominal wall flattens and the ribs fall. Draw an
analogy with the old-fashioned type of fire bellows and imitate the
thoracic and abdominal movements with the hands, finger-tips
touching and palms adducting and abducting on expiration and
inspiration.

The patient may now endeavour to take in a small easy breath,
with his hands at the waist, thumbs behind so that he can feel the

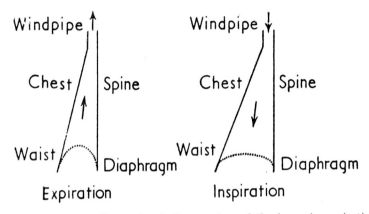

Fig. 30   Diagram illustrating bellows action of the lungs in expiration
and inspiration

forward and lateral expansion of the thorax and at the same time
watch the gap between his finger tips across the solar plexus
increase with inspiration and decrease with expiration. Instruct
him to 'swell up' with air and then to 'squeeze it out'. The verbal
cues are important. The simple instruction to breathe 'in' and
breathe 'out' may produce the exact reverse of the action desired,
pulling in of the abdomen on breathing 'in' and pushing it out on
breathing 'out', known in the trade as 'reverse breathing'. There
is a widespread and firmly held belief that the stomach should be
well pulled in for inspiration, hence the jocular instruction in the
Underground rush hour to 'move up and breathe in'.

Raising of the shoulders and clavicular breathing can be
corrected by practice before a mirror watching movement of the
chest.

Some Exercises for Difficult Cases

It is sometimes extraordinarily difficult in cases of habitual dysphonia to obtain the right response, and especially with unintelligent or older individuals. In such cases the following procedures are helpful.

(*a*) Instruct patient to breathe out, then sigh noisily on the residual air, at the same time giving him a firm push in the midriff. Relax this presure when he gasps for air, then press again as he sighs. Manipulation of the abdominal wall in this way assists establishment of the easy rhythmic swing on inspiration and expiration which it is difficult for some to obtain voluntarily.

(*b*) The patient imitates panting like a dog. He pushes out the stomach wall and then pulls it in. He must not hold his breath, but need not think consciously about breathing until the sharp intake and output of air automatically taking place is heard, then attention can be drawn to it and voluntary control eventually achieved, and the movement slowed down to a normal respiratory rhythm.

(*c*) Breathe out, then pretend to blow out a candle, using residual air; this is followed by rapid ascent of the diaphragm in the need to replenish the lungs with air.

The patient once having correctly performed what is required should be sent away with the instruction to practise several times a day, when possible in front of a mirror so that any movement in the upper thorax can be seen and corrected. A week's home practice may be sufficient time for the individual to learn to produce central breathing when he thinks about it. Frequently he comes back for a second treatment still showing no improvement and having spent a week practising his old method 'because he finds it so much easier'. It is always a mistake to hasten proceedings at this stage. If the patient cannot breathe correctly quite easily and without excessive concentration, he cannot possibly attempt more difficult exercises, and ground gained is immediately lost as soon as he is introduced to a new exercise. For these reasons in the early stages of treatment frequent visits to the speech clinic are preferable to once weekly.

Mention should be made at this point of the portly men and women of Falstaffian dimensions who, unable to obtain any activity in the abdominal wall, rely exclusively upon diaphragmatic breathing. They are often short of breath and generally produce a wheezy or breathy voice. Exercises for toning up the abdominal muscles are necessary. Few will be found to take kindly to the suggestion, though undoubtedly efficacious, of lying on the back and lifting and lowering the legs, or of pedalling an imaginary bicycle in the air. Holding the breath, however, and alternately pulling in and then relaxing the stomach is better received, especially if assurance is given that this exercise will reduce girth and improve health. The panting exercise described above should also be practised regularly.

N.B. Deep breathing when first practised frequently produces giddiness and the patient should be prepared for this and reassured with an explanation of its origin (page 30). He should rest for a minute or two before continuing with the practice and be advised not to practise too long to begin with.

Stays, corsets and any other forms of upholstery must not be worn too tight and they should be discarded if it is at all possible to persuade the wearer that complete corporal disintegration will not necessarily follow their abandonment. The use of abdominal support, of course, is not confined exclusively to women; men have their little vanities too.

Exercises in the Development of Volume of Inspiration and Control of Expiration

In all exercises watch vigilantly the following points:

(*a*) Relaxation: tension generally obtrudes itself at first in every attempt to perform any new exercise demanding concentration and voluntary effort.

(*b*) Central breathing: nearly all patients lapse into old breathing patterns when asked to attempt something new in the way of counting, vocalisation, etc.

(*c*) Posture: any easy stance, feet apart, shoulders back and head up with lower abdomen tucked in neatly should be maintained throughout all exercises when standing, and a good posture when sitting should also be maintained.

(*d*) Oral inspiration: since all breathing exercises are devised to develop the correct breathing habits in speech, and the natural manner of inspiration for speech is through the mouth, this should be practised in all breathing exercises. The nasal passages are too narrow to allow the adequate and very rapid intake of air necessary for connected speech, which should take place imperceptibly between phrases or word groups.

(*e*) Silent inspiration: a loud breathy sound as air rushes into the lungs is an indication of tension in the larynx and some approximation of the vocal cords which should not be present.

(*f*) Avoid the mistake of over-emphasising the need for a *large* volume of air, leading to over-exertion. Small, easy movements of the thorax and upper abdominal wall and effortless *control* of correct respiratory movements is the first objective and *control* of expiration in vocalisation the second.

(*g*) The co-ordination of expiration with phonation should be introduced very early in treatment. As soon as a correct breathing pattern is established a clear well-sustained vowel of appropriate pitch should be the aim.

Breathing Exercises to Establish Diaphragmatic Intercostal Method in Co-ordination with Voice

1. Hand on waist, breathe in slowly and then out, counting in a quiet voice up to four. Practise, gradually increasing the count weekly. No breath should escape between each count. Count in a whisper if the voice is being rested. Count at an approximate speed of one per second.

2. Rib reserve: as counting above ten develops, the patient frequently quite unconsciously holds up his ribs and only lowers them as he comes near the end of his breath. He can be taught to do this consciously if he is a public speaker, actor or singer. A deep breath should be taken, the ribs held elevated up to a count of fifteen and then gradually relaxed. For ordinary purposes a count of twenty should be the target, but for singers and actors a count of thirty is necessary.

3. Breathe in, then count aloud in groups of three, holding the breath for a mental count of three between each group.

4. Breathe in, emit the breath on a loud and sustained voiceless fricative, [ʃ], [s] or [f]. The fricative should be maintained at a steady volume, and not fluctuate, or fade towards the end. Feel the gradual contraction of abdominal wall with the hand as the breath is expired.

5. Practise voiceless fricatives on a crescendo and diminuendo of volume, thus:

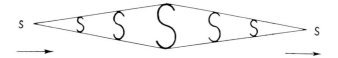

6. Practise voiceless fricatives in rhythmic patterns:

[ʃʃ–ʃʃ–ʃʃ] or [ʃ–ʃʃʃʃ–ʃ]

7. Whispered vowel and diphthong exercises to develop breath control, soft attack and relaxed articulation.

(*a*) Breathe in, then breathe out on a sustained whispered vowel, then voice vowels preceded by h: [hi:], [hu:], [ha:], etc. Work through all vowels in this way.

(*b*) Breathe in, then breathe out on strings of six different vowels and diphthongs. At first do not break expiration; later break expiration between each vowel, achieving a soft attack on each. The therapist must insist upon open articulation and relaxed throat and jaw.

(*c*) Work on whispered vowels, as with fricatives, in different rhythms; repeat exercise voicing vowels.

(*d*) Blow the relaxed lips apart with strong puffs of air and vocalise [bu:] [bu:] [bu:]; the puff of air ensures soft attack.

Teaching the Respiratory Rhythm of Speech, Rapid Inspiration and Controlled Slow Expiration

8. Let the patient breathe in and out slowly several times, then imitate the therapist's demonstration of quick intake and slow expiration. The abdominal wall should jump forward on the intake and subside very gradually on the expiration.

9. Quick intake, breathe out slowly counting six. Correct natural tendency to count fast. Repeat six times, until the new rhythmic swing is performed easily. A suggestion of the movement required may be given by the therapist by a quick hand movement to one side and slow-drawn-out movement to the other.

10. Gradually increase the count on expiration until the patient can inspire quickly the amount of air equivalent to that which he inspires when inspiring slowly for the count of 20.

11. Practise sustaining a trilled [r] at constant pitch and volume—this is a real test of breath control, necessitating a constant breath pressure to maintain vibration of the tip of the tongue and relaxation of the oral musculature. A bilabial rolled [r] is a good exercise also.

THE CHOICE OF OPTIMAL PITCH

Instruction in relaxation, in the control of expiration without tension, and in whispering with a soft attack, generally ensures that the patient when he comes to vocalise in exercises does so in his natural middle range. The therapist is generally able to assess the natural pitch from his voice although dysphonic, and should give him the pitch she wishes him to imitate in all phonation exercises. If, however, he appears to be using a pitch either too high or too low, the pitch of optimal resonance must be discovered by experimenting with the voice, hunting for the middle note up and down the scale on a vowel [u:] or [ɔ:] which the patient finds easy to vocalise. When the optimal pitch is sounded the voice leaps into prominence, being so much more rich and resonant that there is no mistaking its rightness. The resonance change is far more striking in strained than normal voices (Laguaite and Waldrop, 1963) and the discovery of the appropriate speaking pitch is not such a difficult matter; but see Zaliouk's method below. The pitch level agreed upon should be the one now used in exercises and later in speech. The therapist, by constantly bringing the patient back to it, when he strays from it, trains him to listen to himself and thus eventually achieve the automatic auditory control of the voice which is undoubtedly the most important single factor responsible for the maintenance of good vocal habits. A pitch pipe may be used to sound the required note and is especially useful to the patient in his home practice of vocal exercises.

Zaliouk (1960 and 1963) recommends a 'tactile' approach to voice placement which he applied successfully to vocal re-education of deaf children and applies also to hearing individuals with dysphonic voices. We too have found the method very efficacious since our attention was drawn to it. The hands should be placed lightly over the face and nose while humming so that vibrations may be felt beneath the fingers. The vibrations become much stronger when the optimum pitch is reached. The patient should feel the therapist's face and then his own. Another procedure is to place a finger-tip between the lax lips and feel the vibration. This method of tactile assessing of maximum vibration and resonance during production of the optimal pitch for the voice has the advantage of introducing a completely new approach to voice correction. Zaliouk points out that all conventional methods rely upon hearing and a good ear, whereas many dysphonic patients are known to have a poor musical ear and have difficulty in hearing the best resonant tone allied to pitch. Having arrived at the central point, as it were, of the individual's register, vocal exercises should be practised within this natural range.

Humming with the hands pressed over the ears which amplifies the voice is also a useful device for determining the best vocal range, as the harmonics buzz in the ears and are felt in the jaw under the palms.

Use of tactile cues should be made when treating men using habitually too high a pitch and lacking chest resonance. Women with immature voices can also practise feeling chest vibration. The hand should be placed lightly on the throat with thumb and forefinger touching the larynx and the lower edge of the hand resting on the clavicles. Sensation when high and low notes are contrasted should be felt.

RECORDING AND HEARING TRAINING

A recording of the patient should be made at the commencement of treatment, preferably at the first interview, and kept as a check on progress and to provide encouragement when contrasted with voice improvement in the later stages of treatment. Recordings must also form an intrinsic part of treatment and hearing training. Hearing the voice played back gives the patient a chance to listen to himself objectively and critically in a way that is impossible for him when actively participating in voice production. Many people now possess recording machines of their own which can be used at home, following language laboratory methods of instruction.

FROESCHELS' CHEWING METHOD OF VOICE THERAPY

In England the teaching of Froeschels (1948) has never 'caught on' and has few followers. This is probably because his disciples have never settled and taught the method in this island. Consequently tentative attempts at introducing chewing therapy are discouraged by the often marked resistance and even ridicule from patients. This is also the experience of Van Riper and Irwin (1958). These authors have found the method successful in lowering vocal pitch in some cases of boys suffering from pitch breaks and some cases of vocal nodules, when other methods have failed. They comment on the possible psychological value of the method in contra-distinction to its manifest achievement in obtaining relaxation of the vocal and speech mechanism. The technique allows for reversion to an infantile form of behaviour and the oral eroticism of infancy. Some of Van Riper and Irwin's cases improved with practice of vocalised thumb-sucking!

We ourselves are impressed by the enthusiasm for the method evoked in Froeschels' followers. The fact that it is so widely practised in America and on the Continent with such good results would seem to be proof of its value. Practically any technique in teaching, however, will achieve good results in a certain proportion of cases but not in all cases, since no one medicine can cure all ills. Cure depends also upon the faith the therapist has in himself and his method and the faith he can inspire in his patients. Froeschels is not only a great therapist but a great teacher judging by the faith with which he inspires his disciples and such medical experts as Weiss and Brodnitz.

As to the method, we can do no better than quote Froeschels himself from *Twentieth Century Voice Correction* (1948) and advocate study of Froeschels' and Jelinek's book *Practice of Voice and Speech Therapy* (1941). 'Chewing, I am convinced, is the origin of human speech and chewing and talking are largely identical functions. In the chewing of primitive peoples, considerable movement of the lips and jaws takes place and a variety of sounds is emitted at the same time. During the babbling period, infants move their lips, tongues and jaws as if they were chewing, while they in the same way exercise their vocal apparatus.

'Since we can chew and talk at the same time the two functions must be identical.

'The chewing method should be used in the following manner. First an explanation of the identity of chewing and talking is given to the patient. The fact is mentioned that neither he nor any other (stutterer) has ever experienced difficulty in chewing. Then we teach the patient to "chew like a savage".

'Next the patient learns to use his voice while chewing. Although consisting of nonsense syllables, the voiced chewing sounds like human language. (If, on the other hand, monotonous sounds like "ham-ham-ham" are made he does not move tongue and lips as it should be done.) We have the patient chew with voice, do the same ourselves, and so pretend to carry on a conversation. After a number of "chewing conversations" the patient becomes aware of the fact that there is no fundamental difference between this kind of language and his natural tongue, as far as use of muscles is concerned.

'When we finally let the patient talk, we direct him to keep chewing constantly in mind. Every so often during the day he must set aside a few moments for voiced chewing. This is done not as a matter of practice but only to serve as a reminder'.

However, Froeschels does emphasise that in many cases the patient needs a fundamental psychological reorientation, because of the neurotic personality at the basis of many speech and voice disorders.

VOCAL EXERCISES

1. Let the patient work through whispered vowel and diphthong exercises, first whispering, then introducing voice after [h] to ensure a soft attack. Sing vowels singly on an unbroken, evenly sustained breath, then chains of different sounds, later interrupting phonation between vowels. Work on soft attack, soft volume and clarity of tone, also open and relaxed articulation.

2. If avoidance of hard attack is still found difficult, more time must be spent upon whispering vowels and gliding into phonation on the same breath. Vowels may also be preceded by the aspirate [h] or a voiceless fricative lasting three or four seconds. The 'tense' vowels [i:] and [a] cause most difficulty in strained voices, the voice often cracking on these long after all others have become strong and clear. It is sometimes found helpful to preface a difficult vowel with a vowel which is easy for the patient, and then to isolate the difficult one. Examples: [u:i] and [ɔ:a], [a:a].

3. Practise humming, feeling the vibrations on the lips.

4. Practise humming on vowels, gliding up and down the scale covering a third and then a fifth and in varied rhythms.

5. Practise humming and vowels in rapid succession to develop use of nasal resonance (head resonance).

6. Alternate voiceless with voiced fricatives in repetitive strings. Examples: [fv], [sz].

7. Chant and then speak chains of nonsense syllables. Examples: [lim-lɔm-lum; kik-kak-kɔk; pip-pɔp-pʌp]. In this exercise concentrate upon neat articulation as well as clear firm vowels.

8. If the singing voice has to be regained the exercises given so far will have laid the foundations for this, but graded exercises for increasing the range of pitch will be necessary. The exercises of the kind given below are easier than the singing of plain scales. The therapist if not a singer herself need not be alarmed by the prospect of teaching a singer. The patient will be able to compose his own exercises, and her constructive criticism of unconscious

pharyngeal and laryngeal tension, breath control, and knowledge of the need to change the articulation of the vowels by flattening and relaxing the tongue on high notes, for example (see page 80), is entirely adequate for the immediate purpose—but early referral to a singing professor is necessary.

9. Specific work on articulation may be necessary for the patient with slurred speech who talks through closed teeth. Practise consonants in various combinations and rhythms in order to develop co-ordination of fine muscle movements, also kinaesthetic and auditory appreciation.

Examples: [p-t-k, p-t-k, f-θ-s, f-θ-s], or [r-l-j, r-l-j].
[t-tt-t, k-kkk-k], or [kk-kk-kk-k].

Eventually proceed to tongue twisters of the 'Peter Piper picked a peck of pickled pepper' type for developing articulatory expertise.

Speech Exercises

A strong clear voice is achieved first in exercises and only considerably later will this standard of voice production be maintained during connected speech. At first the old speech patterns rule by force of habit, and weeks of practice in mechanical speech must pave the way for automatically good performance in the 'speech of conversation'. An important aim in the latter stages of treatment must be the provision of interest and variety so that the patient's interest is held and his enthusiasm sustained.

1. With a quick inspiration before each line, chant a jingle, concentrating on good tone and articulation. Any doggerel will do, e.g. 'One man went to mow, went to mow a meadow, one man and his dog went to mow a meadow,' etc.

2. Learn to adjust the intake of breath to the length of the phrase. Chant and then speak: '1 is all I need'; '1, 2 is all I need'; '1, 2, 3 is all I need', etc. Increase the count until full capacity is reached. Never let the patient continue to count on his reserve of residual air, for discomfort and tension are immediately felt. The patient must learn to recognise the danger signals, and to replenish his breath supply immediately the necessity arises.

3. Chant and then speak phrases which the patient can compose himself. For example:

   (*a*) It was a cold day
   It was a cold and windy day
   It was a cold, windy and wet day

(*b*) He laughed long
        He laughed long and deep
        He laughed long, deep and heartily

These exercises can be based upon the particular vowels and consonants in which the individual needs special practice. Crisp articulation should be encouraged while the vowels must be 'held' in order to develop their full musical resonance.

4. Vocal flexibility: The prevention of a monotonous and limited pitch range should be an integral part of all vocal exercises. Thus the vowels and humming exercises described under vocal exercises need to be practised with rising and falling pitch. This may be reinforced by visual clues such as moving the hand up and down in a wave-like figure to denote rise and fall and smooth gliding from one pitch to another. The gliding rise and falling pattern may be drawn on paper or phrases marked with the inflection pattern. The same phrase can be spoken with as many different meanings as possible (page 90). The patient must learn to be expressive and animated without relying almost exclusively, as former y, on vocal volume.

5. Practice in repeat reading.

The lines of a poem, or of prose suitably phrased, are repeated after the therapist with careful attention to tone, inflexion, rhythm and pace. The patient's faults should be imitated by the therapist and the patient asked to correct them. When this exercise has been worked through the patient should read the passage himself, attempting to keep the same high standard of performance.

6. Practice in reading.

This is a much more difficult exercise than repeat reading: it should not be introduced too early or else the patient will lapse badly. He should never be allowed to read on in his old customary manner without being pulled up firmly. If he finds it impossible to correct himself he must be drilled further in mechanical exercises with recording and play-back. Reading of poetry and blank verse is easier than prose and should therefore precede it.

7. Exercises for the correction of a considerable drop in vocal pitch at the ends of phrases are often necessary. Although this is a characteristic of English intonation it may be carried to excess, the voice often cracking and losing volume, as breath pressure also drops in sympathy with pitch.

(*a*) Speak the last word of a phrase on an exaggerated rising inflexion. Repeat the phrase omitting the glide and aiming at the apex of the pitch glide

(b) Intone a phrase on a level pitch, repeat, but now speaking the phrase

(c) Speak a phrase with 'and' tagged on to the end as if not the end of the phrase. Repeat, merely imagining the utterance of 'and'

(d) Imitate humming the tunes of phrases hummed by the therapist, then speak phrase with the same tune

8. Spontaneous speech practice.

(a) Short replies to questions, thinking out the answers beforehand and speaking with meticulous attention to the details of elocution

(b) Description of objects or mental pictures: for example, a fountain pen or a rainy day

(c) Prepared talks on any subjects of interest at the moment—film, book or hobby. If the patient is a lecturer or teacher, sections from an address should be rehearsed standing before an imaginary or real audience. If this can be provided in group treatment so much the better

Recording and listening techniques may be introduced when the patient's voice has improved sufficiently or introduced to improve different aspects of voice product on as the need arises.

When a patient's profession needs speaking against a noisy background such as an office, classroom or the factory floor, it is useful for him to practise speaking against background noise. A tape recording of the hubbub at a cocktail party, a class of children or whatever is appropriate, when played back loudly assists the individual to cope with the situation and increase vocal volume without becoming tense and reverting to vocal force.

RE-EDUCATION OF THE ASTHENIC VOICE

Air wastage is the most conspicuous feature of this type of voice disorder. Van Riper and Irwin (1958) stress the irregular respiration of such cases, air being wasted before and after phonation, only using a portion of the air available. This they term 'staircase breathing'. On the continent this air wastage is known as 'wild-air' (Luchsinger, 1962). It is general y accompanied by insufficient approximation of the vocal folds or bowing of the folds due to internal tensor weakness (page 120). The personality, anxieties and environmental difficulties of the patient must be investigated

7

during treatment (page 147). The building of confidence— especially in audience situations where the patient learns to over- come his self-consciousness, diffidence and inferiority feelings— must form an important aspect of treatment.

The general plan of direct speech treatment should follow that for the vocal re-education of the strained voice and include a check on physical health. Voice in most cases will be strengthened by establishing better habits of breathing, increase of lung capacity and control of expiration, and promotion of increased tonicity of the laryngeal muscles so that the vocal folds provide more adequate resistance to the breath stream. This control is best obtained by auditory training, by contrasting weak and clear phonation, and by the imitation of strong and resonant vowel sounds. Through listening to the therapist's and his own voice auditory and kinaesthetic control is established over the laryngeal muscles and develops the necessary degree of tension. Placing the finger-tips on the thyroid cartilage and feeling the vibration in strong phonation is often a helpful measure.

Humming exercises incorporating Zaliouk's tactile method of voice placement are most beneficial in the early stages of treat- ment, also 'ear cupping' (page 171).

If these methods prove inadequate it may be necessary to introduce exercises of greater force, but these must be used with care and discarded as soon as possible for fear of causing laryngitis and strain. It is as well that the patient should practise such exercises in the clinic under supervision and not at home.

Exercises to Increase Laryngeal Tonicity

1. Coughing in order to obtain complete approximation of the folds and to obtain a hard attack can be used to develop kinaes- thetic and tactile awareness of laryngeal tonicity.

2. Follow the above with articulation of vowels preceded by a glottal stop, sustain each vowel clearly for several seconds, then repeat omitting the forced on-glide.

3. Practise syllables with much exaggerated plosives: [pa: pa:]; [bi: bi:]; [ki: ki:].

4. Strings of vowels may also be intoned on one breath, each preceded by hard attack, then repeated while the auditory and kinaesthetic image of good voice is strong but with omission of the hard attack.

5. Singing exercises are useful and also build confidence and help to overcome inhibitions.

6. Reading and speaking to a background of noise is useful. Background noise may be provided by playing music, the clatter of a restaurant or hum of conversation at a party at considerable amplitude. Listening through ear-phones connected to the recording machine avoids disturbance to others in the clinic situation.

Note: In all these methods for obtaining closer approximation of the vocal folds and correction of air wastage in phonation, care must be taken to avoid any increase of generalised tension in the patient and interference with breathing technique. Also the use of hard attack should be discarded as soon as possible, especially with patients who have a history of vocal strain.

THE LENGTH OF TREATMENT FOR CASES OF CHRONIC DYSPHONIA

The aim of treatment is the rehabilitation of the patient in the shortest time possible. The patient, however, sets the pace, not the therapist. Much depends upon the degree of vocal strain originally present, also the age, intelligence and will-power of the patient; his ability not only to apply himself steadily to the practice of exercises, but to transfer newly learned technique into everyday speech. Nine-tenths of the work of re-education has to be done by the patient and unless he is prepared 'to put his back into it' the prognosis is poor. The therapist must, of course, inspire enthusiasm and encouragement; the relationship that is established with the patient is perhaps the most important aspect of rehabilitation and that which most determines its success.

On an average, three months of weekly treatment brings about a great improvement in voice production, but the patient is seldom ready for absolute discharge after so short a period and it is generally a mistake to discontinue treatment so early, though it may now be placed on a fortnightly basis. Very often treatment must be continued for another 3 or 6 months. This is not excessive when we take into account the fact that teachers of speech training and dramatic art consider that two if not three years' tuition is necessary for the perfection of the normal vocal instrument.

Sufferers from vocal strain with difficulties in personality adjustment show a marked tendency to revert after an interval to old speech habits under the influence of environmental stress. The patient who has apparently recovered from dysphonia should be seen at fortnightly and then monthly intervals, and eventually discharged only when good speech is satisfactorily maintained during the period of reduced supervision.

11 Psychogenic disorders: anxiety and hysterical states

It is current practice in psychological medicine to discard the much abused term 'neurosis' for that of 'state' qualified by an accurate descriptive adjective: for example, depressive state, obsessional state, anxiety state. This arises out of the need to distinguish from the layman's use of neurotic, meaning 'difficult' behaviour in people whom we think to react unreasonably and emotionally to events and people. It is also the logical outcome of better understanding of mental illness with more accurate diagnosis and labelling of syndromes. We can therefore use 'neurotic' to describe essentially normal behaviour common to all healthy individuals and characteristic of human beings under stress. We all suffer from periods of anxiety, indecision, depression and euphoria, irritability and outbursts of anger especially in times of ill health, overwork and of family stress. We retain an indubitable normality so far as we recover balance in a few hours or days and homeostasis returns when stress is alleviated. There is a natural buoyancy of spirit coming to one's rescue as surely as a cork rises to the surface after immersion.

A real psychological disturbance or state is recognised when the individual does not recover after a period of time but remains in a prolonged state of imbalance which threatens to become permanent. A mood persists which impairs health and happiness, work efficiency and personal contacts. Henderson and Gillespie (1950) describe the pathology of psychoneurotic reactions as essentially a pathology of interpersonal relationships. Certainly when dealing with patients with voice disorders of psychological origin the trouble is constantly found to be rooted in disturbance of personal relationships and the breakdown in the vehicle of communication, the larynx, is reflecting the breakdown in communication with some particular person or persons.

It is beyond the scope of this chapter, or indeed of this book, to enter into a discussion of the psychopathologies of the voice beyond those of anxiety states and hysteria. The speech pathologist, however, should be prepared to recognise mental illness reflected in the voice if such patients should be referred erroneously to him for treatment. According to Moses (1954) uniformity of intonation and narrow pitch range are always pathological symptoms. Lack of pitch change, 'a limited vocal pattern', is characteristic of depression; excessively wide pitch variations are typical of manic states. Voice disorders occur in obsessional states, and schizophrenia may be characterised by changes in register. Splitting of the personality may even be associated with adoption of female or male voice characteristics (schizophonia). Compulsive neurosis may produce different symptoms such as glottal spasms and prolongation of vowels and constantly repeated rhythmic patterns (well known to the speech therapist in compulsive stammering).

ANXIETY STATES

We have already discussed anxiety in relation to vocal abuse and the psychosomatic symptoms of chronic laryngitis and other lesions of the vocal membrane, so that it is a somewhat artificial frontier that we cross when we come to deal separately with the psychological disorder of chronic anxiety. In this section we will be considering vocal disorders in which there may be symptoms of disordered vocal cord movement and control but in the absence of any evidence of neurological lesion (paralysis) or mechanical trauma. The vocal cords in fact are healthy but present an 'internal tensor weakness' and varying degrees of slackness or bowing. A large proportion of such patients presenting at otolaryngological clinics and passed on to the speech clinic are suffering from an 'anxiety state'. They complain of persisting vocal changes. The voice is weaker than it was and they cannot raise the voice when necessary at a cocktail party, in class or at work. After using the voice much it may become hoarse and breathy. Various disturbing sensations in the throat are described, such as feelings of pressure, of aching, of catarrh and choking or of a lump—the classic 'globus hystericus'.

It is essential to examine the patient for organic signs and to eradicate physical causes for these sensations of discomfort. Malcolmson (1968) found that in a series of 307 patients complaining of lump in the throat 38 per cent had miscellaneous local lesions and 62 per cent distal lesions, of which the most common was hiatus hernia which comprised 69 per cent of the distal lesions. It is interesting and significant that there were only 90 males but 217 females in this series. Delahunty and Ardran

(1970) discovered that 22 out of 25 patients with diagnosis of globus hystericus suffered from reflux oesophagitis resulting in an acid-induced motility disturbance. The feeling of a lump in the throat was eradicated when these patients were placed on an acid-free regime.

It is common experience that females suffer with their throats far more than men and appear to have far more sensitive larynges. Osteoarthritis of the cervical spine is a common cause of referred pain. Pressure symptoms can be caused by a slightly enlarged thyroid gland. Vocal strain can also cause feelings of discomfort especially in individuals who have always had rather weak and ineffective voices—the so called asthenic voice. We have treated many female patients of this character who have developed dysphonia after a period of stress such as family illness when they have been physically overtaxed or after a debilitating virus infection—not always affecting the throat but possibly the stomach. These have been anxiety-prone individuals lacking in confidence and rather unassertive personalities. Anxiety and depression may persist for many months after an acute viral attack (Linford-Rees, 1969) and it is helpful and reassuring to the patient to be shown a connection between vocal symptom and earlier illness and given the hope that it will pass.

Bereavement is another common cause of depression, anxiety and vocal disorder in women. At first the bereaved receives much sympathy but life has to go on as usual and after a while friends and relatives feel it is unwise to encourage expressions of grief and dwelling upon the memory of the loved one. The wife or daughter who has been fully occupied looking after husband or parent is confronted with an aching void of loneliness; guilt feelings and remorse are common, and self-pity develops and the feeling that nobody understands or cares, and then comes vocal failure. This can occur sometimes long after the death of the relative. The voice comes and goes or is weak and cancer fears may grow, especially if the deceased died of cancer, which is often the case in the aged. With these cases of voice disorder the speech therapist can give support by talking things over, and greatly assist in practical suggestions for picking up the threads of normal social contacts and activities.

Linford-Rees (1967c) stresses the multiplicity of factors involved in the aetiology of anxiety states. The intrinsic and constitutional personality of the anxiety-prone patient is inherited and can be traced to one or other of parents and grandparents. There is a predisposition to worry and anticipate difficulties and catastrophes which may occur to oneself or family. Health, work, finances, the future of the children are all causes of anxiety and worry. These people look anxious, having tense facial expressions, bodily postures and gait, they are fidgety and restless and speak very quickly but jerkily. The psychosomatic symptoms are endless. Tension pains of shoulders, back, neck and scalp can produce headache. Cardiovascular symptoms are poor circulation with pallid or blue extremities due to vasomotor constriction of the blood vessels supplying the skin. A rapid heart beat is experienced under circumstances of stress. Breathing may be rapid and shallow with frequent sighing, and breathlessness occurs when walking fast or going upstairs. Gastrointestinal symptoms are dryness of the mouth due to decrease of secretion from salivary glands, and this can be a great inconvenience to singers and actors and aggravate anxiety and vocal disorder. Indigestion, poor appetite, bowel urgency and constipation are further symptoms. Excessive sweating of the brow, upper lip and palms can be observed. Shaking hands with a patient can be revealing; the anxiety-prone individual may have the grasp of a wet fish, not a firm dry hand-shake.

Many women presenting with voice disorder have menstrual and gynaecological difficulties. Endocrine factors play a part and it is difficult to decide which comes first, 'the chicken or the egg'. Hormonal changes after childbirth and during the climacteric produce excessive emotional lability and anxiety in these women who have since puberty shown the pre-menstrual tension syndrome with pain, headache, general malaise and anxiety.

All normal people experience these symptoms of anxiety at one time or another in circumstances which cause fear, such as a narrow escape, addressing a meeting, sitting in the dentist's chair. Bouts of anxiety are normal and anxiety is, in fact, a necessary emotion which increases alertness and releases energy and drive. It is necessary in all competitive activity. It is only when anxiety persists day and night and interferes with the effectiveness of the individual that one can talk in pathological terms of anxiety state. Persistent anxiety produces overwhelming fatigue but also insomnia—a common feature is waking suddenly at 2 or 3 in the morning and being unable to drop off until it is nearing time to get up, when sleep becomes profound. This is not to be confused with similar symptoms in old age, when many people appear to develop a different sleeping rhythm with the need for more frequent but shorter periods of sleep throughout the day and night.

In taking the case history of the anxious individual it is important to discover the precipitating factor which has produced the voice disorder, or the series of health and environmental factors which have led up to a breaking point over a period of time. Indications for successful therapy and quick recovery are the following (Linford-Rees, 1967c):

1. Acute onset
2. Short duration
3. Stable personality and relationships
4. Good work record

Referral to a pscychiatrist is advisable when factors of poor prognosis are discernible, that is, when there is a family history of neurosis and neurotic difficulties since childhood and evidence of unstable personality, disturbed personal contact and poor work record. In the not so severely anxious and disturbed person the laryngologist and speech therapist may together and acting as a team treat the patient with very successful results (Dowie, 1965) and spare the overburdened psychiatrist.

Tension in the throat produces real aches and pains and this becomes a focus of worry, especially as speech is inescapably associated with stressful situations. Voice and throat symptoms can frequently be traced to a family quarrel or argument at work. Cancer fears may develop as a result of a painful throat. The laryngologist can quickly dispel fears on this score but further reassurance is often required from the speech therapist. A course of tranquillisers may be prescribed and help in inducing relaxation and restoration of sleeping habits, besides calming a patient down generally.

For the anxious patient the most important aspect of treatment is the establishment of a sympathetic and understanding relationship with the patient, who must feel able to talk freely to someone who understands how she feels. Discussion with an impartial listener gives the support a patient craves until a degree of security and confidence returns.

It is also most necessary to give practical help; although there may be little wrong with the throat the patient feels there is, and as long as discomfort is felt and an abnormal voice is heard she will remain unconvinced that she is cured and cure will not take place. The symptoms in anxiety-prone patients can be most successfully treated by relaxation. Many patients report on the cure of constipation, of breathlessness, of insomnia and other symptoms once relaxation has been mastered. Patients enjoy this part of therapy very much and learn to rely upon it when under stress. Breathing exercises for the shallow breather can do no harm and vocal exercises for the habitually ineffective or weak voice are necessary. During treatment the patient must be led to gain some insight into the vicious circle which ensnared her, and the connection between vocal symptoms and the stressful circumstances leading up to the 'illness'. It may be necessary to interview the husband or other relatives and to bring in the social worker to help sort out difficulties at work and at home. Most large firms employ doctors and personnel officers who may be called upon to help and give further support. Lonely individuals with no social contacts outside work can be encouraged to join social clubs or join evening classes and develop hobbies which bring them into a sympathetic group with common interests. These activities are not as dreary as they generally seem to be when first suggested to the patient and can lead to a greatly increased interest and enjoyment of life, especially for older patients. Organised holidays and package tours are ideal for people who will not go on holiday because they have nobody to go with. There are a surprising number of lonely spinsters still, despite the tremendous variety of social activities open to the not-so-enterprising individual. These patients cannot summon up courage to break out and undertake interesting activities and need someone to push them out.

Case Histories of Anxiety States

Mrs I., aged 61, was the deputy headmistress of a large junior school. Although she had been trained as a singer and taught singing to immigrant children and sang at charity concerts and to old peoples' clubs, she had for some years been prone to lose her voice—generally with a cold, but latterly for no reason. Her father and mother sang, and her father still sang well after the age of 80. Her mother had died two years earlier and she had then lost her voice twice before concerts and had to cancel her performances. In the past year she had increasing difficulty, becoming aphonic and whispering for a few days but the periods of normal voice were diminishing and the length of aphonic periods increasing. It transpired that her husband who was a Security Express Officer had been involved in a hold-up and severely clubbed outside a bank a year ago. He had been in hospital for some time and on account of an injured shoulder could not carry loads and had to give up his job. He was now unemployed at 62 and had no pension. Mrs I. had to carry on teaching till she had completed a sufficient length of service to receive her maximum pension and be able to retire and live in the style to which they were accustomed. They had no children. Her husband had never been the same since being attacked and was nervous as never before: 'always looking over his shoulder when outside'. She had herself always felt secure and believed in the essential decency of people, but this attack on her husband had changed her whole attitude to life. She was suspicious, critical and resentful and did not feel helpful towards others any longer. She no longer enjoyed singing at concerts, and had not done so since her husband's accident. She was desperately worried lest she should have to give up teaching and the more she worried, the worse her voice became and the more resentful she felt towards society. She did not want to talk about things to her father and had no confidant since her mother died. This was a clear case of a traumatic incident producing an anxiety state and focus on a symptom involving previous functional disorder connected with aphonia after her mother's death. Although some vocal exercises were given to restore her voice, Mrs I. benefited from airing her troubles and the sympathy and understanding she received helped her to recover her equilibrium. She was discharged after four visits and had no trouble with her voice for the next few years, and has now retired.

Sister Maria, aged 66, was a member of a religious community in the City of London whose work was devoted to helping the poor. She worked long hours in slum districts and lived according to her vows of poverty as poorly as the flock she endeavoured to serve. She did her washing, for example, in a public wash-house. She had been trained as a social worker and joined the community after the war at the age of 52. She had always loved her work and been inspired and supported by her spiritual faith. Six months before being referred to us with vocal weakness and an internal tensor weakness she had a bad cold and throat and lost her voice. She then had to attend a retreat and this necessitated reading aloud in a big refectory for half an hour during the one meal of the day which was taken in silence. Her voice became very hoarse and for the past five months she had been obliged to give up an important part of her parish work which was the organising of junior and senior youth clubs. The boys and girls were very obstreperous and she had found difficulty in controlling them before she was allowed to give up the work by Reverend Mother. She was going back to it as soon as her voice was strong enough.

She was run down and had been troubled by high blood pressure. She had a discharging ear after her cold six months before and as she had been deaf in the other ear since childhood she had now to use a hearing-aid. Her eye had also been giving trouble and discharging. She had been put on a nourishing diet by the hospital doctor and told to cut down carbohydrates, but the community's frugal diet did not provide the necessary increase in protein and she did not feel she could ask for more. She had lost much weight.

Even saints reach breaking-point and crack when no amount of devotions and prayer help. This delightful and educated woman filled us with reverence and humility. A special bond of sympathy was established when it was known that her nephew, a medical student, was engaged to a speech therapist; moreover the Father Superior of the Cowley Fathers London House was Chaplain to her Community and had known the speech therapist's godfather, a previous Father Superior. After this it was not difficult to obtain a little more information concerning Sister Maria's anxieties. It seemed that hitherto she had only assisted the present parish sister, aged 40, at the youth clubs; she was now retiring from the work and Sister Maria was to take over. She was really terrified of doing so knowing that with her weak voice she could not possibly control the children and adolescents. Moreover, she felt in her heart that the new strong young curate (probably equally terrified) should be responsible for the youth clubs.

Sister Maria was then told that she could not possibly take over the club work as she might permanently damage her voice and the speech therapist could not answer for the consequences. It was suggested that Sister Maria should tell Reverend Mother about her diet and her anxiety over the clubs and the need for the curate to help her. She was assured that she was not being un-reasonable nor asking too much. This resulted in her being given more cheese and meat to eat and Reverend Mother visiting the curate. It was arranged that he would be responsible for main-taining law and order while Sister Maria would help organise games and dancing and refreshments when she had regained her strength.

This patient's voice remained weak and fluctuating for some

weeks during which time it grew stronger in singing than in speaking. Vocal exercises were given to strengthen the voice. After a couple of months this valiant soul had sufficiently recovered strength and spirits to be discharged with a normal voice—when dysphonia was no longer needed to protect her from undertaking the duties which she feared to embark upon.

HYSTERIA

Hysteria can be defined as a psychogenic illness in which a person develops certain physical or mental symptoms of disorder which are not real. The individual is convinced that he has an ailment but this is entirely imaginary and unconsciously produced for a gainful purpose. The aspect of gain to the patient is one of the most clearly diagnostic characteristics of the hysterical state, and the advantages accruing from the symptom for the individual must be discovered and understood by the therapist before treatment can be effective. This is not always easy. The patient is the one least able to throw light on the subject since he or she is not aware of the motive underlying the symptom. Thus hysterical illness is distinct from malingering. A malingerer professes to have symptoms which in reality he knows are false and has deliberately assumed for gain. The hysteric has symptoms genuine to himself which are incapacitating (Linford-Rees, 1967d), and these may simulate any disease or disorder which the disturbed mind can conjure up.

The exact nature of the mental process which brings about the physical symptom 'that mysterious leap from the mental to the physical' as Freud (1943) called it, is not fully understood. It is only evident that when an individual of hysteric personality finds life intolerable he escapes by a process of mental dissociation and the substitution of some tangible disability in place of insupportable anxiety and fear. The substitute symptom provides a more acceptable focus of attention than the original conflict which is now totally excluded from consciousness. Freud described this symbolisation of conflict as 'conversion' and the individual exhibiting hysterical symptoms as suffering from 'conversion hysteria'.

Forms of hysterical reaction are withdrawal of attention (fugues), loss of memory (amnesia) and twilight states. Conversion symptoms include motor paralysis, abnormal gait, fits, tremor and rigidity. Sensory disorders may be disturbances of sensation (anaesthesia and paraesthesia) or hyperalgesia, besides loss of sight, hearing, taste and smell. Visceral symptoms may be vomiting and inability to eat (anorexia), constipation and retention of urine. All hysterical symptoms are volitional or under control of the will and are not like the symptoms of anxiety states which are mediated by the autonomic nervous system during emotional stress—such as tachycardia, sweating and asthma.

Since conversion symptoms conform to the patient's concept of the disorder it is comparatively easy to ascertain that the disorder is an assumed and imaginary one and not real. A sufferer from writer's cramp only finds his hand and arm going into a spastic and painful contraction when engaged in writing and not in other movements. Paralysis involves movement not the muscles controlled by the motor nerve. An hysterical paraesthesia is found to involve a part of a limb and follows a 'glove and stocking' distribution, not the nervous pathway, and is therefore not neurologically viable.

It is only people of hysterical personality who produce conversion symptoms when confronted with environmental stress. The conversion symptom may be precipitated by some specific trauma or may build up as it were over a period of time during which life becomes intolerable. A belief emerges after a 'period of meditation' and becomes divorced from the main stream of consciousness. Most strikingly the disorder appears quite inexplicable and isolated, to have no logical cause or indeed any connection with the patient's conscious mental life (Yellowlees, 1932).

Because conversion hysteria is an escape into an unrealistic solution, these patients may exhibit a peculiar attitude towards their disabilities. Instead of the acute concern one would expect them to feel over a sudden affliction with paralysis, they may exasperate with their 'calm indifference and inertia' (Janet, 1920). It is just as if they were spectators of disaster rather than vital participants in it (Rigby, 1952). Spiegel (1959) comments upon the horrific accounts a patient may give of his afflictions yet with a certain complacency. The sufferer from a real paralysis strives his utmost to overcome it, the hysteric with a conversion symptom may accept it with remarkable fortitude, even a 'carefully composed martyrdom' (Curran and Guttman, 1949). Other patients, however, complain endlessly and go from one specialist and one clinic to another seeking a cure. If their conversion symptoms change repeatedly, as they often do, they may become real 'cases' well known not only to all departments in one hospital but all hospitals in the locality, constantly under treatment for one disorder or another.

Twin studies indicate that hysteria is not determined genetically and it is now regarded as the product of interaction between personality and environment. Linford-Rees (1967d) describes a specific hysterical personality type who needs to exaggerate and be the centre of attention, wanting constantly to impress others with their ability. There is a tendency to manipulate situations and people for personal gain. Emotional attachments are superficial despite demonstrative, even dramatic and exaggerated loving behaviour. Because of the need to dramatise, exaggerate and present achievements as larger than life-size there is a tendency to untruthfulness and deceit. Many of these people feel they have suffered a raw deal from life in childhood and have been deprived of normal opportunities and affection and have an intense need to be loved and approved of. They may be so demanding that they drive away friends, relations and lovers.

Spiegel (1959) distinguishes between conversion hysteria and anxiety hysteria and in connection with the latter stresses the anxiety felt by the patient which becomes so intense as to be eventually unbearable, and then it is projected on to an outer circumstance. In my own clinical experience it is very difficult sometimes to decide whether a patient is suffering from an anxiety state or an anxiety hysteria and not easy to decide whether there is no gain accruing from the dysphonia in the former for there generally is some form of avoidance present. It is probably less important for the speech therapist to make an exact and refined diagnosis than for the psychiatrist. As a general principle to hang on to, the previous history regarding other anxiety symptoms is most significant for prognosis. In persons who have suffered a series of episodes and symptoms of incapacity for years, vocal recovery from the present episode is to be expected quite soon but permanent cure cannot be expected and recurrence of voice disorder or other symptoms can be anticipated. The speech therapist can often give help and supportive therapy which keeps the patient active and maintaining a useful function in society when otherwise he might be incapacitated by hysterical anxiety symptoms and ineffective, a burden to family and society. Such individuals need help as much as those suffering from episodes of asthma, eczema, or arthritis who are recognised as having pyschosomatic disorders but because the somatic symptoms are more obvious obtain more sympathy and medication. The speech therapist, like the doctor and the psychiatrist, should not feel she is inadequate and failing if she does not 'cure' always. Temporary recovery can mean a return to work or keeping the mother of a family effective and the family happy. Relapses occur but total incapacity does not build up. Some patients need a symptom like Mr X. (page 206) and Miss P. (page 207). In some cases patients carry on despite dysphonia but with regular visits to the speech clinic supplying the need for psychological reassurance and replacing the vocal symptom. The primary aim in treatment should not necessarily be to send the patient packing as soon as the voice returns, which some therapists advocate.

There is no doubt that some so-called hysterics lack moral fibre and crumple up in face of difficulties having discovered long ago, probably as children, that this is an easy way out and of obtaining help and sympathy. But on the other hand there are those for whom it is possible to entertain not only a certain sympathy but even admiration. These are the conscientious and responsible individuals of unstable temperament who suffer torments of anxiety but carry on with a fortitude incomprehensible to the less nervous and the stoic, and only succumb when the burden imposed upon them would try even those made of sterner stuff. In this category belongs a 23-year-old girl entirely responsible for the financial support and material care of her widowed mother, an arthritic and irascible invalid. The girl cleaned, shopped, cooked and held down a full-time job as a typist. Although the reason for this girl's recurrent aphonia was obvious it was equally obvious that the social problems and her reactions to them needed the services of a psychiatrist and social worker or almoner, not those of a speech therapist. A woman of 45 supported an invalid husband by teaching in a modern school in a poor district. Overwork and laryngitis precipitated aphonia due to an hysterical adductor paralysis from which she recovered only after several months' sick leave and speech treatment. Every one of us, it must be remembered, has a breaking-point, though some are tougher than others. Hysterical symptoms may undoubtedly develop in apparently normally-integrated individuals, who have never given earlier evidence of psychogenic disorder, when they are subjected to the stress of war, severe shock or a period of protracted and nerve-racking anxiety (Smurthwaite, 1919). The prognosis in the better-integrated person who succumbs to an isolated attack of illness is better than in the case of one who has all his life resorted to conversion symptoms to extricate himself from difficulties. Broadly speaking, the more prolonged the onset of the disorder the more recalcitrant it will be in treatment, although an isolated attack in all probability will be quickly and permanently cured. The speech therapist will learn in time to recognise clearly those patients whom it is possible to help and those with whom she is obviously wasting her time in face of their need for deeper psychological treatment. The woman, for example, who was 'delicate' from birth, whose voice was always too weak for her to seek employment, who somehow acquired a husband only to leave him because she preferred to live with her mother, presents a deep-seated neurosis which no speech therapist and probably no psychiatrist will cure. The devoted son with a distinguished service record, who became aphonic for a few days during the war and had no further trouble until he developed a ventricular band dysphonia after the shock of finding his father dead in bed, presents quite a different problem. Sympathetic discussion in the speech clinic restored normal voice in a couple of sessions.

HYSTERICAL APHONIA AND DYSPHONIA: REVIEW OF LITERATURE

The most common form of voice disorder of hysterical origin is that of aphonia. It is possible, however, that it has been accorded this distinction on account of the ease in diagnosis, and that hysterical dysphonia is equally common but is more often incorrectly attributed to vocal strain. With hysterical aphonia there is an apparent adductor paralysis of the vocal folds, but there is evidence of normal abduction in deep inspiration and of adduction in coughing and swallowing: only the ability to approximate the folds for vocalisation is lacking. Whispering is generally possible, but the force of expiration may be so reduced that even whispering is scarcely audible. There is often a paraesthesia of the palate and pharynx and absence of gag reflex noted by the laryngologist during indirect laryngoscopy.

Hysterical aphonia is more common in women than men, occurring in the ratio of 7 to 1. Its greatest incidence is between the age of 18 and 34. In children before the age of adolescence it is very rare. Dysphonia apparently unassociated with vocal strain is relatively common in children and may be an hysterical symptom. We have treated several such children in which this seemed to be the case: one of these was a boy of 9 years with a neurotic widowed mother; another, a boy of 10 years, whose dysphonia took turns with a sigmatism and a stammer.

One of the most comprehensive reports on hysterical aphonia and dysphonia is that of Smurthwaite (1919) on the neuroses of the larynx among soldiers of the 1914–18 war. He describes four distinct and recognisable variations in the position of the vocal folds in attempted phonation, all of which should be familiar to the speech therapist in the laryngoscopic mirror.

1. Folds elliptical. A thyroarytenoideus paresis
2. Folds in cadaveric position; folds can be freely abducted but there is no attempt at adduction
3. Both true and false folds tightly pressed together in a spasm of both adductor and constrictor muscles of the larynx
4. Folds approximate in anterior two-thirds, but there is a triangular aperture in the posterior third due to paralysis of the transverse arytenoid muscle

Sokolowksy and Junkermann (1944) also reporting on their war-time (1914–18) experience with hysterical aphonia, comment upon the difficulty of distinguishing between laryngitis and hysterical voice disorders, many soldiers being diagnosed at first as suffering from laryngitis on account of inflammation of the larynx. They describe the diverse symptoms presented by the larynx: 'An entire range of such disturbances came under observation, starting with a complete relaxation of the glottis, as in the paralysis of the adductors, and extending to a clamped closing of the glottis, when the closed ventricular bands scarcely permitted a view of the cords. Between these two extremes (hypokinesis and hyperkinesis) there were to be found pictures which resembled more a paresis of the internal thyroarytenoid, or of the transverse arytenoid muscles or a combination of the two'. A peculiar picture was that of the vocal folds approaching each other without coming completely together. This symptom was found also in the experience of Lell (1941) in describing the aphonias of everyday otological practice.

The voice may be aphonic, breathy, or have a peculiar grating quality in direct relation to the type of pseudoparalysis or dysfunction in evidence. Sometimes both true and false cords participate, giving rise to a double voice (diplophonia), the false cords in this event providing a somewhat deeper pitch than the true folds. When both vocal and false cords are tightly compressed, the voice is high and raucous and this is generally described as the 'ventricular band voice'. Sometimes a male patient produces a pure falsetto or puberphonic voice which arises out of an unconscious desire to revert to the security of childhood and protection and if not a 'conversion symptom' is certainly a cry for help. At different times a single patient may exhibit different vocal variations.

In the great majority of patients the voice can be recovered quite easily at the first treatment. Although there is no uniformity of opinion in the matter, many doctors think it is best to aim at recovery of the voice in one session (Jackson, 1935; Smurthwaite, 1919; Sokolowsky and Junkermann, 1944). Of the 239 cases treated by Smurthwaite only 11 failed to recover and the majority produced voice during the first treatment. Voice returned most easily to those whose folds assumed an elliptical or cadaveric position. Although various methods were used, that of 'moral suasion' was by far the most important aspect of treatment.

A survey of the literature describing the various methods recommended for the recovery of voice in hysterical patients demonstrates forcibly that practically any tactics will succeed if put into effect with sufficient aplomb during the first session with the patient. Barany boxes may be applied to the ears of the patient, who is told to sing while deafened by the racket in his ears. His auditory control of voice being thus removed, his voice returns, the ear-phones are removed and the patient hearing his voice is convinced that it is not irrevocably lost (Labarrague, 1952). This procedure, of course, will not be successful with those patients who do not vocalise with the boxes at their ears. Although the hysteric often does produce voice when deafened in this way, many hysterics do not. The Barany box test is by no means infallible, and dysphonic patients especially are difficult to catch out in this way. The application of a strong faradic current to the larynx is a popular device and generally produces a scream which is convincing to the patient. If there is an associated anaesthesia—and this is possible—the patient remains impervious to the electric shock. Smurthwaite recommended groaning or coughing on a deep breath preceded by breathing exercises, or application of a laryngeal probe to produce a paroxysm of coughing. Pulling the tongue out with the instruction to say 'ah' was also found to be efficacious. Jackson (1949) recommends getting the patient to bring the elbows down to the sides with a thump coincident with a phonatory cough or grunt. If the voice has not been used for months it may be weak and vocal exercises may be necessary, following the return of voice (Smurthwaite, 1919).

Sokolowsky and Junkermann advocate the 'surprise attack',

provoking the gag reflex by probing with the laryngoscope mirror along lines advocated by Lell (1941). Strong verbal suggestion and a confident authoritative manner led to cure in the great majority of their cases at the first session. The administration of systematic voice training techniques which they tried at the outset took time and produced only 60 per cent recoveries of voice.

Recovery of voice, however, is not the sole aim of treatment. Therapy must aim also at removing or alleviating the cause and obtaining better adjustment of the patient to his difficulties by gaining some insight into the connection between the vocal symptom and the precipitating factors.

CHOICE OF CONVERSION SYMPTOM

As can be imagined from the foregoing account there are many symptoms which the hysteric can, as it were, choose from. Sometimes more than one develops at the same time and frequently, with the really disturbed, one symptom replaces another. When this occurs a psychiatrist's help is indicated. Often it is apparent that the patient has focused anxiety upon the voice and throat on account of some real weakness or discomfort. Janet (1920) gives the case of one who was struck dumb by emotion but whose speech was formerly quite inadequate, with an inclination to stammer. Most of the soldiers described by Smurthwaite had been gassed and terrified by the sensation of choking and retained the laryngeal symptom to escape from the terrors of the 1914–18 front and trench warfare. Bangs and Freidinger (1950) found catarrhal conditions to be conducive to the onset of functional disorder. A rhinitis and catarrh can, of course, be a psychosomatic symptom and may very well have been so in those patients described. Lell (1941) noticed that laryngitis and pharyngitis are frequently found to exist in association with hysterical dysfunction. Freud (1938) also remarked on the fact that globus hystericus often stemmed from some real discomfort in the throat. A long uvula, enlarged tonsils, infected lymphatic glands, enlarged thyroid gland and arthritic changes in the cervical spine may all act as triggers to the hysterical reaction. Malcolmson (1968) demonstrated the connection between a lump in the throat and organic symptoms (page 181). Tension in the throat and vocal strain may also play a part in the psychological dysphonias. Under the strain of an emotional scene and laryngeal tension the voice may break and upon this a hoarse voice or voice with rapidly fluctuating pitch changes may become established. Other patients may have their breath taken away by an accusation or shocking piece of news and be rendered speechless and the voice fail to return. Or it may return but after a period of a day or two may suddenly vanish. A delayed shock reaction can take place and dissociation of the frightening or distressful mental awareness of an event from the main stream of consciousness, with appearance of aphonia or dysphonia in its place as a focus for demanding attention and sympathy or a means of escape.

In other patients with no previous vocal weakness hysterical anxiety symptoms of dysphonia can be traced to a traumatic experience in early life or an event occurring some years previously which has some tenuous association with a present anxiety. For example, a woman whose mother died of cancer of the throat twenty years before was depressed by the emigration of her married daughter to Australia. Their departure coincided with a severe cold and sore throat after which she lost her voice and developed a fear of cancer. Aphonia persisted long after she was physically well. When the loss of her mother and her daughter and her cold and throat trouble were all connected in her mind she recovered her voice and began to plan going out to work in order to help her husband save money for the fares to visit her daughter in Australia. A positive and optimistic attitude developed when given guidance. This the patient could not achieve by herself.

From the above remarks it is apparent that all patients need first of all a laryngological check and careful medical investigation into the possible organic cause of the dysphonia or aphonia. This is especially important when inflammation of the cords is present as there is always a possibility of this being an early and precancerous condition, particularly in heavy smokers. It is also important to investigate elderly patients very carefully since the voice may reveal the first signs of an endocrine or neurological disorder. Myxoedema produces voice changes. Parkinsonism and tremor may first appear as vocal weakness; fatigue and debility may be incorrectly diagnosed as 'functional'.

It is a fairly common occurrence in patients referred from the ear, nose and throat department with a diagnosis of 'functional speech disorder', to find the cause of articulation and voice symptoms to be of neurological origin. Several cases of mild expressive aphasia and two cases of early supra-bulbar palsy have been referred to us. One patient who appeared to have a hysterical articulatory disorder of slow onset with scanning speech and aphonia was eventually diagnosed as having a mild cerebellar ataxia following a vascular lesion during pregnancy. Writing also showed severe muscular disorder and the patient was slightly unsteady and prone to fall.

It is a curious fact that the hysterical conversion symptom focuses so often on voice and very seldom upon articulation. We have only encountered one female patient who developed difficulties in pronunciation and a scanning and explosive type of dysarthria with a spastic spasm of the tongue having considerable similarity to the spastic phenomena of 'spastic dysphonia' (page 208). After exhaustive neurological tests this was diagnosed as a hysterical symptom. She was an insecure and timid little woman with an interfering and aggressive mother-in-law from whose dominance the patient's husband had never broken away. The patient developed the hysterical dysarthria after a period of stress and acute anxiety over her son who had left school but was not settling down and changed jobs frequently, but it also coincided with extraction of teeth and difficulty with ill-fitting dentures. She improved with speech therapy but was discharged after a year without having achieved completely normal articulation.

GENERAL PRINCIPLES OF TREATMENT

Linford Rees (1967d) stresses that suggestibility and a craving for attention are important features in the hysterical syndrome which must be taken into account in treatment. They can be utilised to restore the patient to normal function or if mismanaged can delay recovery. If too much attention is paid to the symptom the patient enjoys the interest and concern and wishes to prolong this agreeable state of affairs and being suggestible is encouraged to believe in the seriousness of the ailment. Linford Rees advocates ignoring the symptom and to take no notice of a worsening in the condition while encouraging the slightest improvement and any evidence of attempts to carry on life normally. He writes 'Every effort must be made to make the patient assume responsibility for functional recovery and the more active part he can be made to play in treatment the better'. Consistent firmness is necessary. Sometimes the symptom disappears of its own accord if ignored but sometimes it has to be tackled actively before habit sets in and a way of life builds up around the incapacity rendered by the symptom. The early cure or removal of a symptom makes it more possible for a patient to face the actual life problem and be guided to a better solution than the protective mechanism of the conversion symptom. When this symptom is aphonia or dysphonia and communication is disrupted it is essential that the voice should be restored to normality quickly so that normal interpersonal communication at work and home can be restored.

The most desirable and best method of treatment, it is generally agreed, is to restore normal voice at the first session and this should be the speech therapist's aim also. The psychiatrist has powerful tactical aids such as hypnosis and intravenous barbiturate narcosis not available to a speech specialist. The laryngologist has a probe wherewith a reflex laryngeal spasm and cry may be evoked, demonstrating that the voice has undeniably returned. The speech therapist must exercise the tricks of her own trade. These are a sympathetic but authoritative manner, the ability to elicit a full case history by skilful questioning leading to some explanation to the patient of what has gone wrong, and vocal exercises. The first interview is of immense importance for during it patient and therapist get to know each other and rapport and confidence are established between them, thus forming the basis of treatment. The therapist must give confidence by being herself confident and give consolation by being truly sympathetic. The catharsis of talking things over with somebody who understands is real, and telling aloud what one is thinking gives mental life some objectivity through which a new perspective and sense of proportion may gradually emerge.

Ruesch (1959) in a fascinating account of communication in psychiatry draws attention to the 'metalanguage' and tonal qualities of the voice. He also stresses the absolute necessity of what he describes as the 'feed-back processes in communication' on which the success of all the communication therapies depends. If feed-back, meaning correction and self-correction, does occur the patient is on the road to recovery, regardless of the actual content of therapy. Success of therapy depends on there being another person to talk to who is prepared to listen, understand and respond. Once this feed-back is established the feeling of rapport, of being on the same wave-length, is pleasurable. 'To be acknowledged is pleasant; to be understood is gratifying; to be understood and agree is exciting' (Ruesch, 1959). This satisfaction can then become the impetus for self-improvement. Ruesch points out that understanding is not to be confused with agreeing which involves decision-making and being committed. Linford Rees (1968a) cautions against taking sides, against egging a patient on to take action and advises against giving advice. Obviously, disturbed patients may too easily act impetuously and unwisely and hold the therapist to ransom, blaming him for things going wrong. On the other hand, the thing most often needed *is* advice and if a constructive approach and guidance is not given the patient feels let down and hopeless. Counselling or suggestions can be made to the patient on how to cope with difficulties and this help seems to us most necessary. Commonsense discussion and practical ways in which to manage the daily routine of living, to extend activities and interests and the boundaries of the personality and interpersonal contacts must often be indicated. If suggestions are made, for example, on how a lonely widow can get to meet people in her locality, advice is given only on a principle of action and the possibilities available. The patient must decide whether she wants to do anything along the lines suggested. If she does not want to join a club or evening class but prefers to stay at home she is difficult to help, but often she will think up something quite different and much more satisfactory. It may be learning 'cordon bleu' cookery or helping in the organisation of a jumble sale. Once the principle is grasped the cure is in sight.

TREATMENT

The taking of the case history should be regarded as treatment for the reasons already discussed above. The following lines of inquiry can be pursued: the patient's occupation, family ties, events preceding the onset of aphonia or dysphonia, previous voice trouble and illnesses and attendant circumstances. The investigation should be carried out sympathetically. It is vital to the success of treatment that an understanding relationship should be established between therapist and patient at the outset. No trace of impatience should be shown, nor allusion made to the fact that the patient (if aphonic) could very well vocalise if she had a mind to. The fact is that she has no mind to and until this attitude is changed voluntarily and reaches deeper layers of the personality the voice will not be recovered. Loss of the patient's confidence will only produce an exaggeration of her symptoms in indignant and self-righteous justification of their existence.

It is not necessary to probe deeply at the first interview unless the patient volunteers to unburden her soul, in which case she should be given a patient hearing and allowed a good cry if she breaks down. Many hysterics at first adopt the attitude that 'everything in the garden is lovely' and that they are perfectly content with their lot, apart from the slight inconvenience occasioned by the voice, and even this may be accepted with admirable stoicism.

The therapist having collected what data she can, generally has a fairly clear, if superficial, idea at this early stage of what has precipitated the vocal conversion. A brief explanation to the patient in sympathetic terms can now be given, pointing out that she has had a very difficult time and the stressful circumstances have given rise to anxiety and the loss of voice or dysphonia. The therapist should also assert confidently that this is quite a common complaint, not at all serious and that it can be remedied by appropriate treatment and suitable exercises. If the patient is tense, and the hysteric generally is since this is the armour of self-defence (terrified animals 'freeze' or 'play possum'), relaxation therapy may help. When relaxed a deep breath and an attempt at vocalisation on a vowel may be called for. The therapist may stroke or gently massage the patient's larynx to reinforce the suggestion of what is needed. The confident and convincing manner in which she introduces the exercises are, of course, far more conducive to results than the exercises themselves. Courtland MacMahon, a remedial teacher of speech and voice, the first therapist to work in the ear, nose and throat department at St. Bartholomew's Hospital and the first to work in any hospital in England, is reputed to have had a tall, handsome and imposing presence and had immense success with hysterical patients.

Sometimes an aphonic patient can cough or laugh with voice and this can be utilised in exercises. The patient is asked to cough or laugh and then prolong the sound on a vowel, or hum gently with closed lips. Aphonic patients frequently recover their voices during the first treatment, but should be exhorted to practise their exercises at home, and kept under weekly observation for a short time during which the emotional disturbance and anxiety is more fully explored. Should the voice not return during the first interview, the patient must be told to practise her exercises daily and be assured that her voice will return during the week, and in most cases it does so. No patient should be discharged until she has come to recognise the true nature of her vocal symptoms. She should be helped to interpret her difficulties herself and to recognise that the circumstances of life (together with the emotional reaction these engender) and vocal disorder are closely related, not isolated, facts. The unconscious conflict must be rendered conscious if a cure is to be permanent. The hysteric who is discharged upon the immediate recovery of voice without resolution of the real difficulties will certainly suffer relapse or develop a different symptom. It is too much to expect an individual who has given way under stress to be able immediately to cope with difficulties just because the voice is restored to normality.

The practice sometimes followed by laryngologists of referring aphonic patients to the physiotherapy department for faradic treatment is greatly to be deplored. The practice of sending these patients to a psychiatrist, however, rather than to a speech therapist is an entirely sensible one. Some laryngologists prefer this procedure. The skilled services of a psychiatrist are probably more suitable than those of the speech therapist in many cases of psychogenic disorder, but when it is possible for an ancillary medical service to relieve the overloaded specialist, and release the psychiatrist for the treatment of patients with more serious nervous disorders, it seems economical and reasonable to follow this procedure.

Dysphonic patients produce a wide variety of most interesting and significant vocal symptoms. The voice may rise in pitch and regress to a childish pipe, the voice may break abruptly, shooting up to a childish treble and back to normal pitch, or alternate with aphonia. The vocal symptoms become more acute when talking about or avoiding talking about the most distressing occurrences, the real precipitating factors, so that the therapist knows when she is getting 'near the bone'. The introduction of vocal exercises in order to produce a consistently good and natural voice is easier and more conducive of results with dysphonic than with the aphonic patient, of course. Often a 'good' voice is instantaneously rejected by the patient if it happens by mistake under powerful suggestion from the therapist. A very firm attitude must then be taken and the patient strongly encouraged to persevere and overcome the tendency to relapse. If there is evidence of vocal strain and vocal weakness a course in voice and speech production should be planned. Improvement in projection of the voice will help the individual in social situations and increase confidence, besides providing good opportunity for dealing with personality difficulties over a period of time.

By and large the patient with functional dysphonia appears to be less disturbed than the aphonic, and homeostasis is restored with comparatively greater ease. On the other hand Brodnitz (1969) reporting on 53 aphonic individuals was able to restore the voices of 44 at the first session. It needed 4–6 sessions to stabilise the voice. They responded to a common-sense warm-hearted interest. A large number seemed to have outgrown the initial psychological trauma that had precipitated the loss of voice, but the pattern of aphonia had to be broken by outside help. 34 patients reported regularly for 3 years and only 3 had a recurrence of symptoms, which responded immediately to treatment.

When a patient is referred for treatment after a period of some months as sometimes happens and the aphonia and lack of use of the vocal mechanism is of long standing, the voice will not return suddenly. Brodnitz (1969) comments upon the very white appearance of the cords in such individuals. The reflex laryngeal mechanism presumably suffers from a real disorder of function due to lack of use. We have treated three female patients who had remained aphonic for over a year; it was possible to elicit full histories in which the patients were able to describe the events leading up to loss of voice and its subsequent course with some objectivity. They had in fact adjusted to the original difficulties and were leading normal lives and there was no indication that the symptom was being used to gain sympathy, on the contrary they genuinely found it a nuisance and sincerely wished to recover their voices. A forced tense whisper was used, the anterior two-thirds of the cords being approximated with arytenoids failing to adduct and the typical posterior open triangle maintained. No voice was achieved in laughing or coughing. In such cases vocal exercises must be practised and the habitual forced whisper inhibited in every way possible. Relaxation and absolutely no effort must be insisted upon, then gently, thinking the voice forward and into the nose, right away from the throat, the patient is exhorted to hum softly on a rather high pitch, lips lightly closed. Dropping the head to relax the throat and feeling the vibrations in the nasal bones is helpful. Closing the lips and humming, of course, prevents whispering and completely changes the pattern of motor activity. When the voice returns it is often really weak and tremulous and may come and go in speech. Exercises to strengthen the vocal muscles must be given and attention paid to relaxation and breathing.

Although exercises have been recommended for the hysterical patient, many patients never apply themselves seriously to the methods advocated. This must be tacitly accepted by the therapist and understood in relation to the characteristic detachment the individual shows towards the illness. This attitude to treatment is one of the most important distinguishing features between patients suffering from vocal strain and functional disorder and those suffering from hysterical dysphonia. Diagnosis is by no means straightforward when the paresis of the folds is slight, as with the very common internal tensor weakness which may be due to either vocal abuse or emotional disturbance. Very often the specialist referring the case does not commit himself to a diagnosis of either vocal strain or nervous disorder (Perello, 1962a). In any case he might be wrong and the diagnosis misleading, so he confines himself to a statement on the condition of the folds upon examination. The symptoms of anxiety and tension in both types of disorder are very similar and frequently they overlap. The patient suffering from vocal strain who is too lazy to practise assiduously is sometimes encountered. The malingerer is also, but has the grace to be somewhat ashamed, and responds to correction either by working on his voice or discharging himself when he realises that slacking is not approved. The hysteric on the other hand confesses cheerfully and with disarming frankness that 'he never does a thing' about his voice once outside the clinic. He remains unperturbed by remonstrance or scolding, unfailingly courteous and, paradoxical as it may seem, co-operative and anxious to please. He attends regularly and seldom if ever discharges himself and there is often some difficulty in weaning him from the clinic.

Patients suffering from aphonia and dysphonia which is not of long standing when referred to the speech clinic but persists despite all the therapist's efforts should, of course, be referred to a psychiatrist after a few sessions and treatment not be allowed to drag on without results. Failure to improve is a sure indication of severe psychic disturbance and such patients frequently have a long history of maladaptive personal relationships and other hysterical manifestations. The therapist is not qualified to deal with really severe disturbance. There are different degrees of severity in psychological as well as organic illness and it is only with those individuals whose conflicts and fears are not buried so deep that they cannot be alleviated by common-sense discussion that speech therapy is adequate and successful. When a patient puts up resistance to treatment and it becomes apparent that his emotional instability necessitates deeper therapy, the therapist must never try to trespass across the frontier of that dark continent of the unconscious mind for which she holds no passport. On the other hand, with co-operative patients the temptation and danger of probing too deep must equally be recognised. Not only is the therapist's judgement untrustworthy in psychiatric explanation but transference and counter-transference will be insufficiently recognised and inadequately handled when these mechanisms occur.

CASE OF FUNCTIONAL APHONIA OF LONG STANDING

Miss T., aged 43, had lost her voice with flu and laryngitis 2 years and three months earlier and the voice had never returned. Her mother's sister had lost her voice occasionally and so had various cousins. Between the ages of 20 and 33 she had lost her voice on several occasions and subsequently she had periods of vocal weakness about once a year. At age 26 she had a sub-arachnoid haemorrhage from which she made a complete recovery but was ill and off work for a year. She lived with her mother and was a telephonist and had to leave home at 7.45 a.m. and did not return until 7.30 p.m. Her mother was 68 and not strong; she had a nervous breakdown some six months after Miss T. lost her voice, and used to cry a great deal and was very difficult. She 'deserted' her daughter and went to live with her widowed sister and son for a time. Miss T. had a married brother but she and her mother had little contact with him. Miss T.'s mother had a sister, now a semi-invalid who lived in a neighbouring town and they had felt responsible and visited her every Sunday while her son was in Kenya for 2 years. He had now returned and suggested his mother should come to live with them as they were such friends.

When Miss T. lost her voice she was off sick for 6 months and during this time she was seen by a number of doctors and psychiatrists all of whom told her it was nerves but failed to help her. Speech therapy was never suggested. Eventually a new partner to her general practitioner who had trained at St. Bartholomew's decided to send her to one of our laryngologists whom he had known since medical school, telling her 'they'll put you right', which in itself was a great help.

A direct laryngoscopy had to be carried out because the patient gagged so violently. The larynx was reported normal, the cords adducted satisfactorily as she came out of the anaesthetic. Vocal cords and false cords appeared rather hypertrophied from lack of use. She was seen by the speech therapist briefly before she left hospital and given some vocal exercises. She had no voice and whispered without much tension.

At the first interview for which much time was allowed, the patient was encouraged to talk and a full history was obtained. The relevant facts were as follows. Before losing her voice she had worked happily as a telephonist for 15 years until the exchange was closed and she was transferred to a new and distant exchange where she knew nobody and was alarmed by being put in charge of STD equipment with which she could not cope. She had to wait for trains on cold stations and thus caught cold, lost her voice and so ensured that she was unable to return to that kind of work. When she started work again it was to do clerical work in the telephone exchange in a town on the south coast. She had been engaged to a nice boy before the war and correspondence was maintained but he suddenly stopped writing and later she heard he had married a Belgian. She had never risked being 'let down' again and avoided men. She had seen a psychiatrist four times but he had just wanted her to talk. She complained that he did not tell her what to do and did not help her in any way. She was then transferred to a day hospital group of out-patients who by all accounts were seriously disturbed; the men talked about murdering their wives and the women of their hatred for their husbands, and they discussed sexual details and wept. Miss T. was horrified and shocked and only attended once, moreover she was lastingly indignant and resentful that she should be considered to be like one of 'them'.

The long hours of travel, of work and of domestic duties, and the joylessness of life were obvious. She was conscientious and efficient and had a good work record and an admirable concept of family responsibility. She obviously did not enjoy or need her symptom and really wanted her voice back.

The therapist then explained in sympathetic, simple and understanding terms how stress and too great a load of work and responsibility had served to maintain loss of voice and this had now become habit. Miss T. was praised for courage and fortitude in returning to work and caring for her difficult mother. She must certainly not consider looking after the aunt as well. Her previous vocal weakness had become a focus of anxiety originally and not having used the voice for so long the muscles were weak but exercises would improve the voice gradually. There was no doubt at all that it would come back. In the meanwhile we would have to discuss plans for making life more exciting and enjoyable and a holiday abroad was suggested. Relaxation, breathing and vowel exercises produced a soft voice and Miss T. was told to practise daily and before catching her train, to pop in and collect all the leaflets she could on package tours from the nearby travel agent. She was a trifle anxious about the reaction of her supervisor who was not a sympathetic man and fond of telling her whispering was 'just nerves'. Attendance at a London hospital meant a day off work a week but a letter to the supervisor explained that she had to attend for treatment on doctor's orders, and there was no difficulty. This day off, of course, was very welcome and assisted the cure.

Miss T.'s voice gradually returned, at first in exercises later in speech. Noise masking was used in treatment after four weekly visits as the voice when it recovered went into a spastic spasm, which was no doubt an hysterical symptom. When Miss T. could not hear her voice it was normal as she read and the masking was switched off and on at intervals so that she could hear her normal voice. When she did, she rejected it and the vocal cords and ventricular bands produced a strangulated voice, but when we discussed this she began more and more to use normal phonation. After six weeks' treatment her voice was fully recovered. She was particularly pleased that she could laugh again and enjoyed listening to recordings of herself talking and laughing. She was then seen at fortnightly intervals until she went on the planned holiday and has remained well since, which is now a period of 4 years.

Mr. X., aged **50** years. Diagnosis: 'functional dysphonia'. Voice high-pitched and harsh, produced by compression of both true and false folds. Excessive general muscular tension which did not respond to relaxation therapy. Upper thoracic breathing. This strange voice had descended upon the patient suddenly after a cold three months previously. He said he knew that it sounded painful but he felt no discomfort whatsoever. He was not at all distressed by his voice but he was concerned by the fact that it caused others distress and that people could not sit and listen to him preach.

It transpired that he had addressed evangelical meetings at intervals since adolescence but, a month before this vocal affliction, he had quite suddenly been elected head of the obscure religious sect to which he belonged. His new duties entailed the composition of two or three addresses a week. He was not of a studious turn of mind and had no gift for invention, and after a hard day's work he found that he fell asleep over his Bible instead of composing the inspiring and uplifting homilies it was his joy to deliver. It was obvious that his new responsibilities were too onerous and his vocal trouble provided an escape from office without admission of inadequacy to himself or to his flock. Speech treatment was sought because it was naturally expected of him, and he must show and actually did feel a desire to get well. He admitted he had no faith in speech therapy. He knew a man who had a similar illness which lasted all of three whole years and he was convinced that his illness would follow the same course.

It was impossible not to feel sympathy for this poor man in his dilemma. The recovery of voice would have been the greatest social embarrassment to him, and no happier solution to his problems could be conceived than that which he had himself produced. Treatment was terminated, therefore, with the assurance that speech therapy would not accelerate his recovery, but that he would get better gradually and in the meantime it would be advisable not to tax his voice in any way. A psychiatrist might have explored the life history of this patient and discovered why he had to join this religious sect and why he needed to play a leading role in the group. It is clear that he had to suffer a loss of voice rather than a loss of face. This patient, however, was far too simple-minded and unsophisticated to benefit or even to begin to understand so sophisticated and intellectual a thesis. It was far better to leave him with his own solution. Freud recognised that there are circumstances when it is better to leave a patient with his neurotic symptom than to endeavour to remove it.

Miss P., aged 28 years. A grammar school teacher. She suffered from occasional loss of voice and catarrhal trouble but an X-ray of chest and sinuses showed them to be free from infection. Her voice was thin and high and lacking in resonance, and became hoarse after a day's teaching. Breathing was shallow and high and she was conspicuously tense and nervous. She had been troubled by catarrh for ten years and believed that her nasal passages had been traumatised at school when she had been shown how to blow through one nostril at a time. She sometimes coughed up blood and often woke choking at night. She lived with her mother who was separated from her father; she admitted to much home worry but did not wish to discuss it.

Instruction in relaxation and voice production was given and her voice improved steadily despite the fact that she never practised her exercises. Over a period of 3 months she gradually became more at ease and settled in mind and was remarkably grateful for the sympathy she found in the clinic and especially it seemed for the fact that although she was 'a psychological case' as she put it, she was never pressed for information. The catarrhal complex disappeared and a cold came and went without distress. She then asked to be discharged and on her last visit volunteered the fact that her father had been prosecuted by the police for some infringement of trade restrictions. She had felt acutely that his disgrace reflected on her and that her colleagues and pupils would think badly of her. Her acceptance with kindness and sympathy at the speech clinic had helped her to see her troubles in their right perspective, whereas prior to treatment her judgement had been altogether distorted by anxiety and the fear of ostracism.

The confession of her real problems came in this patient after the voice had become normal and speech therapy was no longer necessary. The positive attitude of the therapist and the exercises were the real healing agents. The unchanged attitude of the therapist after this 'confession' must have given her the final reassurance and security she needed.

CHRONIC SPASTIC DYSPHONIA

Although spastic dysphonia is generally accepted to be a hysterical conversion symptom it constitutes a sufficiently distinct syndrome to merit separate description and discussion. Spastic dysphonia (dysphonia spastica) has been described by laryngologists for many years, the first reference in the literature, according to Arnold and Heaver (1959), being by Traube in 1871. Interest in this rather rare psychogenic voice disorder was re-awakened by the studies published by Arnold and Heaver (1959). The literature is confusing because many speech therapists (Van Thal, 1961) and laryngologists designate the hyperkinetic dysphonia described in connection with vocal abuse as 'spastic dysphonia' (Kiml, 1965; Dowie, 1965). The sphincteric and spasmodic closure of the vocal cords which often involves the ventricular bands is also frequently seen in patients suffering from anxiety and functional dysphonia as well as patients suffering from anxiety and vocal strain (chronic laryngitis). The dysphonia and excessive laryngeal tension in the vast majority of cases is transient and reversible and less severe than the 'spastic dysphonia' described by Arnold and Heaver (1959) in which the characteristic laryngeal spasm is persistent and exceedingly intractable. From the cases we have treated it would seem that chronic spastic dysphonia always starts in this way. Most voice therapists and psychiatrists agree that though sufferers may improve and be supported by therapy, the condition once established is incurable. The extreme laryngeal tension and vocal dysfunction may vary in degree. In the early stages of dysphonia there may be periods of recovery for several weeks. The voice often improves with a change of doctor, therapist or psychiatrist (Heaver, 1958). Aronson, Brown, Litin and Pearson (1968) found the voice fluctuated, being better when relaxed and worse when tired and much worse when under emotional stress. All are agreed that the results of every type of treatment are disappointing: the patient no sooner improves than he relapses again. Patients suffering from the illness should receive psychiatric treatment. Voice therapy may help to alleviate the symptoms especially if psychiatrist and speech therapist can co-operate over treatment, and the patient himself is sincerely co-operative and desires to get better (Bloch, 1965).

Spastic dysphonia develops in psychoneurotic individuals as a conversion reaction. It may develop after a long period of anxiety and especially as a later stage in hyperkinetic dysphonia. It may equally develop quite suddenly after a traumatic experience.

Arnold and Heaver (1959) explain the characteristic laryngeal symptom of spastic dysphonia as an unconscious and involuntary intrusion of a subcortical and primitive mechanism of phonation, after the normal voluntary neuro-laryngeal mechanism is lost, and a shattered personality withdraws from the threats of daily life. The laryngeal spasm and sphincter action of the larynx is clearly visible in the laryngoscopic mirror. The sphincteric closure of the larynx is normally only brought into action in swallowing, coughing and effort which necessitates holding the breath for fixation of the thoracic cage. Its use in phonation must be regarded as a regression to a primitive form of behaviour. Holding the breath and spasmodic closure of the larynx is an instinctive reaction to fright. 'It took my breath away'; 'I was speechless with fright'; 'I couldn't make a sound' are subjective reports of fear so common to humanity that they have become established in recognised linguistic forms or clichés, as Heaver (1958) emphasised.

Patients with spastic dysphonia may be able to laugh, sing, cough and whisper normally, though some cannot. Symptoms are not confined to the laryngeal mechanism; the effort to communicate may strain head and neck muscles. Blinking and facial tics may occur. The muscles of respiration are involved in the tension, the abdominal muscles and diaphragm may go into spasm synchronising with that of the laryngeal muscles.

Until recent years the disorder was considered by the majority of authors to be a psychoneurotic symptom and Heaver's analysis of the case of Mrs Z.A. indicates that it is hysterical although other authorities do not agree. Bastiaans and Groen (1955) draw attention, however, to the inco-ordination between synergistic and antagonistic muscles in hysterical manifestions. Inco-ordination disturbances in the laryngeal and respiratory movements are conspicuous symptoms in spastic dysphonia.

Heaver has described the lack of emotional inhibition in the patient Mrs Z.A. and postulates that during the periods of dysphonia and aphonia which constantly recurred, thalamic emotional influences superseded forebrain cortical control of her speech and voice pattern. This lack of inhibition over her emotions then shunted somatically to the larynx as a symbolic display, leaving only the primitive reflex laryngeal mechanism intact for vocal expression. Heaver stresses the neuro-physiologic regression. In the case of his patient it was synchronous with regression levels of childlike exhibitionism and infantile oral-erotic but forbidden narcissistic demands.

Negus and St. Clair Thomson (1955) describe spastic dysphonia as a phonic spasm comparable to writer's cramp. The symptom of complete arrest or blocking of voice is similar to the speech blocks encountered in some cases of stammering, and spastic dysphonia has been described as a 'stuttering of the vocal folds'. Voice is constantly interrupted by involuntary spasmodic sphincteric closure of the larynx. The voice cuts out during speech, then as air is forced through the laryngeal sphincter a forced and choked voice is produced. The interruption of stressed vowels into two elements is a characteristic symptom. The possibility of real neurological disorder such as disseminated sclerosis and cerebellar degeneration, bulbar palsy and Parkinsonism with essential voice tremor must be considered (Aranson *et al.*, 1968a).

Robe, Moore and Brumlik (1960) described ten patients with spastic dysphonia who were given neurological examinations, and electro-encephalograms were obtained. All these patients had signs of disease in the central nervous system. Nine cases had abnormal paroxysmal discharges generally in the right temporo-parietal region. These authors believe that spastic dysphonia is a symptom of organic neurological disorder. They do not deny that patients show considerable psychoneurotic symptoms and that psychiatric treatment is advisable for them.

A much larger sample of patients have been reported in two

excellent papers by a comprehensive team of speech pathologists, psychiatrist and neurologist at the Mayo clinic which examines 1,000 cases of speech and language disorder per year (Aranson *et al.*, 1968 and 1968a). It was found that 1 in 70 of these patients had spastic dysphonia which indicates the rarity of the disorder. Their study included 34 patients, 20 women and 14 men, the age range falling between 29 and 74 years with an average of 44 years of age. Spastic dysphonia is a disorder occurring in later life, therefore. Of the 34 patients, 27 were given a neurological examination and 20 of these patients were found to have one or more neurological signs; 14 of them were over 50 years of age. The chief neurological symptom was essential voice tremor as described by Critchley (1949). Other symptoms were facial and tongue twitch, head or hand tremor, but 17 out of 22 patients given an e.e.g. had a normal record. Some patients complained of difficulty in swallowing or having pain in the throat or tightness in the chest. The tightly-squeezed voice, a 'strangled dysphonia' with a struggle to force air through the laryngeal constriction was common to all. The psychological evaluation of personality showed these patients to be a remarkably heterogeneous group and only 18 had a suggestion of psychoneurosis. The clinical impression provided three characteristics which were:

1. Compulsiveness
2. Suppressed anger
3. Constant verbal repression

We have noticed the agreeable and co-operative personalities of the few spastic dysphonic patients we have treated and the lack of verbal aggression. But in only one out of six cases we have treated were there neurological signs. This patient had high blood-pressure and suffered a slight stroke 3 years after the onset of dysphonia.

In summary of all the above studies it would seem that the majority of patients have some neurological disorder which provides a physiological basis to the strange vocal symptom. There are, however, without doubt some rare cases where the symptom is not neurological but purely psychogenic and a true hysterical conversion symptom. The dysphonia may start with laryngitis or vocal abuse and recover and then, as stress builds up, dysphonia recurs and can become fixed as a habit or a tic, in the same way as with writer's cramp when muscles go into spasm only in a specific activity. It is necessary to take a careful

history and to seek indications of the gain which accrues to the
patient from the dysphonia, besides making a medical and
neurological check.

The neurologically-based spastic dysphonias can be helped by
conventional speech therapy. Relaxation is very important, also
breath capacity and control and voice production. In the hysterical
types laryngologist, speech therapist and psychiatrist may all
co-operate and, if not cure the patient, at least give support and
reassurance and help him lead a normal and useful existence and
earn his living.

Fox (1969) describes intensive treatment of a woman with
spastic dysphonia in whom there was no apparent psychogenic
disturbance but who had a slightly abnormal e.e.g. suggesting a
diffuse involvement of cerebral function of some unknown type.
Therapy which at first was given three times a day for 10-minute
periods, consisted of teaching breathy voice quality. The failure
of the vocal cords to adduct in breathy vocalisation eliminated the
tremulous and strained quality. The patient learned to use this
new voice 75 per cent to 80 per cent of the time eventually. Fox
believes that spastic dysphonia is an organic disorder which can
be successfully treated and deplores the defeatist attitude which is
generally prevalent that the trouble is incurable. The need for
treatment and supportive therapy is obvious to us, but Fox
admits failure to produce complete cure and the therapist must
accept the fact that it is supportive therapy that is being given.
The use of breathy vocalisation to counteract spasm is in our
experience the most effective form of therapy which we introduce
with relaxation and soft vocalisation of vowels preceded by [h].
These may be followed by vowels preceded by voiceless fricatives,
i.e. [s, ʃ, f]. The nasal consonants and humming are also useful.
Phrases introducing words beginning with these soft breathy
and relaxed sounds follow. Treatment in many ways can follow
that of stammering and the Kingdon-Ward (1941) discussion of
compulsive spastic spasm and habit are relevant to spastic
dysphonia. Her speech sheets introducing syllables and 'easy'
consonants which are then built into words and later sentences are
most useful.

Linford-Rees (1970) has suggested that the spastic dysphonia
which is often seen by laryngologists as an anxiety symptom
which is reversible with voice therapy, may in some hysterical
individuals become established like a tic or habit spasm, in the
same way as occupational cramps (writer's cramp has already

been mentioned). If the individual in time overcomes the need for the gain which derives from the conversion symptom, it is feasible that application of behaviour therapy could effect a cure by drawing upon learning theory and treating anxiety hysteria as a learned habit (Eysenck, 1960). However, no speech therapist has so far as I know worked out a method of reciprocal inhibition on a reward basis or some form of aversion therapy and effected a cure. Tics are notoriously difficult to cure (Ascher, 1959; Spiegel, 1959). Spasmodic torticollis which is a conversion symptom becomes, for example, so intractable and incapacitating to the individual that neuro-surgical operations are performed which may have serious paralytic sequelae but are preferable to the intolerable head movements and wry-neck. Grossberg (1965) applied behaviour therapy successfully in the case of a woman who was terrified of public speaking. This, however, was a phobia, specific and clear-cut. Phobias can arise in non-obsessional and normal individuals by a process of learning whereby fear becomes attached to a certain situation. As long as the patient is not really disturbed, behaviour therapy can be applied successfully to treatment of phobias when psycho-therapy has been found to make no impression at all upon the phobia.

Case Histories

Mr Y. was first referred for speech therapy at age 54 and continued having therapy until he was 60 years old and retired from his job in a bank. He presented first with an acute laryngitis and injected cords which was diagnosed as an infection superimposed upon vocal strain. Medical treatment was prescribed followed by a summer holiday after which the larynx looked healthier but deteriorated upon returning to work. Bowing of the vocal cords and internal tensor weakness were now present besides laryngitis. He was a fit, strong person normally and his only disability a severe deafness in one ear. He was tense and active, always busy and 'could talk the hind legs off a donkey'. He was an expert in the City on imports and exports regulations and currency restrictions and his work at the bank was highly responsible and specialised. He talked all day to customers and had long consultations over the phone, which he found especially tiring for the voice. He was also a lecturer to trainees for higher executive appointments at the Bank School. His hobbies were gardening and decorating. He was efficient and conscientious in everything he did. He devoted most of his holidays to keeping the house in a good state of repair and making improvements; for example, one week he fitted a new sink unit in the kitchen and laid a new floor. He was an active member of his Methodist Church and on many committees and took Sunday School and Crusader classes regularly every week. He was a firm teetotaller and had never smoked. He was rigid in his opinions, especially in religious matters and abhorred the permissive society and the world's depravity. He was very happily married and had three children. The only son became a teacher, and the elder daughter a teacher specialising in religious instruction. The younger daughter was still at school. The whole family was harmoniously united and shared social and religious activities to an exceptional extent. The two elder children eventually married happily.

Mr Y. when first examined in the speech clinic had a hoarse voice with much laryngeal tension, and bowing of the cords appeared to alternate with a spastic dysphonia. He had always, and still had, a high falsetto laugh and could sing falsetto but could not sing in the middle register. His voice had been rather high-pitched and immature. He could always produce normal voice in vowel exercises. During the first year his voice when speaking might be normal for a sentence at a time, but was quickly rejected and followed by spastic voice. Students in training and visiting speech pathologists invariably reported with pride that they had produced a great improvement in the patient's voice, but this was never maintained. Arnold and Heaver (1964) noted this characteristic in spastic dysphonia. After an exceptionally busy day at the bank his voice deteriorated, and also when there were stresses at home and especially if his wife or children were ill. Laryngitis did not return unless he had a cold.

The strangulation of the voice became much more marked when he spoke about topics which were emotionally loaded. During the long talks which constituted the major part of treatment since he resented vocal therapy, it emerged that Mr Y., though superficially happy, was bitterly resentful towards the bank, in which he had failed to get promotion, despite his value as an employee. Younger men had been promoted over him when he came back from the war, yet he was expected to instruct new raw recruits and impart to them all his wisdom and experience without receiving any financial rewards. He could only afford a motor scooter to travel to work and compared his lot with that of the bank manager and the many 'perks' accruing to his high position. Mr Y. felt his lack of promotion and success all the more keenly for the fact that he had a twin brother who had gone into insurance and had in his own words 'always been bigger and better at everything'. This brother was unmarried and lived with three spinster sisters, all of whom had good jobs. They lived in a large house in some luxury.

Mr Y. loved coming to the clinic once a week and the fact that he got away from the bank early and 'left them to it' afforded him considerable consolation; he was thus getting his own back although it was evident he made up the lost time next day. He was always cheerful, friendly and good-tempered, exhibiting verbal non-aggression. Treatment was stopped after 18 months on account of the therapist being absent for 2 months through illness. When Mr Y. was seen again, he had suffered a total relapse and the larynx was again inflamed and congested. In alarm he was referred back to the laryngologist for extensive diagnostic tests, all of which proved negative. The condition cleared once therapy was restarted. After this, supportive therapy was maintained until his retirement but he was now seen fortnightly on the tacit understanding that the bank should not be told and he should still leave early every week and derive the benefit from this mid-week 'rest'. There was never any conflict between his conscience and this deception since he was acting on medical advice. At one time he used an amplifier and head-set at work and enjoyed doing so since it drew attention to his disability without curing it. When this became apparent we advised against using it.

A year before his retirement the bank employees' trades union became active and for a time there was some hope that his case would be reviewed and he might be promoted or given a significant salary increase which would make a great difference to his pension if he did not retire until 65. This hope coincided with success in persuading the laryngologist to refer Mr Y. to a psychiatrist. Mr Y. was willing to co-operate but insisted on continuing his speech therapy sessions and confided to us that the psychiatrist was only asking him the same questions as we had, and telling him the same things. We had discussed many times the reasons for his vocal symptom but the insight he undoubtedly gained in no way persuaded him to discard the symptom. We were not at all surprised to learn quite soon from the psychiatrist that there was a great improvement in the patient's voice and he felt sure he could be cured. Shortly after this he was discharged with a report to the effect that nothing could be done further to help

Mr Y., but had his situation at the bank improved, cure would have been possible!

Actually, the patient was asked to stay on till 65 but since the salary offered would not have affected his pension he refused, being strongly supported in this by his wife. On retirement it was hoped his voice might recover but it remained much the same, the habit having become deeply ingrained.

Student speech therapists in case history discussions often expressed the view that Mr Y. should not be pampered as he was and waste our time, specially as he made no attempt to put into practice the voice exercises. The rationale for giving support for so long was that we kept him reasonably happy and at work and prevented breakdown. The fact was recognised that he needed and used a symptom as an outlet for the aggression which his religion and need for financial security for himself and family did not allow him to express in any other way. This did not seem to be any reason for withdrawing the support he needed and no other department could give.

I am much indebted to Mrs Mary Kirk, LCST, for the following interesting case history of Mrs A. who at first had periods of vocal recovery, presented no neurological symptoms and plainly suffered from a hysterical spastic dysphonia.

Mrs A., aged 50, was first examined by a local laryngologist near her home before being referred for speech therapy at a city hospital clinic. This consultant told Mrs A. that her voice-trouble was psychological but she refused to accept this and was very upset by his remarks. She came to the city hospital complaining of dysphonia and recurrent loss of voice lasting several days. She was examined by a sympathetic elderly consultant who referred her for speech therapy. No progress was obtained and after a period the therapist asked for a neurological assessment but no disorder was discovered. She was then referred to the psychiatric department but did not keep the appointment sent her.

Mrs A. was kept under periodic review by laryngologist and speech therapist for a year, during which time the larynx looked normal with no signs of inflammation. She was now referred to another department of psychological medicine where she attended as a day patient and received suggestion therapy under pentathol and hypnosis. There was a good recovery at first and the voice became normal. Then it deteriorated again. Mrs A. continues to attend this clinic every week.

As regards her personal history she has worked as a cleaner most of her life. Her husband was an alcoholic and physically attacked her and generally treated her appallingly. She left him about 18 years ago. She had 3 children, all by caesarian, and was sterilised after the third. She lost all her hair after this operation and said she kept feeling a choking sensation in her throat, as though she could not breathe, at this time. Her voice became bad after the death of her father, to whom she was very attached. He died of cancer of the lung and larynx and she nursed him through this. She said she never had any fear of developing cancer herself but immediately after his death the choking feeling returned and then she lost her voice. She said she wanted to cry but could not. Mrs A.'s daughter developed hysterical blindness after her grandfather's death. Mrs A. is described in her medical notes as having suffered from various hysterical symptoms for some years.

She presented in the speech clinic with a typical staccato spastic dysphonia. She coughed, sighed and sang normally and her speaking voice was often quite normal for some seconds and then deteriorated. Her breathing was very tense and clavicular. Despite constant work on this her breathing pattern remained very poor—jerky and shallow. She breathed quickly when not using her voice and often a glottal stop could be heard as she breathed out. She found it impossible to breathe in, hold and breathe out, even to a count of 3. Therapy consisted of direct voice work and discussion of what lay behind her dysphonia. She herself told the therapist very little of her personal history, not because she wanted to hide anything but because she didn't think it had much to do with the case. Her sister gave the therapist most of the information. Mrs A. attended regularly but only, it seemed, to please the therapist. She showed no reaction when a tape-recording of her voice was played to her. She did not think it sounded too bad and said that she had got used to it by now. This lack of involvement was a barrier to progress and more than anything else indicated that a cure could not be achieved.

DYSPHONIA AS A RESULT OF PSYCHIATRIC CHEMOTHERAPY

Drugs are used so extensively by general practitioners these days for sleeplessness, nerves, pre-examination jitters and the like that the speech pathologist needs to know a little about drug therapy and to ask anxious and depressed patients whether they are on pills and if so what these are. There are widely different individual reactions to drugs; some people can tolerate large doses while others develop side reactions from small doses. We have had patients complaining of falling asleep while driving or experiencing giddiness or tingling feelings in feet and hands on small doses of librium, which normally have a mildly sedative effect and are frequently prescribed by the otolaryngologist. The tranquilliser helps the patient to relax and also helps speech therapy. Drugs given for depression such as tryptizol have an atropine effect and dry up the mouth, throat and larynx and cause urinary retention. Patients may develop hoarseness and a curious resonance to the voice which can be erroneously attributed to 'functional' or hysterical disorder. The voice recovers when the drug is withdrawn within a few days.

Another group of drugs used for their sedative qualities can produce extrapyramidal side effects and a Parkinsonian syndrome with tremor and rigidity which affects voice and articulation and may be irreversible. We have had one such patient referred to us for assessment of slurred speech who was detected as having an incipient Parkinsonism and was found to have been prescribed stelazine for depression for a considerable length of time.

Androgenous compounds can also cause voice changes, but these are discussed under voice mutation (page 235).

12 Disorders of pitch: abnormal voice mutation

Endocrine imbalance may abnormally influence the progress of sexual maturity in males. Premature sexual maturity (pubertas praecox) can occur in early childhood with increased body growth and premature development of a male voice. Conversely there may be a total failure in development of secondary sexual characteristics in adolescence. Facial and pubic hair fails to grow and the larynx and vocal folds do not attain adult dimensions. Sometimes there is considerable delay in the onset of puberty amounting to several years but subsequently followed by normal development, and this may occur without recourse to hormone treatment (Amado, 1953; Luchsinger and Arnold, 1965g). In our own experience such individuals, though attaining a male voice in their late teens, have remained remarkably immature and naive, with somewhat limited intelligence.

Tuberculosis, tumours and accidents may cause atrophy of the testes before puberty and result in the falsetto eunuchoid voice on account of lack of growth of the vocal folds and development of secondary sexual characteristics. Another feature of abnormal growth is in the long bones of the body, which elongate abnormally and the individual is tall and willowy. This is clearly displayed in the paintings of the famous castrato singer Farinelli (Moses, 1960).

Chaucer's pardoner is a classic example of a eunuch:

> A voys he hadde as small as hath a goot.
> No berd hadde he, ne nevere sholde have,
> As smothe it was as it were late y-shave.

A similar and irreversible condition is obtained by castration of the male child. This was a common practice in the Orient, the eunuchs providing suitably impotent domestic staff for the harem. In the seventeenth and eighteenth centuries the falsetto male singer was much admired, and young boys were again subjected to the barbarous practice of castration in order to satisfy the

219

popular demand for castrati singers, a practice from which the Vatican choir itself was not exempt.

Moses (1960) in an analysis of the psychology of the castrato singer explains the popularity of the castrato singer on the basis of the need in the Baroque period for wish-fulfilment of herma-phrodite dreams and desires in the subconscious. The mystical desire for purity, the unity of male and female in a deity was symbolised in the high voice of those purified by castration and who, therefore, were chaste. Natural tenor singers are occasionally found having a freak vocal range, able to sing with facility in the falsetto register. The peculiar thin and silvery voice of the counter-tenor always has a certain vogue. The fluty, rather haunting quality of voice is due to reinforcement of a limited range of overtones in contrast to the deep baritone or bass voice which is enriched by a wide range of harmonics. Alfred Deller has popula-rised counter-tenor singing in our time. The voice of the male falsetto singer is rather richer in harmonics than that of the boy by reason of the larger adult resonators.

STRUCTURAL ANOMALY

Another rare cause of failure of the voice to break in adolescence is the existence of a congenital web of membrane across the anterior glottis. This may be insufficient to cause difficulty in breathing and therefore may go unsuspected until the restricted length of the vibrating folds prevents the production of a deeper pitch and leads to a laryngoscopic investigation. Division of a simple web or its complete removal will be necessary before a normal voice can be obtained. Speech therapy may subsequently be necessary to establish the appropriate pitch.

Sometimes there are extensive abnormalities in growth of the thyroid cartilage and congenital abnormalities in structure (Arnold, 1958). Division of a web is a simple matter but is best left alone if cartilage is found to extend into the web from the anterior commissure. An infantile larynx is sometimes found in women as well as men and the voice is high and piping. We treated one West Indian woman who lost her voice after an attempt by the surgeon to divide a web which was found, upon exploration, to cover a cartilaginous mass. The voice recovered but no improvement of the abnormally high thin voice was possible, owing to the anatomical structure. Baker and Savetsky (1966) reported on 4 members of the same family with laryngeal webs and noted that congenital partial atresia and web is not a rare occurrence and has a genetic basis. We examined a youth of 18 years who had a husky unbroken voice similar to that of his mother, whom it was thought he had imitated. Laryngoscopy revealed that true cords were absent and in the posterior third of the laryngeal inlet the arytenoid cartilages were absent or deficient. On phonation there was adduction of the anterior cords and triangular posterior aperture.

An unsuspected vocal cord paralysis which may be congenital and have occurred during childhood from an acute virus infection may not be detected until the voice of the adolescent fails to break satisfactorily. He passes through a period of 'stormy mutation' and the voice continues to vacillate in pitch. A male voice does not become firmly established and the voice breaks upwards into falsetto when excited or attempting to sing or shout. A medical student whose voice was weak, husky and prone to abrupt pitch changes but was kept normally under good control began to show deterioration and he was sent to the laryngologist for examination. A vocal cord palsy was discovered and speech therapy prescribed. The case history revealed that he was organiser of a jazz band in which he sang vocal accompaniments most successfully and was as a result suffering from vocal strain.

PSYCHOGENIC PITCH DISORDER (PUBERPHONIA)

Puberphonia is the customary term of reference among English speech therapists to failure of the adolescent male voice to 'break' and acquire male pitch. Mutational voice disorder and mutational falsetto are descriptive terms more popular in America and on the Continent. In the physically normal male puberphonia is always psychogenic. According to Freudian psychology (psycho-analytical psychiatry) the persistence of the boy's voice in maturity is due either to an Oedipus or Narcissus complex (Ferenczi, 1926). In the Oedipus complex the individual's love for his mother is supposed to be of a sexual nature and reaches its full strength in puberty. Since incest is a social crime, the feeling of guilt attached to the fantasy of incest causes its total suppression into the unconscious and with it the denial by the ego of sexual maturity. The family in which the boy is an only child provides particularly fertile soil for the oedipal situation, the boy's relationship to the mother being peculiarly close and often marked by antagonism to the father, which the father reciprocates.

Wolski and Wiley (1965) have reported on a case of aphonia in a 14-year-old boy who lost his voice after laryngitis. Until the age of 12:6 he was very close to his mother. Psychotherapy, amytal injections and hypnotherapy did not bring the voice back. The boy's voice had begun to break and this caused him alarm. He feared he might succumb to temptation and had become antagonistic to his mother. Use of a male voice caused anxiety and the gain in remaining aphonic was obvious. Daily speech therapy was given in hospital and this consisted of humming exercises to overcome hoarseness and the use, when alone, of a tape-recorder. The rapport between the authors, a psychiatrist and a speech pathologist, and the boy was the most potent factor in the resultant cure, it was thought.

In the Narcissus complex the original and universal condition of self-love or narcissism of the normal infant develops along abnormal lines. The adolescent chooses as love object instead of the ego someone who as nearly as possible resembles the self (Freud, 1943). The origin of homosexuality in some cases is thus explained, and the love of man for man not woman. It is an interesting fact that sexual inversion is often accompanied by creative genius, and the cultural heritage of the world owes much to perverted individuals. Shakespeare's exquisite sonnets to his 'lovely boy' have been extensively analysed in this connection by Brown (1949).

> A woman's face, with Nature's own hand painted,
> Hast thou, the master-mistress of my passion,
> A woman's gentle heart, but not acquainted
> With shifting change, as is false women's fashion.

The conflict that tortures the soul of the unconfirmed invert until the 'bad angel fires the good one out' is depicted vividly in that most remarkable sonnet of all, beginning:

> Two loves I have of comfort and despair,
> Which like two spirits do suggest me still:
> The better angel is a man right fair,
> The worser spirit a woman coloured ill.

Many adolescent boys pass through an apparently homosexual phase, though 'hero-worship' in boys nowadays is regarded in a totally different light. It need be no more pathological and dangerous than the 'crushes' or 'pashes' entertained by girls for their female teachers or prefects when confined to exclusive female company—as in girls' boarding schools, for example. The adolescent boy may really fear that he is becoming a homosexual, especially when mutual masturbation is practised, as is often the case. It does not follow that homosexuality will develop, although there is always a danger of the habit becoming established. In the majority of cases these youths do reach normal heterosexuality, though somewhat later than the average youth.

Shakespeare may have passed through such an adolescent phase of homosexual attraction and fear but was certainly no homosexual when he wrote his great tragedies and comedies.

When a man plays the passive or feminine role in the sexual relationship, he develops markedly feminine characteristics, according to Freud (1938). In some cases Ferenczi (1926) explains that this extends to the use of a feminine voice. There appears to be a certain congenital and organic predisposition to the most extreme degree of inversion but in the majority the external influences of life promote and fixate inversion. With psychiatric treatment, the prognosis is favourable in those in whom the struggle against compulsion to inversion is experienced. The majority of homosexuals, however, accept inversion as a natural and legitimate means of obtaining sexual gratification, and since neither guilt nor conflict are experienced, they naturally do not seek psychiatric help.

The Freudian explanations of neurotic behaviour and sexual aberrations are chiefly of historic interest to us since they are now considered unscientific and old-fashioned except by the ever-decreasing number of psychoanalysts. Kinsey, Pomeroy and Martin (1948) showed that there is a continuous gradation in the general population between exclusively heterosexual and exclusively homosexual behaviour. They estimated that 4 per cent of American men were exclusively homosexual. Linford-Rees (1969g) reminds us that homosexuality can occur in apparently normal stable persons free from psychiatric symptoms who are otherwise well adjusted. There are intelligent, happily married individuals with families, in whom homosexuality is latent and well compensated. Masculinity and feminity is not 'an all or nothing affair'. One may meet very masculine females and very female males.

Some of the cases of puberphonia referred to the speech clinic prove intractable for the reasons stated above. Such patients come for speech treatment, being driven by social disapproval of what is often described by them as a 'weak' voice, which may also exclude them from taking up a desired profession such as teaching. The therapist will be able to recognise the existence of deep-seated psychoneurosis by the close ties which bind the individual to the mother, or the pronounced feminine personality and obvious lack of healthy interest in the opposite sex. The only course in these cases is to refer the patient to a psychiatrist, since such problems lie outside the scope of speech therapy.

The speech clinician, however, is often successful with the treatment of voice disorders of a neurotic nature. Therefore ear, nose and throat specialists frequently prefer to send their patients first to an experienced speech therapist rather than to a psychiatrist. The former will explore the possibilities in treatment and request a psychiatric opinion if the need arises during therapy. Physicians with a psychiatric bias like Moses (1954), as Van Riper and Irwin (1958) point out, see mainly the really disturbed patient on account of their known psychotherapeutic approach. They therefore tend to the view that all voice disorders are psychopathological symptoms. It is as well to understand that the adaptation of every individual bears a personal stamp and shows particular peculiarities and insufficiencies of adjustment. We have to regard most patients referred to us as sufficiently healthy mentally to be treated by a speech therapist unless we discover considerable abnormal traits.

For many patients suffering from psychogenic dysphonia, including pitch disorders, the common-sense explanation of difficulties, the cathartic effect of verbalising and of sharing fears and problems with a sympathetic and understanding therapist is adequate. Success in treatment depends upon a combination of sympathetic insight and vocal techniques for voice improvement. In some cases the phoniatric method is the therapist's most important tool; with other patients treatment only succeeds as a result of the interpersonal relationship established between patient and therapist. In every case, we must caution against the real dangers attendant upon the speech therapist attempting to play the part of lay psychotherapist.

Frequently the patient, still with unbroken voice though long past the normal mutation period, appears to have adjusted satisfactorily to his own problems in the process of growing up and obtaining economic independence after leaving school. Van Riper and Irwin (1958) stress the force of vocal habits in dysphonia. Even if the voice symptom started as a psychogenic symptom and the expression of emotional conflicts, it may now have become purely reflex and habitual. Social factors of imitation may have played a part in the development of undesirable vocal habits. Shyness at switching over to a new and more appropriate voice may ensure the perpetuation of an undesirable vocal habit. Sometimes a deeper pitch can be produced quite easily but the patient just lacks the confidence to use this in public, knowing that it will cause comment and possibly 'ragging' and ridicule.

PREDISPOSING FACTORS IN THE ESTABLISHMENT OF PUBERPHONIA

1. Unusually early breaking of the voice which renders the boy selfconscious among his contemporaries leading him to favour the boy's voice until it becomes so habitual that it is impossible to achieve normal voice (West, Ansberry and Carr, 1957).

2. A desire to retain a successful soprano voice which has brought distinction when it is known that loss of this singing voice will mean loss of limelight (Seth and Guthrie, 1935).

3. Fear of assuming a full share of adult responsibility or of losing maternal protection with consequent unconscious assertion of immaturity by means of prolongation of the child's voice, especially when the boy is an only child and there is a strong bond with the mother and the father is unsympathetic. The majority of our patients have been only children and we prefer the above explanation of pitch disorder to the far-fetched and complicated tale of the Oedipus complex.

4. Hero-worship of an elder boy or man by a boy with strong feminine tendencies, if encouraged, may also result in rejection of a masculine voice.

5. The possession of a natural tenor voice or small larynx and short vocal folds would appear to be a predisposing factor in puberphonia, while any of the above can crystallise the condition. A tenor pitch seems to occur more frequently than a baritone or bass in the adjusted voices of puberphonic patients, but in this my observations conflict with those of Weiss (1950) whose experience with many more cases has been the exact opposite.

6. Delayed pubertal development with persistence of childish vocal habits and emotional immaturity having an organic basis (Luchsinger and Arnold, 1964g).

7. Severe deafness with inability to hear own voice or imitate male voice (Greene, 1961, 1962).

8. Congenital abnormalities and asymmetries or paralysis of one fold (Arnold, 1958).

VOCAL SYMPTOMS IN PUBERPHONIA

Although the predominant characteristic of the puberphonic voice is its unnaturally high pitch, there are many variations in the voices of these patients. Sometimes the voice is a true falsetto, high and thin and exhibiting no abrupt vacillation in pitch. It would be logical to assume that individuals consistently using a pitch so foreign to their natural registers would suffer from the added complaint of vocal nodules. This, however, proves to be the exception rather than the rule, and we have encountered only two patients with puberphonia and vocal nodules; one was aged 26 years and the other 69. Excessive tension does not necessarily always exist in association with falsetto voices, and when an individual produces this voice quite easily vocal strain does not necessarily occur.

Most commonly the pitch of the voice is inconsistent and there is considerable variation as the voice constantly breaks and drops down to the natural male pitch and even lower. Some voices drop only 4–6 tones in 'complete mutation' (Weiss, 1950), and may be hoarse and breathy, and this often follows severe strain during the mutation period. Curry (1949) analysed two special cases undergoing voice change, one 19 years old and the other 15 years. The older case was studied because of the lengthy persistence of voice change, and the younger was studied because the breaks in his voice were much more frequent than in the average male voice during mutation. The 19-year-old's voice breaks occurred at the same pitch as the 10- and 14-year-olds' reported in an earlier study (Curry, 1940) but *above* the adult pitch level which was established for him. The 15-year-old's voice breaks were also in an upward direction from the generally lower pitch he had achieved.

In another study Curry (1949a) measured the voice breaks of a 10-year-old and a 7-year-old boy with abnormal voices—the pitch breaks were difficult to measure because so 'chaotic'. The breaks of the older boy occurred within a 3-tone range pitched an octave below normal. This case may have been undergoing early pubescence. Curry quotes Berger who noted that normal mutation shows 'more closely knit vocal behaviour' than the pathological in that the fundamental pitch range does not vary before or after voice mutation, but does considerably in many mutation disorders. This explanation helps to define the often not very clear demarcation between the normal and pathological symptoms of voice break in the adolescent period, though it is perfectly obvious in the adult.

The larynx is generally pulled up high and the throat musculature may be markedly tense. Hoarseness and symptoms of vocal strain and shallow breathing are not uncommon. Sometimes the patient can sing down the scale and reach the tenor register with ease, but reverts to a higher pitch immediately speech is resumed. Others may cough or laugh on a normal pitch. Treatment is very much easier and shorter with cases such as these than when the falsetto is well established. This is presumably on account of the ambivalent psychological attitude towards the choice of voice. It is easier to influence the balance in favour of the low pitch than in those men who are entrenched in a more rigid mental attitude of which the consistent pitch is symbolic.

The treatment of puberphonia is most successful with boys in their teens and men in their early twenties and less successful when older, and most difficult with those described above suffering from incomplete mutation.

Hildernisse (1956) comments upon the advantages of a male therapist with these patients because a greater positive psychic influence can be exerted. Tarneaud (1961) guarantees vocal recovery after eight consecutive daily treatments. Many patients do achieve a normal voice immediately. Whether our difficult patients would have responded more quickly to treatment by a male therapist we cannot judge, of course. Weiss (1955) discussing 'the psychological relations to one's own voice' mentions difficulty in persuading young men with mutational disturbances to give up the habitual voice, and their marked resistance in therapy. Obviously caution must be exercised over making generalisations in this matter, although it must be a factor of importance in treatment of puberphonia of psychogenic orgin. In general, female speech therapists are successful in the treatment of puberphonia provided there is no organic disorder and no deep-rooted psychogenic aetiology.

A laryngologist's report on the growth of the larynx and normality of the vocal cord length and a medical check are, of course, essential before undertaking treatment.

TREATMENT OF THE PUBERPHONIC PATIENT

A careful case history is necessary in an attempt to obtain a picture of the patient's childhood, home background and per-sonality. It is also necessary to gain the patient's full co-operation at the initial interview to make sure he has a sincere desire to improve his voice. This can never be taken for granted though the individual has come for treatment apparently of his own free will. Many boys come unwillingly, sent by headmaster or parents.

Adults may be driven to the clinic by critical comments from their employers or acquaintances. Several patients were embarrassed at being addressed as 'madam' on the phone. Frequently vocal 'weakness' is the patient's complaint and he is apparently quite unaware of the unsuitable pitch of his voice. Hearing training is necessary in all cases so that the patient has a clear idea of the aim of the treatment and is prepared to co-operate and relinquish the hitherto unconscious desire to retain his boy's voice. A recording of his voice should be made and immediately played back to him. The shock is generally considerable and the realisation that his voice is so different from that of the normal male speaker brings with it a whole-hearted desire to be rid of it. If there is no immediate healthy reaction of this nature the prognosis is poor, for it is evident that the individual still fears to face the consequences of sexual maturity and still harbours an unconscious desire to cling to childhood and his mother.

Often when a recording of a deep voice break is obtained it is possible to point out that this deep pitch is the masculine voice most desirable. This commonly produces some comment on the 'horrible noise', clearly showing the man's rejection of the male voice. Such involuntary remarks should be discussed fully and the undesirability of the feminine voice (so unlike the male therapist's or like the female therapist's as the case may be) must be emphasised.

Production of a male voice should be attempted through the various activities mentioned already: laughing, coughing, singing down the scale may elicit an appropriate pitch and this is then prolonged on a vowel sound or in humming. This may be followed by establishment in automatic serial speech, e.g. counting; ABC; days of the week, etc. Feeling chest resonance with the hands is often helpful.

When difficulty is experienced in achieving a deeper pitch, special exercises for the reduction of tension will be necessary. The larynx is elevated in the production of falsetto notes by tension in the suprahyoid group of muscles, while at the same time contraction of the cricothyroid takes place elongating the vocal folds, and the crescent-shaped anterior aperture, viz. the visor action described by Ardran and Kemp (page 38) between cricoid and thyroid cartilages is materially reduced (Stein, 1942; Luchsinger and Arnold, 1965c). The vocal cords are stretched to their maximum length and the intrinsic fibres of the vocal muscles are able to brace themselves against this overall contraction

(Rubin and Hirt, 1960). Patients may be able to sing in the falsetto register accordingly.

Luchsinger and Arnold (1964g) on account of the above laryngeal mechanism in falsetto voice advocate the use of Gutzmann's pressure test to lower vocal pitch. 'The examiner places his finger over the thyroid prominence which is usually well developed. The patient is instructed to hum on a sustained tone while the examiner's finger exerts a slight backward and downward pressure on the thyroid cartilage'. In this manner the habitual elevation of the larynx is counteracted. At the same time the backward pressure shortens the vocal cords and counteracts the pull of the cricothyroid muscle and opening of the visor. As a result the voice suddenly drops by an octave and the male voice is heard. The patient is instructed to press on his thyroid cartilage and practise the exercise himself.

We have never actually been successful with the Gutzmann technique. It may be that here male strength tells and we did not press hard enough.

Suggestion is potent and the real factor conducive to success in most exercises. A description of the mechanism involved in high and low notes may be given and accompanied by a demonstration of the rise and fall of the therapist's larynx—the patient feeling her throat. The therapist at each attempt on the part of the patient to vocalise on a low note should encourage him to do so by herself emitting a note in her lowest range. In fact it is always convincing to point out that the mature female voice is actually deeper than the patient's own.

SOME EXERCISES FOR ELICITING LOWER VOCAL PITCH

1. Hold the patient's head in the crook of the arm, hand under chin, and depress the back of his tongue firmly with the finger. This produces descent of the hyoid and therefore the larynx and lowers the vocal pitch and resonance pitch of the pharyngeal resonator. The patient should emit a groan at each depression of the tongue. For this exercise to be effective the patient must be thoroughly relaxed and there should be no resistance to digital pressure from the back of a rigid tongue.

2. With head dropped forward and neck and shoulders relaxed, phonation is attempted as the patient places thumb and forefinger on either side of the thyroid alae so that he may feel and correct the tendency to elevate the larynx upon phonation. The best sound to use is that non-committal expression of fiction—'hm'.

3. Hold arms out sideways from the body in a horizontal position and drop to the sides heavily while vocalising. The arms must drop through the force of gravity and not be brought down to the sides by the patient.

4. Vocalise on a deep sigh when well relaxed, having prefaced the attempt by a period of deep rhythmic breathing.

5. Sitting with knees apart, drop the trunk forward from the waist and vocalise 'in the boots' as the hands brush the floor.

6. Standing with feet apart and trunk hanging from waist, arms swinging loosely, vocalise on a grunt as the therapist pushes down the shoulders.

7. Impersonate an old man with a cracked voice, a basso profundo or tragedian. The patient may find it easier to speak in a different voice when assuming another identity, just as some stammerers will speak fluently when acting. Also acting reduces shyness and embarrassment.

8. Chin wagging or vibration.

Froeschels (1948) advocates chewing therapy, and voluntary jaw or chin wagging and vocalising when the jaw is thoroughly relaxed. The agility of the mandible of the expert is impressive and probably effective. These jaw gymnastics are difficult to acquire and must obviously be achieved in youth. Dentures, if any, should be removed before such exercises are attempted. Palmer (1949) suggests taking the patient's chin between thumb and finger and introducing a rapid up-and-down shaking movement. If the muscles are relaxed the teeth go 'clickety-clack'. The subject may let his jaw drop and himself flip it up with the back of the hand quickly as it drops back by force of gravity. Certainly none of these exercises can be practised effectively without relaxation having been achieved, and must therefore induce pharyngeal and laryngeal relaxation in the process, which is of course their primary aim.

Establishment of the Masculine Voice in spontaneous speech
As soon as normal vocal pitch is achieved and seized upon with enthusiasm by the therapist it can be developed as described above. The deep voice should be practised assiduously in meaning-less mechanical exercises which will establish the auditory and kinaesthetic patterns desired and enable their effortless recall. Intoning meaningless vowels and nonsense syllables when using the good voice will be found easier at first than connected speech. In most cases the voice is strong and resonant immediately a

pitch appropriate to the adult resonators is used. The contrast in the vocal expression of personality is startling and dramatic for the therapist and highly rewarding.

Sometimes an element of vocal strain with chronic laryngitis is present and in this case a short course of voice production should be given which follows the classic plan of relaxation, breath control and phonation with maximum resonance. If the subject is to use his voice considerably in his profession as teacher or salesman this will be all the more essential.

Very great difficulty is sometimes encountered in persuading the patient to use his masculine voice outside the clinic, since he is frequently convinced that it is more conspicuous and odd than his usual voice. Throughout treatment the deep voice should constantly call forth praise and admiration from the therapist so that confidence in it may develop. If a recording of the deep voice is contrasted with the unbroken voice recorded at the beginning of treatment, it is convincing and helpful to the patient. If it is possible to persuade the teenager to bring his mother to visit the therapist a meeting should be arranged. His mother may then listen to his 'new' voice in the clinic and hear him reading at home. Any awkwardness or embarrassment between mother and son is thus resolved and the voice quickly established.

When self-consciousness is extreme, the individual should be given every bit as much help as a stammerer in overcoming nervousness and shyness. The provision of a variety of audience situations, interviews with hospital staff, and visits to shops is often necessary. A holiday with strangers, if it can be arranged, provides the best opportunity for practising speech without fear of comment or ridicule (Seth and Guthrie, 1943). Normal speech generally comes last with those with whom the patient is most familiar—parents, school fellows or colleagues, and not until the patient can speak correctly in all situations should he be discharged. Occasionally, relapse into falsetto occurs when nervous, but there is actually less chance of relapse than in any other functional voice disorder.

Case Reports

Private J., aged 18, was a new recruit to the army and was referred for speech therapy by the army laryngologist with a report that the larynx was normal and medical tests showed no endocrinological abnormality. However, his physique was that which is typical of the castrato singer, being strikingly tall, slender and narrow. He did not shave and the dimensions of his larynx appeared small with little thyroid prominence. He had a sister who married early and went abroad, whom he hoped later to join, and his relations with his mother were bad. She thought him bad-tempered and he thought she nagged unnecessarily. He was able to obtain a slightly lower pitch of voice and develop a little chest resonance but maintenance of a tenor voice caused discomfort and was well-nigh impossible.

Mr A., aged 18, was apprenticed to a jeweller. He presented with a voice which cracked from falsetto to baritone with great ease and he was in fact able to speak in a male voice at the first interview when merely asked to do so. His larynx was normal but he was stooping and pigeon-chested and breathing was shallow and he was educationally subnormal. When asked whether he was 'tied to his mother's apron strings' he was astonished and replied 'that's what my father is always saying'. He had a clever younger brother who was very much his father's favourite and his father was always 'picking on' the patient and was unfair over everything. His mother was kind and protected him from his father but sometimes he resented her stopping him doing things he wanted— such as taking her car with friends from work to the Continent for a holiday. Both his father and mother came to see us separately, trouble having arisen when the patient reported to his parents that the speech therapist said he must grow up and develop independence. Father was delighted, saying 'At last I have an expert agreeing with me'. Mother was upset. It transpired that mother would never accept that her elder son was a poor scholar and insisted upon his staying at school to pass ordinary level examinations with special tuition until 18 years. He had failed to do so and father had at last been allowed to find him, with great difficulty, a job which was acceptable to mother. Father was a successful self-made man and denied that he favoured the younger son and picked on the patient. He only wanted the boy to be 'tough'.

Although Mr A. switched to a male voice when we insisted in the speech clinic he continued to use the cracking falsetto outside, and as pressure increased to adopt a normal voice he ceased to attend, his mother phoning on his behalf with one excuse after another. She refused to let her son be referred to a psychiatrist, which we thought to be advisable in this case.

Case B.N., aged 16 years, suffering from an unbroken voice. He asked for treatment because his application to become a member of a dramatic society had recently been rejected on the grounds that his voice was unsuitable, and he himself felt that it was not 'strong' enough for dramatic work. He was the youngest of a not very prosperous family. His speech was fast, and accompanied by an extraordinary amount of fidgeting which involved arms, head and legs. He gossiped about his family and friends like an 'old woman' and in manner and dress was what is so well understood in colloquial parlance as 'pansy' or 'cissy'. He had a friend some ten years older whom he admired greatly and with whom he spent most of his spare time. The friend had suffered from a similar voice disorder and had been cured by a speech therapist, and had advised speech therapy for B.N.

The patient was able to laugh on a normal pitch and to sing falsetto, tenor or baritone with facility and had been able to do so since the age of thirteen. He could not speak in a deeper voice because it made him feel 'silly'. When a recording of his speaking voice was played, he could hardly bear to listen to it, however, because it sounded to him 'so girlish'—a healthy admission.

A tenor voice was established in exercises but great difficulty was encountered with speech. The matter was clinched when the good and bad voices were recorded and contrasted, but even then endless discussion and argument was necessary before he could be persuaded to speak normally outside the clinic. He first practised at work on a girl typist, who fortunately was profoundly and favourably impressed, and last of all with the men at the works who had 'ragged' him unmercifully.

This youth showed quite definite homosexual trends but these were arrested in time by speech therapy. The wise handling of the boy by the friend who sent him to the speech clinic was a factor of major importance in attaining adjustment.

FEMALE DISORDERS OF PITCH

The vocal immaturity in women is less conspicuous than in males, as during adolescence the female voice drops 3 or 4 semitones only compared to an octave in young men. However, if the woman's voice does not mature and remains that of a girl it is an indication of an immature personality. Women who shun acceptance of adult responsibility and desire to cling to the shelter and security of childhood may cling unconsciously to the vocal pitch of childhood as a symbolic expression of their unconscious desires (Moses,

1958 and 1959). The immature voice may be accompanied by immature articulation, a lisped [s] or defective [r]. Father's or mother's little girl never grows up and this, of course, may be very appealing to the protective male and has its practical uses. We have treated several women with hysterical aphonia and dysphonia whose habitual voices were inappropriately girlish and immature. In some cases referred with vocal strain and laryngitis there were indications that the pitch disorder was of neurotic origin. In working to produce a lower pitch and improve quality it was also necessary to explore the immature emotional attitudes to people and problems at work and in the home. A common feature was the feeling expressed by these patients of being 'put upon' and being asked to do too much, whereas in reality they were often shirking full responsibility and capitalising out of the kindness and helpfulness of colleagues or relatives, using voice in fact to gain protection, sheltering under the vocal symptom.

Endocrine Dysphonias in women

Endocrine imbalance has already been described as causing huskiness during menstruation (page 183). A slight oedema may produce hoarseness, reduction in muscular tonicity and limitations in pitch. This is not an inconvenience to the average woman but may be troublesome and cause anxiety to teachers, actors and singers. During pregnancy the voice may also be affected by hormonal changes influencing the laryngeal mucosa. Tarneaud (1961) mentions that these symptoms during pregnancy and menstruation cease after childbirth.

Flach, Schmickardi and Simon (1969) reported on 136 professional singers among whom 80 were engaged to sing large operatic parts. Their voices all showed change for the worse in the premenstrual and menstrual period. Two-thirds of the singers becoming pregnant experience vocal deterioration and in a quarter of these cases the voice change persisted after delivery.

Sexual excitement and vocal change was mentioned earlier (page 103). Réthi (1963) explains that the recurrent laryngeal nerves contain both sympathetic and parasympathetic fibres. A vaso-motor rhinitis, hoarseness and catarrhal cough may develop soon after marriage and, with attendant difficulties in establishing the new inter-personal relationship in marriage, the slight dysphonia may become the focus of anxiety. One young woman, an only child who had lived at home and had never had to cook, shop, wash and clean the house, experienced great difficulty in managing her home and full-time job when the honeymoon in Majorca was over. Her voice which was of markedly immature pitch and underwent menstrual changes became permanently weak and husky with a chronic mild laryngitis. Sympathetic discussions of her difficulties and help in planning her daily programme, which included buying a refrigerator to overcome shopping and catering difficulties, reduced her troubles. Vocal therapy formed only a minor part of treatment. The vaso-motor symptoms were part real, part psychogenic.

The climacteric is another period in the life of a woman when vocal difficulties can occur. The vocal cords may become oedematous and this is often accompanied by catarrhal symptoms and the voice may grow noticeably deeper and husky. It is, besides, a time of life when the middle-aged woman often feels ill, irritable and excessively tired with a tendency to nervousness and depression. The most troublesome symptom is the 'hot flush' and sweating at night which disturbs sleep. Short courses of hormone treatment can greatly alleviate the symptoms but if administered for long periods can damage the voice. Women also put on weight and need to diet strictly if they are to retain a fashionable figure. This is another cause of anxiety and also fatigue. Women complaining of dysphonia at this time need sympathy and support, and help from their families must be enlisted. Adolescent children and husbands have little insight into the mother of the household's difficulties until these are explained. The family needs much patience and tolerance to tide her over these difficult years.

Menopausal voice changes may be aggravated by excessive smoking, which produces a chronic laryngitis, cough and considerable drop in vocal pitch. If the woman has to use her voice much at work, it may become a real inconvenience and the laryngeal condition be aggravated by vocal strain. No improvement will be achieved without drastically cutting down the number of cigarettes per day.

Virilisation of the Voice

Gynaecological carcinoma is frequently treated by male hormones (testosterone and its derivatives) and it is to be anticipated that the female patient may develop male characteristics with growth of the clitoris, and hair on the face, legs and arms, and a male voice. These are justifiable hazards in an attempt to control a lethal disease. It is a different matter when testosterone is administered in order to alleviate climacteric complaints. Damsté

(1964) described 6 patients who presented with dysphonia due to administration of testosterone-containing drugs by their doctors who had no conception of the connection between the drugs and the voice. He describes voices as becoming unsteady with fluctuation between chest and falsetto and this may continue for some time before the voice settles into the male register. Damsté (1967) noted a striking difference in the length of the vocal cords on high and low notes, with an increase in extensibility of the connective tissue. The cords also appear greyish. The changes in the larynx are irreversible and treatment with oestrogens (female hormones) does not lead to any improvement. Some patients can be helped, especially the younger ones, by speech therapy and learn to obtain a new balance between glottic tension and respiratory pressure and to use the upper vocal range. Shepperd (1966) reported 5 cases of women who had also been treated for climacteric complaints for periods varying from 6 months to 2 years with commercial preparations incorporating methyltestosterone and oestradiol the presence of which was not suspected by their doctors. All women developed hoarseness and increased growth of hair. Withdrawal of the drugs resulted in disappearance of excess hair but the voice remained unchanged. Shepperd comments on the fact that the voice is not hoarse but strong and deep. This was the case with the one patient we have had referred for treatment. She was a woman of 62 who had been operated upon two years previously for mamillary cancer and had then retired from teaching and removed to the coast to live with her sister. This had not proved a happy arrangement. She was referred for speech therapy with a diagnosis of functional dysphonia, the larynx appearing normal. The masculine character of her voice led to the enquiry whether she could be on testosterone. This proved to be the case and she was switched to oestrogens, but no improvement in pitch was achieved. Vocal exercises and hearing training did, however, help her to speak in the upper limits of her chest register.

Myxoedema

Myxoedema is a condition produced by undersecretion of the thyroid gland. It causes cretinism and mental defect in childhood if not diagnosed in time. Myxoedema can occur in normal individuals in old age. The skin becomes rough and dry and the hair thin and the individual may gain weight and become slow in movements and thought. An early sign is a slowly progressive deepening of the voice and a slight huskiness or blurred quality. This is less conspicuous in men than in women. The vocal cord movements remain intact but the cords increase in bulk due to deposition of mucopolysacharides in the submucosa. Ritter (1967) advocates stripping of the vocal cords. He also mentions that patients may develop deafness. Heinemann (1969) investigated 42 cases of hypothyroidism and stressed the fact that if the voice is allowed to deteriorate substantially, administration of thyroxin will not improve the voice. The difficulty is that old people do not realise they are going downhill and a diagnosis is often only made when the myxoedema is well advanced.

Ficarra (1960) draws attention to the usefulness of voice change and myxoedematous hoarseness as a diagnostic tool after thyroidectomy. The voice may give the first indication of hypothyroidism and develop as quickly as 36–48 hours after operation before generalised signs appear.

13 Disorders of nasal resonance

Disorders in nasal resonance can be divided into two chief categories, one characterised by too much nasal resonance and the other by too little. The terms hyper- and hypo-rhinolalia have been used in the past, also hyper- and hypo-rhinophonia, and rhinophonia or rhinolalia aperta and clausa. 'Excessive nasality' and 'insufficient nasality' have been approved by the British College of Speech Therapists (Terminology for Speech Pathology, 1960). 'Nasal speech' and 'denasalised speech' are other terms in use.

There is a great deal of confusion over the question of nasality in speech for although the fact that 'something is going on in the nose', to quote Froeschels (1957a), is perfectly apparent even to the lay ear, it is often exceedingly difficult to define what exactly this is, and to explain its physical origin. Before modern instrumental techniques were introduced there was no great problem. The traditional view was accepted that nasality was produced simply by sound waves passing through the nasal cavity when the palatopharyngeal sphincter was open, as in the case of [m], [n] and [ŋ]. Clinical experience, however, did not support this view because every now and then a rare individual would demonstrate acoustically normal speech in the presence of unquestionable nasal escape. In our own experience, a girl aged 9 years, for example, whose cleft of hard and soft palate remained unrepaired because of residence in Kenya during the second world war, was found to have normal tone and excellent articulation except a glottal substitution for [k] and [g]. Such cases rendered the simple principle of rhinolalia aperta and clausa—i.e. prevention or otherwise of entry of vibrated air into the nasal cavity—as the only factor involved, no longer entirely acceptable. The introduction of X-ray photography and acoustic spectrographic analysis followed the work of model experimentalists like Paget (1930) and threw fresh light on old clinical problems.

Various spectrographic analyses of the acoustic components of nasality have been published but there is much disagreement in the literature concerning what constitutes nasality. Van den Berg (1962) summarising knowledge up to date states that there is now relative agreement with Delattre's (1955) findings, that the nasal formant is in the region of 250 c.p.s. accompanied by decrease in overall intensity of sound waves and especially of the first formant of the vowel. Thus there is an imbalance in the relative prominence of the vowel formants, the higher formant appearing stronger than the lower.

It is clear that deviation from normal tone depends upon imbalance of the overall harmonic spectrum of the voice. Certain deviations in size and shape of the resonators, the size of their orifices, the flexibility of their walls, the energy and fundamental pitch of the laryngeal note, can produce an infinite variety of acoustic results all grouped together by the human ear as having some deviation from the normal voice and indicating something going wrong in the nose.

Speech may be characterised by 'mixed nasality' as Morley (1966) explains, the vowels having a hollow tone without nasal resonance and consonants articulated with audible escape of air down the nose. This is often given a Latin name, rhinolalia mixta.

A great variety of disorders of resonance is possible in cleft-palate speech but difficult to define by any means. In general *nasality* refers to nasal tone of the voice in articulation of vowels; *nasal escape* or emission refers to the audible friction of air escaping down the nose through the nasopharyngeal sphincter during consonant articulation. Consonants may be correctly articulated as far as actual tongue contacts are concerned in the presence of some nasal escape. Nasal escape may occur also in conjunction with incorrect articulation of the consonants, the fricatives may be produced by contact of the back of the tongue with the pharyngeal wall producing pharyngeal fricative substitutes for [s], [z], [sh] and [ch] characteristic of cleft-palate speech.

The patency or otherwise of the naso-pharyngeal sphincter determines whether air escapes down the nose or not, but nasal escape of air has no absolute correlation with nasality or lack of it in vocal output as assessed by the ear of the listener when the sound waves have travelled through a number of acoustic filters to the outer air. The spectrographic analysis is apparently of little help since it provides too much information (page 110). Van den Berg (1962) says 'Nasality is immediately recognised by the human ear, but the acoustical correlate is difficult to describe exactly. . . . This might seem to be unimportant for the phonetician and not for the phoniatrist, but this would be a mistake . . . nasal qualities, at least qualities which are interpreted as being nasal, may arise without *participation of the nose*, by too large damping factors at other places of the vocal tract, primarily in the vicinity of the larynx . . . the clinician needs to be aware of this'.

In the first edition of *The Voice and its Disorders* this chapter was entitled 'The Nasal Dysphonias'. This was, and is, an accurate term since resonance cannot be divorced from any consideration of voice (any more than stress and inflexion can, since they involve temporal and pitch factors). But I have been told by lecturers in speech pathology and therapy that my original term is confusing to students. I have therefore in deference to their experience changed the title to 'Disorders of Nasal Resonance' which is also accurate and perhaps will avoid confusion. Nevertheless, reference in the above quotation from Van den Berg to the 'vicinity of the larynx' illustrates the accuracy of the term nasal dysphonia. Nasality in this chapter will be considered mainly in relation to the nose and palatopharyngeal competence but it should not be forgotten that nasality may also be imparted to the voice by muscular constriction in the laryngeal cavity and the relative positions assumed by the ventricular folds, aryepiglottic folds and epiglottis, also elevation of the larynx by the suprahyoid muscles. This is why relaxation of muscular tension in voice therapy is a constant theme in this section.

The most important factor in the production of excessive nasality appears to be, therefore, not the degree of nasal escape of air, but the degree of tension existing in the nasal and oral pharynx and laryngeal cavity, and the size of the orifices leading into the nose and mouth in relation to the size and shape of these air-filled cavities (page 70).

Paget (1930) in his celebrated experiments with the reproduction of vowel sounds by artificial resonators, discovered that when a vowel resonator formed by a rubber tube was attached to an organ reed, and the tube was pinched in the vicinity of the reed, a distinctly nasal tone was imparted to the vowel. He concluded that nasality depended upon the constriction of the pharynx in a certain way. Modern research largely confirms Paget's experimental findings.

West (1957), a sound practical clinician, in discussing dyslalias caused by nasal obstructions, has explained the principle of 'cul-de-sac' resonance in connection with the oral and nasal cavities. The oral and nasal chambers may be linked 'in parallel', as in the artistic production of a vowel sound, with palatopharyngeal sphincter slightly open (page 73). In this event the harmonic overtones of both cavities are delivered to the outer air as separate tones and reach the ear of the listener in a blended tone, of pleasing quality (Fig. 27).

When, however, the two cavities are linked in such a way that one has no outlet to the outer air and forms a cul-de-sac, then the resonance characteristics of both chambers are blended and possibly distorted before they reach the outer air. West says 'the acoustic phenomena of adding cul-de-sac resonance, when such resonance should be absent, or of subtracting it, when it should be present, are conspicuous even to the lay ear'.

Nasal consonants are produced with soft palate depressed and the closed oral cavity acting as a linked resonator giving the characteristic nasality. Vowels produced with the obstruction of the naso-pharynx by adenoids, lack the quality of the linked nasal resonator.

The presence of enlarged tonsils which obstruct the oral pharyngeal outlet, demarcated by the pillars of the fauces, further modifies the vocal tone. A deflected septum or polyp causing anterior nasal obstruction again alters the nasal resonance and reduces what we identify as nasal tone. So also does nasal catarrh.

It should be remembered that linguistic factors and emotional reactions to speech enter into the judgement of what is acceptable or not. To the Dutch all English vowels sound nasal, to the English all American vowels have a nasal twang and when we are told this is not so we find it hard to believe. Nasal consonants [m], [n] and [ŋ] and nasal vowels in French are acceptable when used as linguistically determined phenomena, but nasal vowels in English are not acceptable and [b], [d] and [g] when substituted for their usual counterparts, as in 'by dose is ruddig', are objectionable.

If an individual has a good ear, a good kinaesthetic sense and co-ordination it is possible to produce a very acceptable quality of voice perceived as normal although the palatopharyngeal sphincter is 'incompetent', that is to say incapable of complete closure and prevention of escape of air down the nose. It is a question of regulating articulation and voice to produce the right harmonic recipe, which is dependent upon auditory, tactile and kinaesthetic feed-back, besides such factors as the speech of the home and environment of the child as well as his emotional stability. Speech which is free from tension, produced without excess air pressure, with open-mouthed articulation so that more air waves escape through the mouth than down the nose, thus avoiding formation of cul-de-sac resonance, may be so harmonically balanced that it is perceived as normal though nasal cues are clearly discernible in the spectrograph (Van den Berg, 1962).

It is not contended that speech can often be normal in conditions of real incompetence of the velopharyngeal sphincter nor that secondary surgical procedures are not necessary when primary repair has failed to produce normal speech. Although tone may be good with some nasal emission of air, a considerable degree of closure is obviously necessary to allow the adequate compression of air in the oral cavity on which the correct articulation of the consonants, especially fricatives and plosives, depends. For the average child the competent management of speech is far too difficult in the presence of an incompetent mechanism. Disorders of articulation ensue, such as palatopharyngeal and glossopharyngeal fricative substitutions for [s] and [ʃ] and glottal stops for plosives which compensate for lack of oral air presure, and are so common in defective cleft-palate speech. It is contended, however, that the total avoidance of nasal escape by trying to develop complete palatopharyngeal closure should not be one of the chief aims of speech therapy for the individual with incompetent closure. This is the chief aim of the plastic surgeon and must be left to him to achieve, if possible.

McDonald and Baker (1951) have reported upon the successful treatment of 200 cases of children with repaired cleft of the palate who developed normal speech without the aid of blowing exercises, which may build up tension in the pharynx with a resultant increase in nasality. These children were taught to discriminate between nasal and non-nasal vowels and to articulate with open mouth and relaxed tongue. In this way, no nasal pocket resonator was allowed to develop.

Goda (1966) describes working mostly on voiceless consonants for direction of breath pressure orally, and also on nasal consonants to improve nasal tone with patients suffering from velopharyngeal inadequacy.

Calnan and Renfrew (1961) decided that the use of blowing tests to assess palatopharyngeal competence in speech was not justified. McWilliams and Bradley (1965) compared cine radiographic ratings of velopharyngeal closure in blowing and speech. They found that out of 37 patients who had undergone cleft-palate surgery, 26 achieved more adequate closure in blowing than in speech but 8 achieved better closure in speech than blowing.

It appears entirely logical that treatment of nasal speech should concentrate upon hearing training and auditory control of nasal escape, rather than upon attempts to promote elevation of the palate by specific exercises such as sucking and blowing which often develops a 'nasal grimace' (constriction of the nares). The palatopharyngeal musculature is given constant and adequate exercise in the natural functions of yawning, crying, and above all swallowing. Moreover, the mechanism for blowing is somewhat different from that for speech, and to cultivate movement not normally associated with speech patterns would seem to be both physiologically and psychologically unsound. When palatopharyngeal closure is potentially possible but undeveloped, as in the case of paresis following poliomyelitis, immobility of the palate following adenoidectomy or secondary repair of the palate, then artificial stimulation of palate movement by blowing exercises may be necessary, and no objection can be made as long as there is no direct attempt to transfer these muscle patterns or co-ordinations into speech patterns.

CLINICAL COMMENTS

In our review of several hundred cleft-palate patients (Greene, 1960) attending the Plastic Surgery unit at Stoke Mandeville Hospital under the direction of Kilner, various observations were made by the whole team which emerged out of the great difficulty in assessing which voices fell 'within the bounds of normality'. This is a difficulty of which every experienced clinician is only too aware and is described clearly by Renfrew *et al.* (1957), who noted also the disturbing discrepancies in judgements of the speech therapists involved in their study.

Some of our cleft-palate patients suffered obviously from insufficient nasality due to deviations in the nasal septum or deformity of facial bones, though frank nasal obstruction was not present. Patients with a competent sphincter after repair of cleft of the soft palate only, produced better vocal tone than those with complete bilateral and unilateral clefts because there was no associated oral and nasal deformity. The few adults with unrepaired clefts of hard and soft palate had better tone than those with badly scarred tight and immobile palates who had not enjoyed the advantages of plastic surgery in infancy (Reidy, 1958). Another factor which was obviously significant but which we had no facilities for examining scientifically was the pitch of voice in relation to the abnormal resonator system, and the subjective impression of nasality. The high-pitched voice of females might 'get away with' more nasal escape than deeper male voices, a fact also noted by Renfrew *et al.* (1957). When the boy with an unrepaired cleft and normal vocal tone, reported in the first edition of *The Voice and Its Disorders* (page 132), grew up with voice mutation and development of a deep voice it became distinctly more nasal when recordings were compared with those made earlier. He and his family, however, considered his speech sufficiently normal not to warrant surgery and refused it. A lad of 19 years with unilateral total cleft of the palate repaired in infancy, referred from another department on account of a falsetto voice (puberphonia) and slight nasal escape, developed more pronounced nasal characteristics when a male tenor voice was established. Searching the American literature for possible confirmation of these observations it was satisfying to find Froeschels (1957a) advocating judicious experiment with elevated pitch and increased intensity on account of the lesser degree of perceived nasality at higher pitch levels. A later study by Hess (1959) into pitch intensity and cleft-palate voice quality was also revealing. In this research project, speech pathologists assessed recordings of fifteen cleft-palate speakers for (*a*) severity of nasality, (*b*) breathiness, (*c*) harshness and (*d*) hoarseness, when vowels were produced at two different pitch levels and two different intensities. Results of this investigation led to the following conclusions:

1. Nasality, harshness and hoarseness are less severe at the higher pitch level than habitual pitch.
2. Breathiness is unaffected by pitch level changes.
3. At more intense levels of phonation there is less nasality, less breathiness, less hoarseness, but more harshness.

CAUSES OF VELOPHARYNGEAL INADEQUACY

Inadequate velopharyngeal closure can be caused by a variety of factors. These can be classified as (1) structural abnormalities, (2) neurological disorders congenital and acquired, and (3) psychogenic disorders.

Structural abnormalities

Cleft palate is the commonest congenital deformity which can cause velopharyngeal inadequacy even when repaired in infancy.

It is due to various degrees of the failure in the two halves of the lip, alveolus, hard and soft palates to fuse during the first 3 months of foetal life. Clefts can be unilateral or bilateral of the lip and alveolus and partial or total of hard and soft palate. In the British Isles the conventional and almost universal procedure is to close the lip of the infant at about 3 months and the palate at 6 to 12 months of age. A V.–Y. Wardill four-flap operation is used to close the palatal cleft and is described with great clarity by Morley (1966). An improvement on the Wardill operation has been devised by Braithewaite and appears to produce even better speech results (Braithewaite and Morley, 1963). In a series of 343 children nasopharyngeal closure was considered adequate for articulation in 98 per cent. Normal resonance was found to be closely correlated to good movement of the lateral pharyngeal walls. Morley says 'as spontaneous development of articulation towards the normal is now usual following operation on cleft palate in infancy the work of the speech therapist in this respect has become that of assessment'. McWilliams (1960) reported on cleft-palate management in England and compared a group of English children who had a mean age of operation of 15·6 months with an American group and mean age of operation 3·48 years. She found that the speech of the English children was superior to that of the American and concluded that 'it would appear from the evidence presented that English writers are not exaggerating when they claim relatively normal speech as the expected outcome of early surgery for the repair of cleft palate'. As the American children underwent a variety of different surgical procedures from a variety of surgeons it would appear that early repair is the chief factor contributing to superiority of English speech results. American surgeons work more closely in a team with orthodontists than in England and have been impressed by the skeletal facial and dental abnormalities which develop in cleft-palate children and are preoccupied with the dangers of impeding bone growth by very early surgery. British surgeons have always put speech first and—except for the cosmetic appearance of the lip—dental and jaw anomalies last. Thus little encouragement has been given to orthodontists, and surgeons are so confident of their results that in the British Isles it is virtually impossible to have made an obturator or prosthesis which will function adequately on adults with velopharyngeal insufficiency. In the small percentage of cases in which velopharyngeal incompetence exists after primary repair of the palate, a Hynes pharyngoplasty is carried out (Hynes, 1954). The salpingopharyngeal muscles are dissected and sutured in a bar across the posterior pharyngeal wall above the level of the Atlas. The soft palate has to be split to gain access to the pharynx. The bar brings the posterior wall of the pharynx forward and the edges of the raw areas left by elevation of the salpingopharyngeal flaps are sutured together thus decreasing the lateral dimensions of the pharynx. The superior constrictor and the levator palati function well and as long as the original gap in the nasopharyngeal isthmus is not too wide the results of this pharyngoplasty are excellent (Fig. 31). At first, tone of voice may be denasalised due to oedema of the operated area but this subsides during the next three months and tone will become normal. Articulatory typical cleft palate consonant errors will have to be corrected by the speech therapist and will not be cured by prevention of nasal emission alone. New tongue contacts have to be learned laboriously.

In America pharyngeal flaps have become increasingly popular as a primary or secondary operation of choice in cases of velopharyngeal inadequacy after primary repair. Stark (1960) after studying for a period with Kilner at Oxford was not as entirely satisfied with the Wardill palatal repair as British surgeons. He performed in New York in 1954 his first Langenbeck palatoplasty combined with a pharyngeal flap attached to the soft palate and forming a permanent bridge across the nasopharyngeal isthmus. He reported his surgical procedure, 'the addition of a pharyngeal flap to primary palatoplasty' in 1960 (Stark and De Haan, 1960). A report on the speech results and the dental occlusion in 81 patients (Stark *et al.*, 1969) is now available. The conclusions arrived at are that the Langenbeck palatoplasty (Morley, 1966) which requires minimal surgery over the hard palate does not interfere with bone growth. Early surgery ensures development of normal speech: the speech in the series was rated as average or above average. Early closure appears to minimise middle ear disease.

There is a considerable body of evidence from electromyographic and cine radiographic studies that the superior constrictor and palatopharyngeal muscles are active after the pharyngeal flap operation and not disturbed by it. (Broadbent and Swinyard, 1959; Isshiki *et al.*, 1969). The flap itself reduces nasal escape and the lateral wall to mid-line (mesial) occlusion replaces the velopharyngeal approximation of the Wardill and Braithewaite palatoplasty (Stark, 1960). There is some discussion as to whether inferiorly or superiorly based flaps provide the best results. Hamlen (1967) came to the conclusion that there was no difference in the speech results. Stark (1960) favours an inferiorly based flap but situated high and above the adenoids. Isshiki *et al.* (1969) say that the flap should be at the site of maximum mesial movement and that high attachment as advocated by Owsley *et al.* (1966) produces excellent results.

Bzoch (1964) a speech pathologist, has produced a well-documented report upon the effects of a specific (superiorly based) pharyngeal flap operation by one surgeon upon the speech of 40 cleft-palate patients aged 4–45. Speech was assessed under 8 categories and a 5-point scale. All patients had hypernasality before operation, 3 remained nasal immediately after and none after 2 years. Hyponasality developed in 29 cases, with complete obstruction of nasopharynx and distortion of nasal consonants. Twenty of these patients could only breathe through the mouth. Nasal breathing and normal resonance developed later in 9 cases and improved in 20 but did not become entirely normal. The posterior end of the flap can be expected to shrink gradually and this happened in 30 of the 40 cases with thinning to the extent of 1–3 mm. It is apparent that over-correction of nasal escape with transposition of too wide a pharyngeal flap is a hazard with this operation as it is also with the Hyne's pharyngoplasty.

Hamlen (1967) reviewed 677 patients over a period of 10 years who underwent primary palatoplasties at the Toronto Hospital for Sick Children. The majority achieved normal speech with or without speech therapy. However, 101 patients (50 boys and 51 girls) with incompetent velopharyngeal closure underwent a pharyngeal flap operation (65 superior based and 31 inferior based). The age range was from 4 to 19 years with average age 11 years. The speech results, with very little speech therapy as compared to British standards, were highly satisfactory. All Hamlen's patients had hearing tests, intelligence and personality tests. She found a strong correlation between speech attainment and intelligence and to a lesser degree with hearing—that is an intelligent individual was not handicapped by a slight hearing loss. The operation cured excessive nasality and the chief problem in speech therapy was (as always) to correct cleft-palate sound substitutions. The intelligent cases were successful in learning new speech patterns but those with IQ 80 and below found it very difficult. Hamlen concludes that prognosis for ultimately normal speech is poor for those of subnormal intelligence.

In summary, one can say that the Wardill or Braithewaite palatoplasty is the procedure of choice for British surgeons on account of the excellent speech results. The question of whether the degree of skeletal deformity and dental mal-occlusion is increased by this form of operation is an important one. Not only may the cleft-palate individual suffer from a facial abnormality but orthodontic treatment may be long, tedious and costly, besides which many patients with competent velopharyngeal closure but malocclusion suffer from lateral lisps (Greene and Canning, 1959; Greene, 1960). As a secondary operation for patients in whom primary palatoplasty has failed to achieve velopharyngeal competence, the Hynes pharyngoplasty (again the procedure of choice for British surgeons) is successful when the palatopharyngeal gap is small, but unsuccessful when the palate is short and immobile (Greene, 1960). In such cases a pharyngeal flap operation seems to be the logical solution.

Fritzell (1960) has described a palatoplasty operation with elongated pharyngeal flap devised by Bengt Johnson in Göteborg which has been used in adults with extensive palatal defects in whom an orally raised pharyngeal flap would not provide sufficient material to close the gap. It can replace the difficult and long multiple-stage procedure of tubed pedicle flap for reconstruction of the palate which is sometimes carried out on patients when they can no longer wear an obturator or denture which has to be attached to teeth. The Johnson flap has its lower margin at the level of the cricoid cartilage and can be made to reach the alveolar process. Speech may also be much improved after this operation.

Sub-mucous Cleft of the Palate

Sub-mucous cleft of the palate describes a condition in which the mucous membrane is entire, thus concealing failure in union of the two muscular halves of the soft palate beneath. It can be partial or complete and the cleft extend into the bony palate. The uvula is frequently bifid. The cleft may not be detected in infancy and only be diagnosed when speech fails to develop normally. The soft palate may fail to elevate or elevate partially and there may be an associated deep pharynx. The condition should not be confused with congenital paralysis of the palate and movement of the lateral pharyngeal walls should be assessed (*see* supra-nuclear paresis). The bifid uvula if present is always a suspicious sign, but further confirmation can often be found by feeling for a notch in the centre of the posterior edge of the bony palate. Also a translucent line may be visible down the centre of the soft palate when illuminated from above, giving proof of failure in union of the muscular halves.

Surgical treatment is on the same lines as cleft palate, the mucous membrane having first to be divided. Patients who have developed normal articulation and suffer only from slight nasal emission are generally cured by palatoplasty. Patients who develop typical cleft-palate articulation in our experience have more serious velopharyngeal inadequacy and require a pharyngoplasty as well as palatoplasty.

Congenital Short Palate

Incompetent palatopharyngeal closure and nasal speech may also be caused by a congenital short palate with the associated deformity of an unusually deep and wide nasopharynx (Fig. 31). This may only become evident after removal of adenoids which have hitherto reduced the dimensions of the nasopharyngeal cavity, and made closure by the palate possible. Damsté (1962) says that the condition though rare is, in his experience, twice as frequent as sub-mucous cleft. In Utrecht a Wardill-Kilner combined with a Savenero-Rosselli pharyngoplasty is performed, usually with success. Speech therapy is prescribed, not to improve velopharyngeal competence but to correct articulatory errors.

In England a Hynes (1954) pharyngoplasty is generally per-formed as well as a palatoplasty, which performed alone is generally unsuccessful. The palatopharyngeal gap as shown in cine radiography should determine choice of surgery.

Many children with apparently short palates and nasal escape following adenoidectomy soon recover normal speech (see 'Adenoid-ectomy' below) and care over too early diagnosis of short palate after adenoidectomy must be observed. Other possible factors contributing to nasal speech must be excluded, such as emotional disturbance, hearing loss, low intelligence and temporary paresis associated with generalised poor co-ordination in a child.

The Hynes pharyngoplasty does not always produce adequate closure, although it may appear to do so immediately post-operatively when oedema and swelling is present. After an interval of three months, which is the interval necessary before a true assessment of speech results can be made, nasal escape may return. A pharyngeal flap operation has a better prognosis when the nasopharyngeal gap as shown by lateral X-rays is such that it cannot be anticipated that a pharyngeal bar will provide velopharyngeal competence.

Adenoidectomy

Development of nasal emission following adenoidectomy in children with previously normal speech is not uncommon. Linden

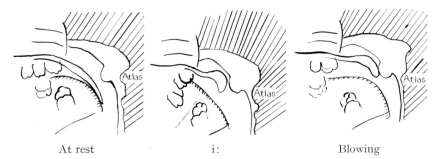

At rest   i: Blowing

FIG. 31A   Lateral X-ray tracings showing improved closure of naso-pharyngeal isthmus after Hyne's pharyngoplasty operation on the same child, who obtained normal speech after a period of speech therapy

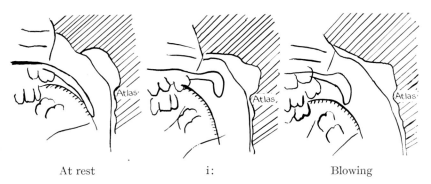

At rest   i: Blowing

FIG. 31B   Lateral X-ray tracings showing incompetent pharyngeal closure in the case of a child of 8 years with congenital short palate or deep nasopharynx
(By courtesy of Stoke Mandeville Hospital)

et al. (1968) report transient nasal emission in 26 out of 29 children investigated. Frank (1969) found that nasal emission disappeared after a week and he found that there was an actual shortening of the palate due to oedema immediately after adenoidectomy. Nasality can persist for several months (Greene, 1957). Nasality is due to a number of factors post-operatively. Linden *et al.*

(1968) mention the altered spatial relations after removal of the adenoidal pad and need for greater elevation of the palate and pharynx and soreness as contributory factors. Articulatory defects do not develop but owing to nasal emission consonants now lack force and the voice is muffled rather than nasal. In an endeavour to prevent nasal escape a nasal grimace may soon develop and with it an increase in nasality. As movement of the palate recovers, speech gradually reverts to normal, although this may take as long as three months. It is often advisable to arrange an interview with a speech therapist in order to reassure parents and child. A hearing loss of conductive type which is not uncommon, on account of the growth of adenoid tissue round the eustachian orifice accompanied by middle-ear infection, will naturally make the recovery of normal speech more difficult. Nasal speech may also be exceedingly intractable in children suffering from a disturbed relationship with the mother, the child being infected by his mother's anxiety concerning his speech, or the child discovering that nasal speech is a means of obtaining extra attention. Very careful examination of the palate is necessary, however, before this diagnosis can be made, in case organic causes are present.

In the event of a congenital short palate (see below) being proved, a pharyngoplasty will be necessary but surgical inter-vention should not be considered for at least a year after adenoid-ectomy. We assessed at one time a girl of 14 years who had a pleasant singing voice and was in demand at local charitable concerts. She had developed excessive nasal escape after a recent adenoidectomy and after 6 months' duration of the symptom, clinical and lateral X-ray assessment showed without doubt that this girl suffered from a short palate in relation to a deep pharynx. The surgeon in charge fortunately decided to postpone carrying out a Hynes pharyngoplasty. Three months later speech and singing reverted to normal quite suddenly. In this patient one can only conclude that there was some psychogenic reason for long-lasting nasal escape. It also shows that lateral X-rays are not entirely reliable.

Adenoidectomy in Cleft Palate

The removal of adenoids in children with repaired cleft and normal speech may produce nasality if the palate is short and naso-pharyngeal closure has hitherto been obtained by contact of the palate with the projecting adenoidal pad (Fig. 32). When removal of adenoids is recommended in patients with cleft palate it is advisable to remove by curette that part of the adenoid tissue which impinges upon the eustachian orifice and to leave the central mass intact. In the normal course of events the adenoids atrophy during adolescence. Children with short cleft palate and enlarged adenoids appear not to lose their good speech as they grow up, even though incompetent closure may develop as the adenoids atrophy, because this takes place by imperceptible degrees and the child automatically regulates speech production to conform to his already established auditory patterns. At

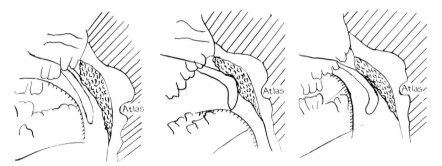

F𝚒𝙶. 32   Severe nasal obstruction by adenoids in 5-year-old (stippled areas). Typical adenoidal speech (insufficient nasality)
(By courtesy of Stoke Mandeville Hospital Radiography Department)

Stoke Mandeville Hospital Plastic Surgery Unit we followed through to maturity several children in whom the anticipated nasal speech did not develop. Probably movement of the pharyngeal walls compensates for velar insufficiency.

In cleft-palate children whose speech remains nasal after adenoidectomy, surgical procedures as for children in whom primary repair has failed to produce competence will be necessary.

NEUROLOGICAL DISORDERS

Supra-nuclear paresis

An isolated paralysis, either unilateral or bilateral can occur, though rarely, as a congenital defect. Generally there is involvement of pharyngeal, lingual and laryngeal muscles and besides nasality due to palatal paresis there is attendant dysarthria, drooling, and dysphonia. The condition is known as congenital supra-nuclear paresis or congenital supra-bulbar palsy. It is a form of cerebral palsy and a feature of 'spastic' children with extensive motor involvement. Wynn-Williams (1958) carried out a Rosenthal pharyngeal flap type of operation in which the flap was lined by mucosa in order to avoid shrinkage of the flap which takes place in the simple Rosenthal procedure. His primary aim was to assist swallowing and cure drooling, and in this the operation proved successful. Speech with speech therapy and correction of nasal escape improved most in children with least neurological impairment, and especially when the palate alone was involved. Grady (1958) described speech results and treatment of dysarthria in Wynn-Williams series.

It is difficult to persuade British surgeons to perform a pharyngeal flap operation of any sort on any type of case, therefore we have ample evidence that Hynes pharyngoplasty with or without a palatoplasty is not successful as a remedial procedure for nasal escape due to congenital palatal paresis. On the other hand a pharyngeal flap is more successful in our experience. As Isshiki *et al.* (1969) point out, movement of the pharyngeal walls is diagnostic for pharyngeal flap procedure and patients with poor pharyngeal motility have a poor prognosis. A careful radiographic neurological assessment is advisable before operation is decided upon, as well as a speech assessment by a speech pathologist.

Hamlen (1967) reports good results in 6 patients of good intelligence with neuromuscular disorder and palatal involvement who underwent pharyngeal flap surgery. Hardy *et al.* (1961) reported on results of pharyngeal flap surgery on 3 cerebral palsied children and on a further three in 1969. Only 3 children benefited from surgery followed by speech therapy—the other 3 'did not try'. They conclude that prosthetic management is the procedure of choice in cerebral palsy and found a 'palatal lift' of special design helped 5 children and a bulb-type obturator another. The general consensus of opinion is that surgery is unsuitable for cerebral-palsied children with extensive neuromuscular involvement.

Nuclear Lesions[1]

A focal lesion following bulbar poliomyelitis resulting in paralysis of the palate in the absence of any other symptoms is exceedingly rare, but possible. The muscles of deglutition and phonation are in most cases also involved. Many of these patients make a good

---

[1] Upper and lower motor neurone lesions are described in connection with dysarthophonia in Chapter 14.

recovery and it is largely a matter of time before function returns to impaired muscles. Speech therapy is helpful in maintaining the patient's morale. Blowing exercises and also gentle massage of the palate from side to side with the finger, which the patient can perform himself, may be beneficial. The Lubit palatal exerciser (Lubit and Larson, 1969) might be used. This consists of an acrylic biting piece and an inflatable latex bag which is inserted in the mouth and massages the palate on inflation, and is said to produce good results in cleft palate incompetence. Open articulation and reduction of force in articulation will also reduce nasality.

Peripheral Neuritis

The palate is sometimes paralysed temporarily after diphtheria on account of a peripheral neuritis which prevents conveyance of nervous impulses to the muscle. Movement of the palate is soon recovered and speech therapy should not be necessary, but anxiety with regard to impaired speech and a superimposed neurotic disorder and prolongation of nasal speech is possible. In this event speech therapy will be necessary.

Patients suffering from diphtheric palatal neuritis are now exceedingly rare since infant immunisation is generally practised. However, in a local outbreak in 1963 of diphtheria among children who had not been immunised, speech was assessed. Two children had gross nasal escape which was far more conspicuous than in any case of cleft-palate or post-adenoidal nasal speech we had encountered. Speech therapy was not given in these cases and speech recovered with the movement of the palate and subsidence of the illness.

Myasthenia Gravis

This is a disease of unknown aetiology in which the normal chemical changes necessary for conduction of the motor nerve impulse at the neuromuscular junction are lacking. The disease may produce weakness in the whole muscular system and extreme fatigue, but the first signs may be heard in slurred articulation and nasality due to weakness of the palate (Wolski, 1967) and nasal escape. The disease itself must be treated by the administration of neostigmine or by thymectomy. Since muscular movements revert to normal during alleviation of the illness, speech therapy is not indicated and in any case rest is essential.

Deafness

Children with congenital severe global hearing loss acquire speech with great difficulty which is characterised by nasality comparable to that of cleft palate.

Neurotic Disorder

Finally, nasal speech can also be due exclusively to emotional disturbance in the presence of a perfectly competent speech mechanism. Speech in these cases is generally *variable* and characterised by excessive nasality rather than nasal escape. It can be a hysterical manifestation of sudden onset and it can persist after adenoidectomy in disturbed children (see 'Adenoid-ectomy' above), and it occurs occasionally in stammerers. A differential diagnosis between congenital short palate and psycho-genic nasality can be very difficult. A decision to operate to cure velopharyngeal insufficiency should never be made hastily. Diagnostic speech therapy in doubtful cases should be given over a period of time during which the child's emotional stability should be explored, as well as the mother-child relationship. An attempt must be made to gain the child's confidence and establish security so that the need for the symptom to gain attention is undermined.

The following case histories demonstrate the complexities of differential diagnosis.

Psychogenic disorder

B.I. Tonsils and adenoids were removed from this little girl at the age of 7 years 9 months. Her parents declared that speech was entirely normal before the operation but that when she arrived home from hospital, suffering from a severe cold and high tempera-ture, her speech was almost unintelligible.

When examined in the speech clinic three months later there was gross nasal escape and grimace throughout speech and she failed to displace even one cubic centimetre in the Windsor measure. There had been no nasal regurgitation at any time, which the ear, nose and throat surgeon described as 'phoney'. Nevertheless the palate appeared to be paralysed and did not rise when touched or in articulation of the vowel [a:].

Speech therapy and blowing exercises were commenced and after a few weeks the palate showed a flicker of elevation on vowels. In the meantime, a plastic surgeon had examined the girl and suggested that she had contracted a focal attack of

poliomyelitis following tonsillectomy, with paralysis of the palate
as a result. She was accordingly examined by a neurologist who
found no grounds at all for confirming this diagnosis and stated
that since the palate was beginning to move the prognosis for
eventual recovery was good.

Speech therapy continued and it was noticeable that nasality
and nasal grimace, although always present, varied greatly in
degree from week to week. The child, once shyness wore off, was
discovered to be seriously maladjusted. She was unco-operative
and wilful in the clinic. She drove her parents to distraction at
home by her disobedience. She was the only child of elderly
parents, whose relations were far from harmonious and whose
business commitments provided constant anxiety and overwork.
Nerves were frayed and little time or patience were left for a
troublesome though much loved and spoiled daughter.

Seven months after the commencement of speech therapy it
was possible to take lateral X-ray photographs of the palate.
Previously the little girl's nervousness had debarred this procedure: the sight of a new recording machine, for instance, had
at one time thrown her into a state of terror. The X-ray pictures
were instructive. Although the palate failed to elevate in blowing
and articulating vowels, the camera had by chance caught a
photograph when crying, and this showed excellent elevation of
the palate and complete occlusion of the palatopharyngeal
isthmus.

These X-ray studies confirmed the suspicion which had been
steadily growing that nasal speech, though originally due to
post-adenoidectomy palatal weakness, was now a psychogenic
symptom. Her parents, when this was explained to them, were
most resentful at the suggestion that their daughter was 'playing
them up' and alternately demanded surgery and hypnotism
which were not provided.

Speech exercises were early discarded because resented, and
play therapy alone was given, through which B.I. developed a
strong affection for the therapist. As confidence and co-operation
increased, she would sometimes speak without a vestige of nasal
tone, especially if she were 'top dog' in a game and issuing orders.
Nasal tone and grimace returned dramatically as soon as she
was returned to one or other parent in the waiting-room.

A change of school at 8 years 5 months and a new uniform and
friends produced normal speech, even at home, for a week, then
something upset her and she developed a non-inflammatory

earache, followed by mysterious tummy-aches which the doctor pronounced to be 'psychological'. Speech, of course, deteriorated. After three weeks she returned to school and gradually settled down happily. Speech six months later was normal. The resemblance of these nasal symptoms to hysterical symptoms is an interesting feature of this case. When we last had news of this child, though, she was attending the child guidance clinic on account of 'night terrors'.

A.C. Boy of 9 years who had always stammered but had been diagnosed by various doctors and surgeons as having a 'breathing difficulty' on account of clonic expiratory spasms. He also suffered from variable degrees of nasality 'according to how he felt', as his mother accurately expressed it. His mother had twice been admitted to a mental hospital for treatment of depressions. Her extreme anxiety found an outlet in alternately abusing and beating the boy for his naughtiness or insisting something should be done about his speech.

He was eventually referred to the plastic surgery department; lateral X-rays revealed (naturally) incomplete nasopharyngeal closure and pharyngoplasty operation was performed. We were not in agreement in this case that the palatopharyngeal mechanism was incapable of competent closure, although we agreed that its actual function was incompetent but could be explained as a neurotic symptom. The boy was much upset by hospital and his speech was more nasal after operation. His palate appeared paralysed but this was a hysterical manifestation and it recovered function during his first visit to the speech clinic as an out-patient. His speech after six months' speech therapy was on the whole no longer nasal, also his stammer improved. Nasality and stammer both returned whenever he was upset at home or at school.

Congenital Palatal Paralysis

Miss A., aged 50, a cook by profession, had been born, as far as could be ascertained, with a paralysed palate. Her speech had always been typical of a cleft palate, with excessive nasal escape and glottal and pharyngeal consonant substitutions. She had served in the army during the second world war and with the money she had saved she paid for private speech therapy upon discharge, which improved her articulation. She had always been desperately unhappy about her abnormal speech and when she read a newspaper article describing the wonderful advances in surgery for cleft palate she decided something could be done for

her case. She was now 45 years of age. She had great difficulty in
persuading anybody to 'operate on her voice' and became increasingly disturbed although she was referred to various specialists
by her doctor including an orthodontist who did not think a
prosthesis would help, and a psychiatrist who could not persuade
her to accept things as they were. Eventually, by sheer persistence,
she persuaded a plastic surgeon to place her on his operating list
and after waiting three years, during which time she became more
disturbed, he reluctantly performed a Millard palatal push-back
operation with island flap procedure (Millard, 1960), declaring
quite correctly that it would probably be of little use. It is not the
slightest use making a paralysed palate longer, in fact it may
make things worse since there is more muscular tissue to lift to
close the nasopharyngeal gap. Miss A. was nevertheless, much
happier immediately after operation as it was easier for her to
speak, on account of the oedema and swelling present, but she
became exceedingly upset when no speech therapy could be
obtained and her speech began to deteriorate. When a speech
therapist was at last appointed to the vacant post in her district
7 months later Miss A. felt it was too late to benefit from therapy
and failed to attend. The fact that speech began to deteriorate
around the crucial 3-month post-operative period which is the
known period of time for transplanted tissue to settle down and
shrink fully, was important. It indicated that benefit might be
obtained from a procedure which could permanently reduce the
nasopharyngeal aperture—a pharyngeal flap, in fact.

Miss A. eventually appealed to the Patients' Association for
help, which asked us to see her and advise whether any further
treatment could help her speech.

Examination of palatal function showed a complete paralysis,
no sign of elevation or lateral pharyngeal wall movement. Speech
was grossly nasal and very difficult at times to understand.
When speaking carefully she was able to achieve correct articulatory tongue positions but [s] remained a pharyngeal fricative.
Her tongue movements were clumsy and there seemed to be a
dyspraxic element in attempting to imitate speech sounds. A
cine radiographic study was obtained which confirmed total
paralysis of the palate but a flicker of mesial pharyngeal movement. Miss A.'s doctor who had been sympathetic and helpful,
and an angel of patience throughout her long and stormy battle
for treatment, agreed to refer her to a surgeon who could be
relied upon to perform a pharyngeal flap operation. This he

carried out when she was 51 years old. Nasal escape was considerably reduced after this procedure and oral tone improved. There was no nasal obstruction and the patient breathed freely through her nose. Comparison of recorded speech before and after operation showed a dramatic improvement in clarity and intelligibility. This patient of poor education and temperamental stability was too old to benefit fully from the operation, however. Though her speech with weekly therapy continues to improve she feels herself that she has derived little benefit from surgery. The difficulties with articulation persist and seem insuperable. She will never achieve the perfect speech to which she aspires and so overcome the humiliating abnormality which she cannot accept on account of a rooted conviction that people despise her for it.

Acquired Palatal Paresis

Mr P., a man of 46, was referred by the laryngologist for treatment of nasal escape which had suddenly developed 8 weeks before and was thought to be a neurotic symptom. The patient certainly had a neurotic personality which was confirmed by his doctor whom he had constantly consulted for years over one vague symptom after another. He was often severely depressed. The onset of nasal speech coincided with disappointment over promotion. The palate showed no signs of paralysis and elevated adequately on [aː]. Speech improved considerably with hearing training and use of open articulation during long discussions of the patient's personal difficulties, and was sometimes normal.

After two months the patient complained that he still could not blow up balloons and that crème-de-menthe stung his nose (it was Christmas-time). These observations did not appear to be those of a neurotic imagination but valid to the therapist who promptly re-examined the patient's palate. This time a unilateral paralysis was obvious on elevation, the palate deviating strongly over to the unaffected side by the unresisted pull of the healthy levator palati. It was concluded that the patient must have had a mild attack of bulbar poliomyelitis originally. The neurotic personality structure of this patient aggravated nasal escape, as he focused all his anxiety upon this new symptom.

Congenital Short Palate

Miss B., aged 22. The mother of this young woman first wrote to us on the advice of the speech therapist who had given her daughter speech therapy for six months while at boarding school when aged 8 years. Therapist and mother had met quite by chance these many years later. Miss B. had spoken normally until 7 years old when her tonsils and adenoids had been removed on account of infection and deafness. After this her speech was unintelligible and nasal. She had various ear, nose and throat check-ups and it was reported nothing was wrong and that the trouble would clear up in time. At age 15 years she had more speech therapy and after a lateral X-ray investigation, her mother was told that she had 'a lazy palate' and that probably when she got a boy friend she would take more trouble and speak normally. Her mother said she had not only no boy friend but her speech was interfering with her career and social life, could it be habit or nervousness? I agreed to see Miss B., then learned from Mrs B. that she would have some trouble persuading her daughter to come to see me but hoped I would not mind a delay. Eventually, after a year, Miss B. telephoned quite late one evening, obviously in the hope that nobody would be in the speech clinic—her speech was so nasal there was no need to be told her name. Asked where she was, it transpired she was outside the hospital and saying I had waited for over a year and could wait another five minutes for her to find the clinic, I told her to come straight in. A drab, nervous little person arrived. At first she was on the defensive and rather aggressive, making it quite plain that she had come only to pacify her mother, to whom she was devoted, and that she resented any further attempts to put her speech right. She did not mind it herself and her friends never noticed it. She had become a committed Christian recently and was planning to go into the mission field. Gradually she relaxed and spoke of how hard she had tried despite being told she was lazy, and especially by her father, who blamed her for not speaking well. It was then not difficult to persuade her to agree to an assessment from a really expert plastic surgery team. It was obvious that pharyngoplasty operation would improve her palatopharyngeal closure. On saying [aː] the palate elevated well, but just did not reach the posterior pharyngeal wall. Her facial bones were rather broad with eyes set wide apart, which may be associated with a wide pharynx. Articulation was good and when pronouncing single words with open articulation vocal tone was normal.

Miss B. was referred to the Plastic Surgery Unit at Oxford. Dr Ardran on cine radiographic data reported as follows:

> The line of this patient's hard palate is level with the arch of the atlas or even slightly below it. The first three vertebrae

of the cervical spine show some congenital abnormalities, the spine's number 2 and 3 being fused. Aednoidal mass small: pharynx large. Superior dental plate in situ.

On saying 'ee' the palate elevates well though it is rather thin but fails to make contact with the posterior pharyngeal wall by about $\frac{3}{4}$ of a cm.

Counting 4, 5, 6, 7 the palate remains elevated and the gap is considerably reduced and momentary contact may be made with the posterior pharyngeal wall, though this is not complete.

Blowing was effective with no evidence of nasal escape, partly with the aid of a diffuse Passavant's ridge.

Swallowing: no significant abnormality. The palate does not, however, make closure with the posterior pharyngeal wall until finally pushed up by the tongue at the end of the swallowing act.

Conclusion: I would have thought that a pharyngoplasty would have produced a good result.

Mr Eric Peet performed a Hynes pharyngoplasty and immediately afterwards as is usually the case, speech was denasalised and there was some nasal obstruction but after 3 months speech became entirely normal. This transformed the patient's personality—she left the secretarial work she had kept taking up and dropping, and took a job in the accounts department of a large London women's clothing store. Here the girls took her in hand, persuaded her to have her hair re-styled, use make-up and dress fashionably. When last she called in at the hospital to pay me a friendly visit she was scarcely recognisable, looking happy, smart and beautiful and on her way to a party.

This patient's problem was not a difficult one to solve, it is only sad that help was provided so late owing to the sheer lack of experience or ignorance of those who had tried to rehabilitate her.

Psychological Considerations in Treatment of Cleft Palate

Because cleft palate is organic, consideration of the personality structure of the cleft palate patient with abnormal speech and facial disfigurement has been much neglected. This appears to us strange when speech pathologists are so orientated to 'therapy' and treatment of the patient 'as a whole'. Although familial neurotic reasons for maladjustment may not be present, there are considerable repercussions of abnormal speech and personal appearance on development of the personality. This is emphasised

in other speech and voice disorders—laryngectomy, for instance—
yet scarcely at all in cleft palate.

The sensitivity over speech and appearance was most conspicuous in adolescents and adults attending the Stoke Mandeville
Plastic Surgery and Jaw Injury Unit for secondary corrective
surgery. These patients were happy to undergo operations for
improvement of the relationship of the lips (Abbé's flap operation;
Morley, 1966), reduction of the maxilla to correct relative prog-
nathism, reconstruction of the palate by tubed pedicle flap, bone
grafts to the nose and correction of deviated septum. A most
necessary aspect of the speech pathologist's work in the rehabilitation centre is an interest in the cosmetic operations and positive
encouragement and reassurance after operation when the patient
is in doubt of the ultimate improvement while oedema is present
or scars conspicuous. Advice over make-up should be given or
consultation with a beautician arranged. The co-operation of the
nursing staff is also necessary. I was in the habit of stressing this
aspect of patient management in lectures to postgraduate nurses
in this plastic surgery centre. It often caused surprise and discussion and nurses confessed frequently that they thought cleft-
palate patients, especially women, far too demanding in their
requests for cosmetic operations. They did not appreciate the deep
feelings of inferiority engendered by abnormal appearance and
speech and the great need for moral support and sympathy both
before and after operation.

Speech Prognosis when velopharyngeal incompetence is incurable
It is surprising how good speech can become despite a patent
nasopharyngeal gap and unavoidable nasal escape, and entire
failure to displace water in a Windsor manometric measure or to
blow out a carnival blower. Such exercises, though testing the
efficiency of nasopharyngeal closure, require far greater breath
pressure than is actually necessary for good articulation. If a
patient can blow a fair blast on a whistle, and I have yet to meet a
patient with an incompetent mechanism who cannot, then oral
breath pressure is adequate to obtain correct articulation of all
consonants and intelligible, even pleasant, speech. The patient
need not be highly intelligent: some of our best results have been
with rather dull but hard-working individuals. A good speech
sense and keen co-operation are necessary to master and remember
correct articulatory patterns. In these circumstances speech can
become good but, on account of the necessity for quiet unforced

speech, it may lack projection (carrying power). Though adequate for ordinary social purposes, speech may not be adequate for public speaking or teaching.

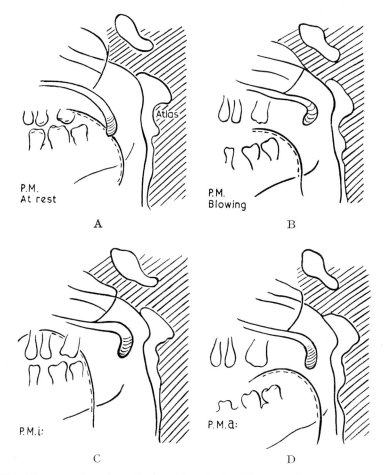

Fig. 33   A and B: lateral view of patient with unrepaired soft palate. C and D: lateral views of same patient with repaired soft palate and remaining palatopharyngeal gap on elevation

Fig. 33 shows the outlines of lateral X-ray photographs of a patient with a cleft of the soft palate, unrepaired until the age of 18 years. The palate is obviously too short for the capacious pharynx and there is poor occlusion on vowels and blowing. It is interesting to compare these diagrams with those of the normal palate, and also with the congenital short palate in Fig. 34, which shows an even greater degree of incompetence.

Treatment of the girl of 18 years (Fig. 34) along the lines described below was given a 3-months' trial, during which period her speech improved so considerably that the intention of performing a pharyngoplasty operation to provide a competent sphincter was not put into practice. Speech became almost normal after a year's treatment despite the original typical cleft-

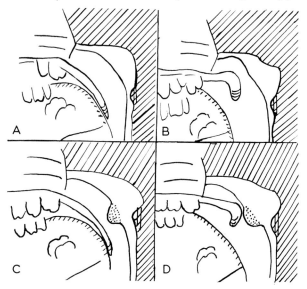

Fig. 34   A and B: lateral views of patient with repaired cleft of soft palate (Group II) and nasopharyngeal gap. C and D: improved naso-pharyngeal closure after Hynes pharyngoplasty; palate now reaches muscle transplant (stippled area)

palate speech in which tone was hollow and there was glottal substitution for [t], [d], [k] and [g] and glossopharyngeal scrapes for [s], [z] [ʃ], [tʃ], [dʒ].

Case History

A girl aged 15 years suffering from a complete cleft of the soft palate was referred for speech therapy upon the insistence of the headmistress of her grammar school. Her parents were both nurses and the father especially was averse to surgical repair of the palate. Speech therapy had been avoided hitherto because the parents feared that this would lead to an operation on their only child. When first examined, articulation of consonants was poor, all plosives substituted by glottal stops and fricatives and affricates by glossopharyngeal scrapes. Tone was nasal accompanied by a nasal grimace. Speech was very rapid and difficult to understand. She was unable to blow with any force or suck up paper on the end of a straw. Despite the unrepaired soft palate, exercises such as blow football and sucking up peas with a straw were prescribed and assiduously practised. At the same time the correct tongue positions for the articulation of defective consonants were taught. The girl was highly intelligent, co-operative and hard working.

After nine months' speech therapy all consonants were correctly articulated in spontaneous speech and palatal exercises had resulted surprisingly in improved oral pressure and reduction of nasal escape. This had, however, been achieved only by considerable increase in nasal grimacing and nasal tone. When observed on the fluoroscopic screen, it was noticeable that reduction in the size of the pharyngeal cavity was obtained by forward movement of the posterior pharyngeal wall and bunching of the lateral pharyngeal walls.

Although the intelligibility of speech was much improved by correct articulation, the grimace and nasal tone were severe and rendered speech far from satisfactory. It was obvious that the effort to produce nasopharyngeal closure and prevent nasal escape was too great, hence the nasal grimace and increased nasality. Accordingly it was decided to discard blowing exercises and to correct the nasal grimace by practising before a mirror. Immediately it was noticeable that although nasal escape increased it did not become more audible and articulation of consonants remained satisfactory, while vowels lost their nasality with the exception of [u:], [au], [i:], [ei] and [ai]. The results of this change in treatment were so encouraging that speech therapy now concentrated upon the method described below, which was largely evolved during treatment of this patient. After a further year's treatment speech was so good that her parents now refused even to consider fitting of an obturator and she was eventually discharged with speech which was clear and acceptable if not altogether perfect.

TREATMENT OF THE PATIENT WITH NASALITY AND
CONSONANT SUBSTITUTIONS

1. *Relaxation.* The need for a relaxed speech mechanism must be emphasised from the outset and specific exercises for relaxation

of lips, tongue, jaws and throat given when necessary. *A quiet voice and slow speech* free from all tension and stridency should be cultivated. Most patients in their anxiety to be understood put far too much effort into speech production. Van Thal (1934) in her practical little book on cleft-palate speech is found cautioning the patient over the dangers of trying too hard.

2. *Hearing Training.* A simple auditory discrimination test should be given first since many cleft-palate patients have reduced hearing acuity. If deafness appears to be present, referral to an otologist is necessary.

All teaching of vowels should be prefaced by hearing training, contrasting nasal and non-nasal vowels until the patient can clearly discriminate the difference. Hearing training lays the foundation for correct imitation of sounds and is especially necessary in the reduction of nasality in vowel sounds, which these patients at first find more difficult to appreciate than consonants which provide stronger kinaesthetic and tactile feed-back.

Vowel sounds must be contrasted until the patients can clearly differentiate between the good and the bad tone in the therapist's voice and then in his own. Tape-recording is essential during treatment. Consonants must also be contrasted in the same way. The therapist presents the correct form and then the patient's substitution so that again he can detect good and nasal tone in the therapist's voice and then his own. It is extraordinary how often cleft-palate patients are unaware of their faults in articulation and voice. They can be unhappy about their speech, realising it is 'different' but remain unaware of how different it is. Because of this lack of awareness and because these patients are hypersensitive, care must be taken over playing back recordings until some positive improvement in speech has been obtained in order to avoid the shock of hearing speech at the beginning of their treatment. I have never forgotten the painful experience of playing back a recording to an intelligent young man of 23 with unrepaired cleft, who promptly burst into tears. He had unintelligible speech and though he had taken a good Advanced Level School Certificate he had a frustrating and menial job in an office. His parents had refused to have the cleft repaired in childhood. This story has a happy ending, however; after repair of the palate he became a ward orderly in the hospital and received intensive speech therapy. When speech was normal after six months he entered university and took a degree in economics.

3. *Correction of Excessive Nasality.* The jaws should be well

separated for production of vowel sounds with the back of the tongue, the pillars of the fauces and the pharynx all relaxed. This ensures an increase in the total volume of the oral and pharyngeal resonators and at the same time provides an ample orifice of communication between the oral and pharyngeal cavities.

It is generally the case that some vowels are more nasalised than others. The vowels [u:] and [i:] for instance are often excessively nasal on account of the back of the tongue's natural position in articulation being lifted upwards and forwards. This creates a large pharyngeal resonator with small oropharyngeal opening which favours the passage of sound waves up through the nose.

The vowels [a:] and [ə:] on the other hand may be little nasalised because the tongue is flat, the pharyngeal resonator small and the oropharyngeal orifice wide (see Fig. 27 for contrast in tongue position in [a:] and [i:]). The non-nasal vowels can be utilised to decontaminate the nasalised vowels in the following exercises consisting of artificial diphthongs and triphthongs:

(*a*) [a:i:a:] [a:i:a:]—isolate [i:] or [i:ə:i:ə:]—isolate [i:]
(*b*) [u:ə:u:ə:]—isolate [u:] or [ə:u:ə:u:]—isolate [u:]

Non-nasalised consonants may also be used with the same purpose of reducing nasality in vowel tone. If [p] and [t], for instance, are produced with no audible nasal escape it will be found helpful to practise exercises such as these:

(*c*) [pu:p], [tu:p], [tu:t], [tu:tu:], etc., then isolate denasalised [u:] and incorporate in words: 'toot', 'too, hoot, who', etc.

4. *Correction of articulation and Reduction of Audible Nasal Escape (Emission) by Reduction in Breath Force.* Nasal escape of air is accepted as unavoidable and no attempt is made to prevent it and no palate exercises are given. If there is any nasal grimace this, of course, must be corrected and the patient instructed not to attempt to *prevent* air coming down his nose. All that matters is that nasal escape should not be *audible*.

Practise before a mirror to watch and inhibit any excess muscle tension may be necessary. The teaching of correct tongue positions in the articulation of defective consonants and reduction of nasal escape are best developed concurrently and, in fact, *articulation exercises used as a means of directing air through the mouth instead of through the nose.* When glottal substitutions for plosives and pharyngeal fricatives for sibilants are used the tongue does not participate in speech and is held more or less flat in the floor of the mouth. It is important in this 'typical cleft-palate speech' to teach the patient to use the tongue tip in articulation as soon as possible and to start with 'cooling' the tongue tip held lightly between the teeth as for [θ] and sucking air in and out.

Exercises in Breath Direction and Articulation

(*a*) Blow softly through the lips then practise interrupting the breath stream by gently closing the lips with a soft [p-p-p]. Follow this with the voiced counterpart [b-b-b]. Teach each fresh consonant as far as is possible from one already mastered.

(*b*) Practise blowing air through the upper teeth and lower lip, then interrupt with [f-f-f]. Follow with [v-v-v].

(*c*) Sigh breath over the tongue held between the teeth and obtain [θ], follow with voicing and [ð].

(*d*) Control nasal escape on [t] by prefacing with [b].

(*e*) Teach [s] and [θ] emphasising the need for air to flow over the tongue tip.

(*f*) Sigh a prolonged [ʃ] and interrupt with [t] to improve [tʃ].

As in the case of vowels it is also found that some consonants are produced with less nasal escape than others and the principle of decontamination can again be used to improve nasal consonants by placing good consonants adjacent to bad. If, for example, fricatives are good and plosives poor then exercises such as the following can be devised:

(*g*) sp-sp-sp—isolate [p] or st-st-st—isolate [t].

(*h*) spat-pat, spit-pit, spy-pie.

(*i*) steer-tear, store-tore, stow-toe.

Recording techniques described on page 152 are very suitable in treatment of cleft-palate children and adults.

GENERAL OBSERVATIONS ON TREATMENT

In a short time the patient can be given for home practice lists of words incorporating only those sounds which he can achieve well and with ease. The consonants [w], [l], [r], [j] are useful for inclusion in words since they are generally easy sounds for the patient with nasal escape to articulate. It is important that he should practise at home only those words and exercises which he can produce correctly in the clinic, otherwise the correct auditory and kinaesthetic patterns are soon lost, the patient continues to practise articulation at home in much the same old way and more harm than good comes from his home work.

The consonants [k] and [g] are the most difficult for these patients to achieve but even these can sound normal if contact is made by the tongue against the palate farther forward than is usual in normal individuals. This is best accomplished by holding the front of the tongue down firmly with a spatula and exhorting the patient to say [t] or [d] according to whether [k] or [g] is required.

Consonants [t] and [d] may be very difficult to elicit in place of a glottal stop. In order to get plosion in the right zone of articulation it is often helpful to imitate spitting out pips with a sharp contact of the tongue against the top teeth. Alternatively small pellets of paper may be used. The sucking sound as the tongue tip pulls off the alveolus in the interjection of impatience, [tch-tch], may also succeed in producing the right results. Or [t] may be taught from [s] after [θ] has been mastered. The patient blows an [s] and then taps the alveolus or teeth with the tongue tip gaining the desired plosion.

Besides the necessity for careful analysis of each patient's speech, and the listing of nasal and non-nasal sounds, the therapist must use her ingenuity in discovering which combinations of sounds the patient finds most easy, and so help him over many obstacles which might otherwise dishearten him. For example, a patient may have learned the correct articulation of [k] and [g] in place of a glottal plosive but find extraordinary difficulty in joining these to a vowel without reverting to the old substitution. He may, however, find the combinations [cr], [gr], [cl] and [gl] easy, in which case such words as 'crew', 'grey', 'claw', and 'glow' can be mastered before proceeding without difficulty to the correct articulation of 'cod', 'gay', 'caw' and 'go', and omitting the consonants 'r' and 'l' which act as glides on to the vowels. These speech glides are of very great assistance to the patient with an incompetent palate and it can be understood, for instance, from the phonetic point of view why [k] is easier to achieve after [ŋ] (think) than after [s] (skewer).

It is best not to include nasal consonants too soon. If introduced too early, they release reflexly the old muscular and auditory patterns, and just one nasal consonant in a phrase is sufficient to disrupt the good, but as yet poorly canalised speech. The attempt to elicit non-nasal vowels after nasal consonants, e.g. [mmm-a:] or [ŋ-i:], which is sometimes advocated is generally inadvisable until the patient has made considerable progress in hearing training and nasality has been much reduced. Then such exercises can be given to good effect, together with other voice production exercises for the development of forward resonance and good tone, including singing and intoning (pages 175–8).

In fact the therapist will not go far wrong if she leaves competence of the palato-pharyngeal mechanism to the plastic surgeon and treats the patient as one who suffers from dyslalia and a disorder of voice and refrains from becoming obsessed with the idea that she is treating a disorder of nasal escape exclusively.

'Speech should be improved by horizontal strata rather than vertical sections' (Greene, 1960). It is a mistake in my opinion to concentrate too long upon any one aspect of treatment and to concentrate upon the perfection of one sound after another. The improvement of tone can proceed concurrently with the correction of articulation, forming two separate lines of work at each treatment. The consonants can be taught in isolation one after the other in rapid succession, while those mastered first can be in process of inclusion in all positions in words. It is important to give patients over the age of ten, who are generally very depressed and hopeless about their speech, a sense of achievement and progress. We have found that intensive speech therapy, seeing the patients two or three times a day for a few minutes over a course of a week or two while in hospital, produces excellent results. Patients having learned correct speech production in set exercises may then return home to weekly speech therapy having been given a flying start in rehabilitation. It is a pity intensive treatment cannot be arranged in all hospitals to which patients with cleft-palate are constantly returning for cosmetic procedures or orthodontic treatment. Because speech therapy along the lines described here actually requires less muscular activity than normally employed by the patient in his speech, treatment can be commenced as early as a week after secondary repair of a palate or pharyngoplasty, and as soon as the patient feels well enough to co-operate. While in hospital not a moment should be lost. In the past, when blowing exercises for improvement of palatal competence were given, surgeons were in the habit of postponing speech therapy for three months. This tradition may unfortunately still persist in some units. In our case it was found that when an explanation of the aims and methods of speech therapy were given and the bogey of blowing exercises and palatal breakdown expelled, we were permitted to start speech therapy as soon as the anxious patient showed an interest in starting treatment.

INSUFFICIENT NASALITY

The voice suffers from insufficient nasality when there is an obstruction of the nasal airway which renders nasal breathing difficult or impossible. Lack of adequate nasal resonance destroys the bright ringing quality which is so characteristic of head resonance. Vowel sounds are far from normal and the voice is dull and muffled, but lack of nasality is most evident in the articulation of the nasal consonants. Inability to breathe through the nose renders mouth breathing necessary and probably habitual. The nasal consonants, which are continuants, cannot be adequately maintained but resemble their plosive counterparts, [b], [d] and [g], mainly on account of the precipitate release of the organs of articulation and opening of the oral cavity.

Because the nasal consonants are frequent in the English language, their denasalisation renders speech distinctly abnormal and even unpleasant to the listener who associates the lack of nasality with nasal obstruction. Reduced nasality in speech is as objectionable as nasal speech because of this. Severely denasalised speech is fortunately rare and a certain degree of nasality is possible for most speakers even when considerable obstruction of the nasal airway exists, provided the airway is not entirely closed. An individual is frequently able to compensate for lack of nasal resonance by increased pharyngeal constriction and deliberate prolongation of the nasal continuants.

CAUSES OF INSUFFICIENT NASALITY

A deflected septum is a common cause of reduced nasal resonance. It can be a congenital malformation and often occurs in association with cleft of the palate. It can also follow an accident causing a broken nose if it is not corrected surgically before healing takes place.

Nasal obstruction after pharyngoplasty and pharyngeal flap operations have already been described in connection with surgical correction of velopharyngeal incompetence. Bzoch (1964) found this to be a greater problem than excessive nasality after operation.

Nasal and nasopharyngeal tumours in adults are rare and require immediate investigation and treatment by surgery and/or radiotherapy if malignant.

Chronic inflammation of nasal mucosa (rhinitis) accompanied by constant nasal discharge (rhinorrhoea) is a common and troublesome cause of insufficient nasality. Inflammation may involve the laryngeal and pharyngeal membranes and produce chronic hoarseness. Catarrhal conditions are very frequently associated with enlarged adenoids in children. Adenoids alone do not cause complete nasal obstruction and mouth breathing. The chronic catarrh may persist after adenoidectomy unless appropriate medical attention is given to the microbial infection remaining after adenoidectomy. Nasal speech is not the only possible sequel of adenoidectomy: reduced nasality is equally possible and may persist through force of habit in a child until he is given speech training.

Chronic catarrh may apparently also be induced by damp climatic conditions, the population in certain areas being more afflicted with the troublesome complaint than others. In Liverpool, for instance, chronic catarrh is so prevalent that the most pronounced characteristic of the local dialect is its reduced nasality. Individuals speak as if they suffer from a severe cold in the head, which in many cases is true. The dysphonia, however, is mainly imitative. The low-lying Vale of Aylesbury also produces a climatic denasalised dialect.

Another form of rhinitis which is often intractable is due to perennial nasal allergy which assails the sufferer at all times of the year and is not confined to the seasonal exacerbation of 'hay-fever'. The condition is often associated with asthma and eczema. House-dusts, the spores of fungi, feathers, the fur of particular animals—cats, dogs and horses—and also certain foods may start the antagonistic reaction. New antihistamine preparations alleviate the rhinitis in some individuals but do not provide a cure. Antibiotic inhalations are sometimes prescribed, as also is vitamin therapy, such as the administration of large doses of ascorbic acid. Systematic skin tests may trace the individual allergy to specific cause. If a food, this can be omitted from the diet; if a dust, immunisation by an autogenous vaccine may successfully cure the rhinitis. The general health of the patient appears to be of some importance, sudden attacks of sneezing with streaming nose and eyes, and headaches, being reduced in times of fitness and well-being (Craddock, 1949).

Polypoid growths in the nasal passages sometimes occur and may be related to conditions of chronic allergic rhinitis. Polyps should be removed surgically in order to facilitate nasal breathing and improve nasal resonance. They have a habit of recurring and also may recur in the larynx (page 124).

The psychogenic origin of rhinitis, asthma and eczema is also well recognised, many psychiatrists maintaining that these conditions are always of functional origin even when a specific allergy is proved. It is probable that in many individuals hypersensitivity to certain agencies is the primary cause of disorders of the respiratory tract, but that emotional factors later become attached to the original physical reaction. It is difficult to understand how babies who suffer from eczema and asthma from birth, could have acquired these symptoms through emotional trauma. Only when allergy is not proved, and this is frequently the case, is it at all likely that the symptoms are purely psychosomatic in origin. The number of sufferers from these distressing complaints of hay fever is apparently on the increase as a result of the strain imposed upon human beings by the pace of modern civilisation (James, 1952). It has been suggested by Wolf (1952) that acute fears and anxieties, frustration and guilt produce symptoms of rhinitis through the unconscious desire to wash away the conflict, a desire which is given the concrete symbolism of hypersecretion of the nasal mucosa. Rhinitis can be invoked in these individuals by deliberate lack of sympathy on the part of an interviewer in a clinical situation and in the total absence of an allergic irritant. Similarly, it may be allayed by an atmosphere of ease and sympathy even in the presence of a high concentration in the atmosphere of the specific irritant to which the subject is supposedly allergic (Wolf, 1952).

Insufficient nasality and hoarseness stemming from catarrhal conditions or other obstructions should be thoroughly investigated by an ear, nose and throat specialist and receive appropriate medical treatment before speech therapy is attempted.

Lack of nasality is not entirely related to the degree of nasal blockage present. Obstruction always causes the voice to be deficient in nasal resonance but does not necessarily exclude the possibility of nasality, which is dependent upon the size of the nasopharyngeal resonator and the relative sizes of its orifices. If the resonator is not properly adjusted to produce nasality, insufficient nasality may persist after removal of nasal obstruction. The voice of a man of 18 years, for instance, continued to lack nasal tone after the complete removal of a large tumour which extended from the nasopharynx into the nasal cavity. His speech responded quickly to speech therapy. It is noticeable also that many of the children with cleft-palate who suffer from insufficient nasality on account of nasal obstruction and malformation of the septum, still continue to speak in the same way when the septum has been straightened and the airways freed. A further illustration is that of a child who suffered from severe nasal escape after adenoidectomy, but as movement of the palate developed she gradually reverted to her habitual denasalised speech, although she could now breathe through her nose without any difficulty.

In these instances habit is the cause of persistent lack of nasality. The individual continues to apply the same auditory patterns to speech production after the actual removal of the cause of insufficient nasality and obstruction in the nasal resonator. He produces the sounds he is accustomed to hear, probably unconsciously and at a reflex level but effectively adjusting articulation and resonance to compensate for lack of nasal obstruction, and will continue to do so unless speech therapy is given.

TREATMENT OF DENASALISED SPEECH

When catarrhal conditions produce hoarseness and lack of nasal resonance, it is found that an improvement in voice production generally alleviates the hoarseness but the reduced nasality persists. This is on account of chronic inflammation of the nasal mucosa and although the nose may be kept free by constant blowing the nasal resonator acts inescapably as an acoustic filter to those frequencies so essential to normal vocal resonance. Direct speech treatment can do little to help such patients unless the rhinitis is of psychogenic origin, in which case it may just conceivably respond to sympathetic treatment and reassurance. When the nasal consonants are defective, however, speech therapy can in most cases achieve considerable improvement. Nose breathing and adequate nose blowing must be encouraged. Hearing training which teaches the patient to discriminate between [b], [d], [g] and [m], [n] and [ŋ] and to recognise the faults in his own production of these sounds is essential. Humming on [m], [n] and [ŋ] should then be practised placing the hand over the mouth and nose and feeling the vibration. Cupping the hands over the ears also gives a subjective impression of increased vocal amplitude and is a useful adjunct to development of vocal tone. When sufficient nasality is achieved these sounds should be linked to vowels and nasal syllable drills composed. For example: [mim-mam-mɔm], [nin-nun-nan], [ŋaŋ-ŋɔŋ-ŋiŋ]. After this, words and sentences liberally peppered with nasal consonants can be given. At first the patient, with his proclivity to enunciate plosivies in place of [m], [n], [ŋ], will clip the nasal consonants short, but must learn to prolong and exaggerate them until they are well established in speech. As a result of this tendency to substitution, he will at first also find the common combinations of nasals and their plosive counterparts in English, difficult to manage. Such words as 'meant', 'hand', 'camp', 'linked', and the very common abbreviations 'won't', 'can't', 'isn't', 'mustn't', 'don't', will be the last to be corrected and will need considerable attention in the latter stages of treatment.

Case Report

C.Z. A girl of 9 years, severely reduced nasality as a result of chronic catarrh since the age of two years; [b], [d] and [g] sub-stituted for [m], [n], and [ŋ]. Adenoidectomy at 6 years had not made the slightest difference to the catarrhal condition or speech. Every examination possible had been made without revealing the cause of rhinitis and the speech specialist was the last in a long line of specialists who had endeavoured to help the child. The oral structure was normal, but the nose and cheek bones were flattened, exhibiting the typical skeletal structure of the adenoidal facies. The soft palate surprisingly showed *no* movement at all in the articulation of vowels. The child kept her nose clear by constant blowing and did not breathe through the mouth. She was tense, holding her thin little shoulders high, and her breathing involved the upper thorax almost entirely. She was of nervous temperament, and so conscious of her speech that she was unable to read in class without stumbling over every word, although in the clinic she could read adult material fluently. Although not an only child she was extraordinarily staid and polite, and so quaintly old-fashioned that the school staff invariably referred to her as 'great-grandmother'. Her speech was, with its penned-in and clipped characteristics, somehow in keeping with her personality.

Despite the catarrhal condition, which did not improve during treatment, she was from the first able to hum with normal nasality and to produce perfect nasal consonants in isolation. She enjoyed humming tunes and practising 'playing on her trumpet' as we called it with hands over the nose or ears. Great difficulty was experienced in obtaining normal nasal sounds in nonsense syllables and speech; she had a good ear and was able to recognise good and bad sounds quickly and was distressed by hearing a recording of her speech. Articulation suddenly improved when it was suggested that she should relax, and not try so hard with nonsense syllable exercises but speak lazily and easily, drawling and prolonging the nasal consonants instead of cutting them off short and sharp and producing plosives as was her custom. Not only did nasal consonants now become normal, but head resonance and vocal quality improved and speech became both good and pleasing. The soft palate, which was unusually immobile at first, appears to have provided insufficient nasopharyngeal closure to cause nasality. As speech improved movement of the palate increased and elevation on vowel sounds became normal.

14 Dysarthrophonia

The term dysarthria denotes defective articulation due to lesions in the nervous system which cause motor disorders of the muscles of articulation (impaired neuromuscular function). Anarthria denotes absence of articulation due to loss of neuromuscular function.

Dysarthria is always associated with dysphonia if we include disorders of resonance in our concept of voice. If the tongue and/or palate are affected by paralysis the quality of vowels and vocal resonance will also be impaired. We have described fully the inseparable relation between voice, articulation and resonance elsewhere (Chapter 4). It is permissible to speak here of disorders of resonance of neurological origin to distinguish these disorders from those in which the vocal folds alone are involved, giving rise to aphonia or dysphonia. In the more severe cases of paralysis with ataxia and hypermotoricity, the palatal, pharyngeal, laryngeal and respiratory muscles may be involved. The type of motor disorder and its extent will determine the type and degree of dysphonia. Peacher (1949a) suggested that dysphonia associated with dysarthria should be called dysarthrophonia. This term we favour for it appropriately labels voice disorders due to a neurological lesion. It reminds us, as speech therapists, not to concentrate upon one aspect of defective speech to the neglect of another but to treat the problem of respiration, voice and speaking as a holistic entity.

We refer the student to Berry and Eisenson (1962) for a clear and simple account of the neuroanatomy and neurophysiology involved in the neurological speech disorders outlined below.

UPPER MOTOR NEURONE LESIONS

The upper motor neurone paths concerned with speaking arise in the cells of the precentral convolution of the motor cortex adjacent to Broca's area. Their axons descend forming the fronto-bulbar portion of the pyramidal tracts. They synapse with the nuclei of the peripheral motor nerves situated in the bulb (medulla

277

oblongata) which is continuous with the mid-brain and the spinal cord below. The upper motor neurone does not govern movements of isolated muscles but groups of muscles. Moreover, the fronto-bulbar portions of the pyramidal tracts, which connect with the bulbar nuclei of the motor nerves responsible for articulation, respiration and phonation, come from both hemispheres. Since the bulbar nuclei are connected with the left and right cortex, lesions in the fronto-bulbar tracts must be bilateral to affect the muscles of phonation, respiration and articulation. When bilateral damage of these connections occurs the speaking disorder is severe. The

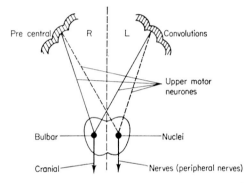

FIG. 35   Double connection, from both hemispheres, of upper motor neurones with bulbar nuclei

muscles are affected by a spastic paralysis. No wasting in the muscles follows.

Such lesions occur in adults suffering from widespread cerebral arteriosclerosis who sustain vascular accidents (c.v.a.). The condition is known as supra-bulbar or pseudo-bulbar palsy. Swallowing is generally severely impaired besides speech but the reflex movements of swallowing may be hardly disturbed as contrasted with the voluntary movements for speaking. Slow recovery of muscular function may take place, during which speech therapy may help the patient to improve speech. In patients suffering from vascular accidents the disorder is progressive. Further accidents occur and the chance of recovery lessens with each.

In cerebral palsy (encephalopathy) motor disorders are a common symptom. They may either be congenital or acquired at birth or soon after from anoxia, kernicterus and virus infections. The maturation of muscular function with increasing age is an important factor in the development of motor control in these children with co-ordination disorders. Improvement in co-ordination can be anticipated with advancing age and renders speech prognosis more optimistic but somewhat unpredictable.

A congenital or acquired supra-bulbar paresis involving only the muscles of tongue, lips and palate may occur (Wynn-Williams, 1958), but such selective evidence of brain damage is rare. Careful neurological examination generally reveals some involvement of other muscle groups in larynx, pharynx or limbs and a slight generalised inco-ordination may be revealed when careful psychomotor testing is carried out. Intelligence is often low in these cases. Wynn-Williams has advocated a Rosenthal type of pharyngoplasty to cure the severe drooling which results from difficulty in swallowing and is such an embarrassing and socially unacceptable symptom of the syndrome. The operation is apparently successful in its primary aim. Grady (1958) has reported some speech improvement and a reduction in nasality following operation. The degree of benefit to be anticipated from surgery is dependent upon the nature and extent of paralysis and the intelligence. A careful neurological and psychological assessment is necessary beforehand. Often the lingual and labial paralysis is so severe that the child cannot benefit from provision of a permanent bridge between palate and naso-pharynx. (See also under disorders of nasal resonance, page 253.) Many children with slight impairment of oral muscles and tongue thrust are found to improve spontaneously by the age of 8 or 9 years as maturation takes place.

VOICE THERAPY FOR SPASTIC DYSARTHROPHONIA

Voice therapy for adults and children suffering from supranuclear palsy aims at helping the patient to make the best use of existing muscular function. Articulation is slurred and slow and vowels distorted and the voice lacks projection and resonance. There is considerable nasal escape when the velopharyngeal mechanism is involved. Pitch change is difficult and inflexion monotonous and droning; the voice may be harsh and spastic and overloud at the beginning of a phrase, then become breathy and fade away. Respiration is shallow and not co-ordinated with voice on account of spasticity in the muscles of respiration. It is a mistake to work upon improving articulation alone in these cases for concentration upon a well-articulated word and tongue contacts may increase muscular tonicity and involuntary spasms of the head, neck and limbs. The need for development of speech and rhythm is emphasised by Peacher (1949) and Butfield (1961). Voice therapy must emphasise co-ordination of respiration and phonation with speech phrasing, stress and melody. Speech therapy which emphasises the need for correct word shapes alone is too limited in its approach for the needs of most patients. Mysack (1959b) emphasises the need for development of acoustic temporal features of speech.

Relaxation forms an important and essential basis for voice therapy. Co-operation with the physiotherapist is essential so that she can work upon posture and advise the speech therapist how to manage the patient physically. Adults are tense and anxious, the more especially because intelligence is unimpaired in dysarthria. They are fully able to verbalise their plight to themselves and to worry in a way in which the aphasic patient often apparently cannot. Nervous tension tends to aggravate the muscular spasticity.

Once a degree of relaxation is achieved rhythmic breathing may be emphasised and volume of inspiration increased. Expiration must be controlled and co-ordinated with the production of humming, then with vowels singly, then in various combinations, rhythms and inflexions. Imitation of short phrases may follow in which speed, stress and inflexion are preserved without too great emphasis upon articulation. Practice of consonants and word drills may be carried out as a separate activity. Scanning speech, the utterance of one carefully articulated syllable at a time, can be practically unintelligible whereas speech which achieves a certain fluency and melody may be easily intelligible though articulation may deviate considerably from normal patterns. This is because we rely in listening upon many cues and deeply ingrained linguistic patterns against which we watch the incoming speech signals and identify them. These are acquired in the first year of life and speech which lacks these normal linguistic traits is exceedingly difficult to understand even though articulation is accurate. (Refer back to Chapter 5, 'Vocal Synthesis', pages 88 and 90 in particular.) Communication theory, evolving in phonetics laboratories has engaged itself extensively with what makes speech intelligible and how much information can be excluded from communication networks (telephone, radio, etc.) before speech becomes unintelligible. Fry (1963) gives a clear account of the information necessary to comprehension by the listener in ability to code and decode. Connected speech is understood from articulation features but also from intonation, stress and rhythm and also familiarity of phrasing. Much of what we say consists of automatic, well-worn phrases or clichés, so much so that people working or living together using the same personal and professional language need not listen to half of what is said as they fill in the gaps mentally. The speaker need not finish his sentences and can jump from one facet of his theme to another. This is why a tape-recorded lecture cannot be written down to provide an article for a journal unless it has been written first and read. In order to appreciate the argument fully, we have only to consider the ease with which we understand a chatty conversation over the telephone and the impossibility of hearing or identifying an unfamiliar name. An isolated signal given outside a linguistic context generally has not only to be spelt but each letter given a label (i.e. A for Andrew, J for John), although the actual amount of physical acoustic information transmitted over the line (telephone circuit) remains constant.

All this does not exclude the real need for tongue, lip and palate exercises when necessary. A patient who has been unconscious and then fitted with a feeding tube for weeks or even months will have difficulty in chewing and swallowing and articulating. Often only after the feeding tube is removed is the speech therapist called in because the patient is not articulating intelligibly, although he is swallowing minced foods. Reflex and primitive crude movements may be achieved laboriously in deglutition but can be almost impossible in speech. Nursing staff and even doctors do not always appreciate this. An important aspect of assessment should be watching how the patient feeds himself, masticates and swallows. Specific exercises for developing and strengthening tongue and palate and vocal exercises are helpful when muscles have been long inactive; they aid recovery and not least give encouragement. Promotion of tactile and kinaesthetic awareness and oral spatial relationships is needed. Many individuals have loss of sensation in the lips and tongue and drool for this reason after swallowing has improved. They need to be reminded to keep the lips shut and to hold their heads up. Use of a mirror is helpful. Stroking the lips and tongue with a spatula often promotes some reflex movement and revives kinaesthetic and tactile awareness of oral lingual spatial relationships. Stroking with ice cubes (or, much more pleasant, a fruit lolly) is also often beneficial and ice therapy is advocated by many physiotherapists.

Elderly patients sometimes appear to lose the ability to monitor their speech after some months of severe illness and remain fixed at a poor speech level from habit. Such patients benefit quite rapidly from the hearing, kinaesthetic and tactile training involved in the speech and voice training described above. Often it is a question of maintaining a certain standard without further improvement but also, and more importantly, without further deterioration.

In the field of geriatrics, the speech therapist must be aware of wider possibilities of deterioration than speech alone. Patients may be confused, amnesic, disorientated, severely depressed, irritable and suspicious. It may be necessary to win the individual's co-operation and make friends long before any speech correction can be attempted. The possibility of dysphasia must be excluded. Hearing impairment is very probable and enquiries must be made as to whether the patient has a hearing aid. Often he has one at home but does not use it because he is not sure how to, or is unconvinced it helps, or it may not work. Often new batteries are the only thing needed but nobody has thought of this! An audiologist or teacher of the deaf should be called in which also ensures an extra visitor for deaf patients. Eyesight needs to be assisted by spectacles: the patient generally has them already but needs to be reminded to wear them and it is necessary to see they are *clean*, especially with hemiplegic patients Finally, we must remember to persuade patients to wear their dentures, even though there is generally some difficulty in retaining them in position when dysarthric. The hospital dental department may have to be consulted. It is mportant to get all the necessary aids for living (teeth, eyes and ears) 'seen to' before the patient leaves hospital. Once he is an out-patient it is far more difficult to make appointments for patient and family. (Fawcus, 1964 and 1964a; Butfield, 1961; Grewel and Greene, 1968.)

Butfield (1961) says that the therapist should listen to the patient and that encouragement to speak is the best therapy of all. Nevertheless, ability to write needs also to be tested and a patient may be allowed to write when he cannot make people understand. He is thus spared the frustration and upset this often engenders— even to the extent of giving up all endeavour to communicate. The patient who cannot control pen or pencil can be given a spelling board, or an alphabet clock with hand attached may be easier to manage. Pictures of things a speechless patient may need can be made available for the severely ill.

Patients below retiring age, who have made a good recovery

do not need speech therapy so much as to be incorporated in a group and Butfield (1961) advises placement in a rehabilitation centre. If returning home sufficiently alert and physically able, the patient can practise reading aloud with a member of the family, or if a tape-recording machine is available, the speech therapist can provide suitable master tapes with empty spaces during which the patient can repeat after the therapist, or read simple passages, with master tape and written text. Hearing the deviations between his own speech and that of the model or 'master' stimulates automatic self-correction or 'monitoring'. A patient must also be encouraged to make recordings himself and play them back listening critically, that is if manual control allows. Many language-laboratory techniques may be adopted to the needs of patients of all types. It must be remembered that all Comprehensive Schools in England and many evening institutes have language-laboratory facilities and speech classes might be organised at convenient times for suitable groups of patients. Programmes can be devised in collaboration with the heads of language departments or with teachers of speech and drama, many of whom have taken a 'speech option' in colleges of education during their training and are interested in deviant speech.

The problem of speech and the patient's articulatory proficiency should be kept in mind in synchronous speech practice. If brady-lalia (bradyarthria) are severe the patient will be unable to keep pace with anything like normal speech. The speech model must therefore be suitably slow and adjusted to the needs of the individual. Supervision is necessary in the early stages of repetition or synchronous play-back and speaking practice, in order to ensure that the patient's speech is actually synchronised with that of the model and also follows approximately the same pattern of stress and melody.

Use of a speech amplifier (see under Parkinson's disease) is also a useful aid to self-monitoring voice (page 152).

STRIATAL LESIONS

Lesions involving the caudate and lenticular nuclei in the corpus striatum affect the synergic movements of expression, postural adjustment and locomotion. Damage to these nuclei produces the characteristic involuntary writhing, gesticulation and grimacing of the athetoid or choreic and may profoundly disrupt speech co-ordinations with regard to respiration, phonation and articulation.

Athetosis may be acquired by adults through disease. In children it is a common type of lesion occurring in cerebral palsy, though often combined with wider involvement of the nervous system, as described by Grewel (1960) and Ingram (1960).

Articulation and voice may be disrupted continuously or sporadically in athetosis. Explosive voice with sudden increase of volume or aphonia are associated with arhythmic breathing and involuntary adduction or abduction of the vocal folds. Speech may be preceded or interrupted by 'wild air' and involuntary grunts or vowel sounds. Pitch and stress are also necessarily deviant. Inspiratory voice (stridor) occurs. Nervousness and tension aggravate the symptoms. Relaxation, rhythmic breathing and controlled expiration and phonation are the aims in treatment. Physiotherapy should also aid establishment of correct breathing patterns.

Chorea is characterised by rapid jerky movements of the body. The muscles of face, tongue, palate and larynx may be involved. Involuntary sighs, clicks and pitch changes are heard. Speech symptoms may be similar to stammering or cluttering. Chorea is thought to be due to lesions in the corpus striatum and follows acute rheumatic fever in young children and adolescents. Thanks to improved methods of treatment, 'St Vitus's dance', as it was called, is seldom seen nowadays. The involuntary tongue, lip and jaw movements can be mistaken for stammering. Chorea can occur in adults but chiefly in pregnant women and in a severe form. Rest and sedation are essential and it should not be confused with a hysterical manifestation.

PARKINSON'S DISEASE

Lesions in the globus pallidus and substantia nigra (basal nuclei) in the corpus striatum are responsible, it is thought, for the rigidity and tremor which is characteristic of Parkinsonism. A cog-wheel movement can be felt if the patient's elbow or wrist is manipulated. The pill-rolling movement of thumb and finger with bent arms and forward posture and festinating gait are also typical. There is a mask-like rigidity of expression and often a head tremor. If the patient is asked to tap a rhythm with his hand he may not be able to do so—his movements 'running away with him' and festinating as with gait and also speech. There is in advanced cases great difficulty with writing. The fingers are incapable of effecting the delicate co-ordinations necessary in maintaining the constant changes in direction. Writing becomes smaller and smaller until it is too small to read. Drawing a spiral of convolutions is another test and reveals the hand tremor present.

In advanced stages of the disease articulation, speed of utterance and volume of voice are affected owing to tremor and rigidity of all muscles.

Paralysis agitans is the name given to the ideopathic form of Parkinson's disease. There is also a post-encephalitic form which

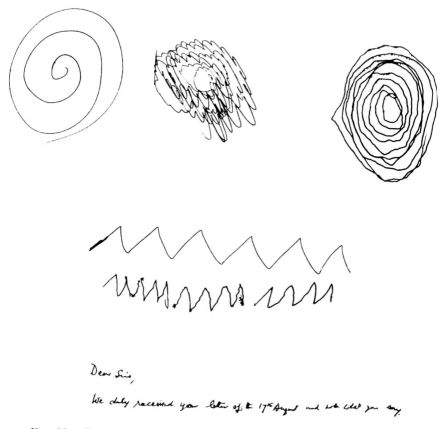

FIG. 36   Example of Parkinson patient's writing and copying of patterns

may develop as long as 20 years after the original illness and in this form there are ocular gyri and a greater degree of rigidity than tremor. There is also an arteriosclerotic form which develops in older patients and there are generally other neurological symptoms of degeneration. Drug therapy is the usual treatment for arteriosclerotic Parkinsonism.

Parkinson's disease often develops unilaterally and some time before involvement of the opposite side. Such cases are the least crippled in the early stages and speech is never impaired. The disease is slowly and steadily progressive and speech therapy is of limited value and is chiefly supportive when speech and voice begin to deteriorate.

In the early stages relaxation and reassurance and encouragement to speak and maintain a good standard of performance is very helpful and can inspire a patient to make the best use of residual function. Grewel (1957a) says that lack of speech propulsion or initiative is characteristic of the disease in its advanced stage. Butfield (1961) stresses the need to encourage and keep alive the desire to communicate.

An increasing number of patients are referred for speech therapy as a result of a more positive attitude to rehabilitation following advances in surgery and pharmaceutical therapy. Patients who have refused surgery may be brought into hospital for trials with new drugs and referred for physiotherapy, occupational therapy and speech therapy in a concentrated rehabilitation drive. Speech therapists need a more positive attitude towards speech treatment. The problem is enormous. Canter (1963) quotes an estimate of one million to one and a half million in the United States suffering from Parkinson's disease in 1958. In England there are an estimated 20,000 Parkinson cases (Greene and Watson, 1968). Many of these patients are house-bound or in institutions, gradually deteriorating, receiving the same drug therapy for years and no speech therapy or physiotherapy which can keep patients mobile. The formation in 1969 of the Parkinson's Disease Society of the United Kingdom Limited, a charitable organisation, is a step forward in attempts to help these people and to promote research and also awareness of sufferers from the disease by the community. The address of the Society is 11 Girdwood Road, London SW18.

SPEECH SYMPTOMS IN PARKINSONISM

There is considerable individual variability in voice and speech symptoms and these have little if any correlation with severity of general physical symptoms. Speech deterioration may be the first symptom of disease. Patients with severe paralysis may speak quite well. We have not found that speech correlates with varying degrees of tremor and rigidity and the reasons for speech deterioration varying from patient to patient remains obscure when degree of tremor and rigidity appears similar. Of course, in advanced stages of Parkinsonism all movement is severely impaired, including swallowing and speech.

Speech is described as slurred with lack of inflexion, and a tendency to accelerate as utterance proceeds (i.e. festination, from 'festino', I hurry), added to which the voice loses volume and speech trails away into an unintelligible mumbling or murmur. The extension of movements of articulation and phonation are reduced by rigidity and at the same time movements of articulation festinate just as the gait festinates with an uncontrollable propulsion. The patient on the level may run forward with shorter and shorter steps until he grasps an object or dances a tattoo on one spot, especially when needing to change direction and turn a corner. The patient may become aphonic and block in speech, being unable to initiate movements it is believed on account of akinesia described by Luria (1961 and 1966) as akinetic mutism. There may also be rapid repetition of phrase or last word (palilalia). These symptoms are reminiscent of cluttering.

Apart from the subjective impressions of experienced neurologists and speech therapists recorded in the literature, the voice and speech symptoms have been examined very little on a scientific basis. The research of Canter (1963, 1965, 1965a) is a welcome exception. Canter (1963) examined the three parameters of intensity, pitch and duration in 17 ambulatory males with Parkinson's disease and no other disorders. All patients had had normal speech, none had received surgical treatment and all had anti-Parkinson drugs *withdrawn* for 48 hours prior to testing. These patients were matched with a similar age group of normal subjects in order to distinguish between speech in Parkinson's disease and in the normal ageing process. The Parkinson and control groups read a passage which was recorded and subsequently analysed. Canter surprisingly did not find any significant differences between volume of voice between the two groups. There were marked differences when vocal pitch was evaluated in the two groups. The Parkinson subjects' range of frequency used was smaller than any of the ranges of the control group. Eight of the controls used a range of an octave or more, but not one of the Parkinsonian subjects had a range of this magnitude. As regards duration, on average there was little difference between the groups but two Parkinson patients spoke much slower than the normals 60–70 words per minute compared to the slowest normal speaker at 140–159 w.p.m. One Parkinson patient spoke at an extraordinarily rapid rate of 249·6 w.p.m., whereas the fastest speed in the normal subjects was 200–219 w.p.m. (3 subjects).

Canter (1965) advocates work on sustained phonation for 'weak' voices and increased pitch range and in his third paper based on the same study (1965a) he examines articulation and diadochokinesis. The Parkinson patients were unable to perform rapid movements of the tongue-tip particularly, and clarity of articulation was more highly correlated with overall speech adequacy than were vocal pitch, duration and volume. Pitch limitations did not influence intelligibility as evaluated by listeners. It is in fact speed and stress, in our opinion, which are the two factors which contribute most to incomprehensible utterance and it is these factors which are the most difficult for Parkinson patients to control and monitor in their speech.

Surgery for Parkinson's disease aims at severing the connections between the thalamus and basal ganglia by a stereotactic procedure with electrocautery (thalamotomy). It is executed under local anaesthesia so that the patient remains conscious and can talk, and the probe is removed when tremor ceases and rigidity disappears. It is a hazardous operation and not always successful and occasionally a patient is dysphasic and even hemiplegic afterwards, although in most cases they recover from the dysphasia. The operation does not cure the disease but arrests it for a time in its slow inexorable course. Physiotherapy is necessary after operation on account of an akinesia which makes initiation of movements difficult and often the patient has to learn to walk again.

A great advance in surgical technique was achieved by the introduction of cryogenic surgery by Cooper (1962) which is far less dangerous and produces better results than electrocautery. Refrigeration by liquid nitrogen from a cannula inserted into the basal ganglion creates a safe haemostatic lesion. This technique has the great advantage of making possible the application of moderate cold and a temporary lesion as a test to identify the locus of abnormal neural activity. This is reversible if necessary before permanent necrosis is produced by application of intense cold. The procedure is called cryothalamectomy. Because of its increased safety, treatment can be extended to both younger and older patients.

In our experience (Greene and Watson, 1968) speech is in general neither improved nor rendered worse by thalamotomy but remains very much the same as before. Sometimes the voice is weaker owing to the patient forgetting to breathe and inspire an adequate volume of air especially immediately following thalamotomy. This we attribute to general akinesia and the condition responds quickly to physiotherapy and speech therapy. Fluctuations in speech performance occur and speech can deteriorate and tremor return when the patient is upset and tense, as when he is asked to perform before a crowd on a ward round. This makes assessment of pre-operative and post-operative results extremely difficult.

Patients are generally much happier after surgery and are especially glad to be relieved of tremor, about which they are sensitive and embarrassed, besides which the fatigue of trying to control tremor and a body which is never still is considerable. They increase in confidence and often talk more and make better social contact, so that in this important respect one can say communication improves. Another important gain is that facial expression may return and the face light up with recognition more easily, so that people are less put off by an unresponsive expressionless and unwelcoming stare.

Allan, Turner and Gadea-Ciria (1969) have reported on their investigation into speech disturbances following stereotaxic surgery in 118 patients over a two-year period (1963–65). They measured voice volume with a sound-intensity meter and articulation, grading dysarthria mild, moderate or severe. As regards voice volume they found that voice deteriorated more frequently with left operations, 25 out of 37 (67 per cent) compared to 16 out of 44 (36 per cent) of right operations. Patients undergoing bilateral operations showed a high incidence of impairment of voice volume—30 out of 53 (56 per cent). As regards articulation: 20 out of 37 patients (54 per cent) with left operation deteriorated; 16 out of 44 (36 per cent) with right operation; and 35 out of 53 (66 per cent) with bilateral operations. Assessment of the patients was made early after operation; also it is not stated whether drug therapy had been suspended or not when the patients were tested; presumably it had been pre- and post-operatively but this is a very important factor both to control and confirm in any research project. We found failure to ensure drug withdrawal (on account of purely practical nursing reasons) in our own efforts to tape-record patients before and after thalamotomy rendered our comparative speech assessments invalid. Particularly was this so when we endeavoured to record patients on follow-up 3 months after operation when attending hospital as out-patients.

Drugs offer the most optimistic means of control of Parkinsonism for the future. Two new drugs—L. Dopa and amantadine—

are now being used. We have little experience of patients on L. Dopa but with amantadine we found speech improved considerably at first with two patients then reverted disappointingly to its original state. L. Dopa is reported to improve the speech of some patients. William Lipton, the American author, in a radio interview described his fight against Parkinson's disease and the benefit he experienced from L. Dopa. He described vividly the trammels imposed by the disease—the helplessness and futility of life, the feeling of being trapped shamefully in a cage and the constant fight against immobility. It is a slow, insidious disease which requires great courage to combat. Lipton's speech was affected and he mentioned particularly the fact that concentration is lost while speaking so that the afflicted individual forgets the end of sentences. Once the ill-effects and nausea produced by L. Dopa had worn off and the benefit of the drug was felt, Lipton described the intense relief and freedom experienced, comparing this to a fly being lifted out of jam or honey and able to take flight again.

Administration of L. Dopa is proceeding rather cautiously in Britain and it is too early to report upon the speech benefits; our own study is only just beginning with the first patients placed on L. Dopa therapy. Rigrodsky and Morrison (1970) have reported their preliminary findings concerning speech changes during L. Dopa therapy. They evaluated speech of 21 Parkinson patients before and during various dosages and generally after a period of one month, but not all were on maximal dosage. A difficulty is that on account of side effects maximal dosage may be held up or vary with individuals, and the authors realised the need for longer follow-up. Their findings concerning speech were not so dramatic as the general physical improvement. The speech parameters evaluated were as follows: (1) overall adequacy; (2) clarity of articulation; (3) normalcy of nasal resonance; (4) the time factor in speaking, i.e. overall rate, appropriate phrasing, pauses, fluency and rhythm of speech. The patients were tested on oral reading and picture description. They were able to report statistically significant improvement in one parameter only— that of the time factor. In our opinion, covering as it does features of considerable importance in communication and those which are much affected in Parkinsonism, their cautious report is in fact rather encouraging. The neurologists in charge of these patients were of the opinion that speech was better after long periods of maximal dosage.

Psychologically Parkinson patients appear surprisingly stable and depression is only in reasonable proportion to the health, incapacity and financial and social problems attendant upon the disease. Warburton (1967) who examined a group of individuals after thalamotomy and a control group of physically handicapped for other reasons, concluded that depression was not an integral part of the disease and on the Maudsley Personality inventory ratings found that the incidence of depression was similar in both groups. Social isolation and poverty were important causal factors in Parkinsonism depression, however, and were more often the result of this disease than were other physical handicaps. This does not change the fact that Parkinson patients are often very anxious and very depressed. On the other hand, the majority battle on with great courage and cheerfulness. Every individual has a breaking point and when a patient breaks down and gives up it is because he can stand no more. Canter (1965) comments on the concentration by therapists on 'motivation' whereas patients may be using their 'maximum reserve function'. Rehabilitation centres, as Butfield (1961) points out, are ideal for these patients and for boosting morale, which can bring about astonishing physical improvement. The London Camden Medical Centre, for instance, provides facilities for re-admission of Parkinson patients when social workers report the family needs a rest or the patient is deteriorating. These facilities should be available to all Parkinson patients, but rehabilitation centres are few and have long waiting lists and give priority to the young and the newly disabled rather than providing refresher courses for the chronically disabled.

Patients who cease to try and give up hope become chair-bound or bedridden early, and utterly dependent upon their families. We had a patient who made a splendid recovery after his second thalamotomy and was walking well, helping to serve tea on the ward and speaking well. He was discharged home and three weeks later was re-admitted on account of a reported sudden deterioration in physical state, speech and personality. After a week of the three revitalising therapies and heartening encouragement from nursing staff and neurosurgeons, the patient was back to his previous condition. He was discharged and within a week had again collapsed. This was a social problem and perhaps a psychiatric one.

Patients with frank organic disease are in general very much easier to understand and manage compared to patients with psychosomatic disorder and anxiety. Whereas the Parkinson patient has incurable and handicapping illness and difficulties of adjustment, more severe in some individuals than others on account of personality and degree of family support, their difficulties are as a rule logical and comprehensible. But with patients with psychogenic disturbance it is a mystery to discover what the illness and physical symptoms are all about, requiring careful search and patient imaginative handling.

VOCAL FAILURE IN PARKINSONISM

The voice may be lost entirely after thalamotomy but can be restored by vocal exercises. Butfield (1961) recommends forcing exercises (see page 331). A patient who suffered from aphonia after thalamotomy and was not given speech therapy for two years, recovered his voice when he moved south from the north of England. He was helped by humming and vowel exercises with hard attack, relaxation and breathing technique.

Patients whose voices are weak benefit greatly from breathing exercises especially after stereotactic operations. Physiotherapists should be asked to include diaphragmatic breathing in their physical training programme for these patients. Amplification of the voice is also helpful for those still at work and a selection of pocket amplifiers are now available (see pages 293 and 422). (Greene and Watson, 1968.) First, an amplifier reduces tension and anxiety which arises over the fear and frustration of not being audible in an office or factory or round the committee table. When relaxed a patient speaks far better. In most cases patients are able to discard the device after a time or use it only occasionally. Secondly, there is an automatic tendency to raise the voice to the same level as that when amplified as soon as the aid is turned off. Patients who are too elderly to manage an aid themselves can practise with the therapist, who switches on for a period of conversation and then off. In all cases amplification helps a patient to monitor his speech and highlights feed-back (Watson, 1967).

Amplifiers are available with hand microphone or throat microphone and with speaking tube, head-set or spectacles attachment for those unable to hold the hand microphone on account of tremor. A box loudspeaker for placing on a desk is useful for addressing meetings and can also be run off the amplifier. (See page 392 for illustrations and page 422 for a commercial list.)

Hand-microphone and speaking-tube attachments give good

reproduction of speech according to the quality of the instrument. The 'throat microphone' (or transducer), which is held under a collar or on a band round the throat, picks up vibrations from the thyroid ala and though giving the voice a tremendous boost rather distorts the consonants and overall speech. Although satisfying to the speaker he may not be so intelligible to his audience. Careful evaluation of speech with different accessories to an amplifier is necessary.

Auditory speech-training units as used in education of the partially-hearing child serve the same purpose as pocket amplifiers, and being bigger have far better reproduction. However, these instruments cannot be carried around on the person and are expensive.

Some recording machines have a device which allows immediate play-back of speech with volume control. This is possible on the Uher 4000 Report-L., which is in every way an excellent, reliable and really portable recording machine strongly recommended for all purposes.

Electronic speech amplifiers using batteries are available from Lustraphone Limited and S. G. Brown with hand microphone, throat transducer, speaking tube with head-set and table loud-speaker accessories (pages 392–3). George Washington also produces an amplifier with hand microphone and a battery charger unit which runs off the electric main. For addresses and details of equipment see list of electronic speech aids (page 422).

The 'Sama' instrument has the best reproduction but is bigger than Lustraphone and S. G. Brown amplifiers and also more expensive. It has two controls: an off-on switch and a volume control so that volume can be set at the required level and the instrument switched on and off as needed. The Lustraphone switches on when the microphone jack is plugged in and the volume control can remain set as required, but plugging in the jack can be difficult for a Parkinson patient. The S. G. Brown has one switch which controls off-on and volume, so that volume has to be regulated each time the instrument is switched on. It is cheap, small and reliable.

All electronic gadgets have their idiosyncrasies and so has each patient; the difficulties may combine to defeat the patient using an aid altogether. In most cases a considerable amount of patience and perseverance must be practised by the patient, while the therapist requires patience and perseverance in her instruction. We advise that all speech aids should be tried out under the supervision of a speech therapist so that the patient can receive maximum benefit from the aid and speech therapy. If an individual requires an aid it is pretty certain he requires speech therapy too. We deplore the purchase of instruments by patients, who are then disappointed and have wasted their often depleted funds, these instruments not being available on the state Health Service in England as are hearing-aids, spectacles and dentures (see page 417). Every hospital should run an advisory service and have speech aids available for demonstration and loan to patients —the equipment being the property of the hospital. We have instituted such a service at St. Bartholomew's Hospital and have been able to advise and help many patients not only from Britain but from many parts of the world.

Finally, in connection with amplification, we must mention the amplifier attachment available for telephone users at work and at home (Telephone amplifiers, 1963). The nearest telephone sales department should be consulted. The telephone number for this will be found in the telephone directory under 'Telephone Sales' in the section 'Facilities and Services' at the beginning of the directory. It is not generally any use enquiring for information over the post-office stamp counter.

DYSARTHRIA IN PARKINSONISM

So far we have discussed the vocal problems of Parkinsonism and these are the most responsive to help and treatment. When dysarthria and speech propulsion have developed it is a far more serious and difficult condition to alleviate. Amplifiers may help the patient to monitor his speech and can be tried, but since an amplifier only makes speech louder it does not spontaneously give benefit in the same way as when voice alone is lacking adequate volume. If vocal volume is a problem in severe cases of speech deterioration, which Canter (1963) did not find was so, then an amplifier is likely to prove of some benefit. The rapidity of utterance is of enormous difficulty for the patient to control in spontaneous speech and must be sensitive in some way to cortical and linguistic thought processes. Patients perform beautifully if asked to count, to say the days of the week, repeat short phrases after the therapist, to read a passage marked with pauses, even to answer questions mechanically and briefly with a pause between each word. It is common experience (Allan, 1970) that there is very little carry-over from clinical practice and performance into everyday life. As soon as the patient is liberated from the vigilant supervision of the therapist, speech festinates again. We have treated patients, recovering from thalamotomy, in hospital daily for months and tried every conceivable speech training and recording technique imaginable. We have included rhythmic training and tapping in time to control speech festination. We have tried electronic metronomes as recommended by Wohl (1968, 1970) and by Allan (1970) for stuttering, and allowed patients to practise at home with them. We have also used syllabic speech (Andrews and Harris, 1964) and we have treated highly intelligent, well-motivated patients still at work, but with the same poor results. As Allan (1970) truly says, 'Those of you who embark on group treatment for patients with Parkinson's disease must reconcile yourselves to running such a session for evermore. It seems to be impossible to discharge such patients. While they are having regular therapy their speech remains relatively intelligible—discharge them and even with promises to continue daily practice at home, they will have deteriorated in no time at all'. This sad state of affairs she attributes to lack of initiative to help themselves, but after treating many patients who try desperately hard to make themselves intelligible I do not think this is entirely true. It is the nature of the disease and the neurological damage sustained by the higher centres of speech organisation, in the realm of praxis and not paralysis, which is responsible for the uncontrollable features of speech festination in normal situations of communication.

The parallel between certain features of Parkinson speech and cluttering provides considerable fascination to treatment if the speech pathologist has both types of patients under her care. The tachyphemia and uncontrollable speech propulsion is the common factor, not the tremor and rigidity, of course. For further reading on this subject see Arnold (1960); Shepherd (1960); Moravek and Langova (1962); Böhme (1968).

Weiss (1960) describing therapy in cluttering gives many exercises which may be used in speech training for Parkinson patients. The writing symptoms are also similar: if a Parkinson patient can write he misses out small words and syllables frequently. The thought processes bear some resemblance to each other. William Lipton drew attention to the trailing off in thought and the inability to finish sentences. Clutterers also ramble on in a confused way. This may be due to the feed-back of inaccurate and distorted speech patterns. Hughlings Jackson long ago wrote, 'We speak not only to tell other people what we think but to tell ourselves what we think'. Henry Head (1925) discussed the importance of this statement in his approach to aphasia and disorders of rhythm, stress and syntax. In more recent years there has been an upsurge of interest in the influence of feed-back of one's own speech following on the discovery that delayed auditory feed-back produced stuttering. Postman and Rosenweig (1957) have also shown the close relationship between sensory and motor performance in speaking. They found in their experimental research that the recognition of verbal stimuli is influenced to an important degree by the *verbal* (speaking) habits of the speaker. Recognition of speech signals was improved by strengthening and differentiation of verbal habits, i.e. the saying over of what was heard.

Libermann (1957) in his important research into how the individual perceives and discriminates speech signals, found that the individual has to say over to himself what he has heard when learning new and unfamiliar speech patterns. Libermann states: 'Speech is perceived by reference to articulation—that is, that the articulatory movements and their sensory effects mediate between the acoustic stimulus and the event we call perception'. The individual mimes orally what he hears, then responds to his articulatory movements and the proprioceptive and tactile stimulus. Libermann reverses the long-accepted view regarding the primary importance of acoustic stimuli in recognition of speech and suggests that perception is actually more closely related to articulation than is the acoustic stimulus itself. The speech therapist who doubts this may recall his difficulty as a student in perceiving the strange sound combinations of his phonetics instructor and the need to say these over to himself or mime the necessary articulatory movements. Visual cues from watching the instructor's mouth were also important for identification. Anyone who invigilates at a written phonetics examination must be amazed at the sight of the examinees mouthing to themselves as they write their phonetic transcriptions and descriptions. The sight calls to mind forcibly the oral gesture theory of the origin of language put forward by Paget in 1930.

When a Parkinson patient is in the dilemma of being unable to hear his speech or control his speech organs on account of akinesia, an amplifier which raises vocal volume to the threshold of audibility must help him to recapture auditory control. Thus phrasing and speed of utterance can improve in intelligent and well-motivated individuals. In fact amplification appears on the whole the most promising and logical approach to the Parkinson patient's speech problems.

PSYCHIATRIC CHEMO-THERAPY

Sedative drugs given to disturbed patients can have harmful side effects and produce Parkinsonian symptoms. (See page 218.)

SENILE TREMOR

A tremor occurs not infrequently in old age. It is finer and more rapid than Parkinson tremor and is not accompanied by muscular weakness or rigidity. Brain (1941) describes it as not being present in the limbs at rest and says it occurs first only in voluntary movements. It is even more marked in the upper limbs and especially the head. The tremor of the laryngeal muscles may be heard in the voice of senile patients.

FAMILIAL TREMOR (MINOR'S DISEASE)

Familial tremor may occur in several members of the same family and in successive generations (Critchley, 1949). It may occur in infancy and generally develops in the first twenty-five years. The fine tremor is increased in voluntary movements but remains constant generally throughout life. It can be generalised or be especially conspicuous in hands, tongue, lips and also larynx. It is increased in voluntary movement and therefore speech, and is aggravated by emotional disturbance. We have had experience of two such cases, both women, referred to the speech department from the laryngologist with diagnosis of 'functional' disorder. There is need for a neurological examination to exclude other forms of tremor which may arise in hysteria, hyperthyroidism, toxaemia, disseminated sclerosis, Parkinsonism, bulbar and supra-bulbar palsy and cerebellar ataxia (Aronson *et al.*, 1968). The developmental history, however, will give a clear indication of its familial nature. In both the patients referred to above, the vocal tremor was of long standing but emotional disorders had suddenly exacerbated the symptoms and the voice disorder became the focus of anxiety. Reassurance and instruction in relaxation and exploration of environmental difficulties helped these patients.

In non-familial cases of generalised tremor the necessity for a neurological assessment is all the more important. The fact that the voice is so markedly affected by tremor is a positive sign that it may not be a psychogenic symptom.

LOWER MOTOR NEURONE LESIONS

Bulbar Dysarthria

The lower motor neurones have their origin in the motor nuclei of the brain stem (bulbar medulla) and grey matter in the anterior horns of the spinal cord, and are distributed to groups of muscle fibres in particular muscles. Lesions in the bulb produce a flaccid paralysis and wasting in the muscles of deglutition, articulation and phonation in proportion to the nuclei involved. Fibrillation of the muscles of the tongue can be seen. The cranial nerves involved are all or some of the following:

> Trigeminal (5th) to face;
> Facial (7th) to face and lips;
> Glossopharyngeal (9th) to tongue, pharynx and palate;
> Vagus (10th) to larynx and respiratory muscles;
> Hypoglossal (12th) to tongue.

In adults a progressive bulbar palsy may develop as a complication of bulbar disease. The distribution of muscle atrophy varies according to the nuclei involved. As the disease is progressive, speech therapy cannot benefit the patient. Speech is slow and laboured, the voice hollow and uninflected and the muscles tire quickly so that isolated words may be just recognisable but a phrase deteriorates into laboured phonation with such severe dysarthria that articulation can hardly be said to exist and eventually the patient is anarthric. Deglutition becomes increasingly difficult. The patient can resort to writing for purposes of communication when speech is no longer intelligible and intellect remains intact.

In children bulbar paralysis is often caused by poliomyelitis. The disease may be restricted to the anterior horns of the spinal cord but may include, or be confined to, damage to the motor nuclei of the bulb and involve facial, lingual, pharyngeal and respiratory muscles (Bulbar poliomyelitis). Rarely the palate alone is paralysed and nasal speech may be the first and only symptom noticed (pages 253 and 259).

A considerable degree of muscular recovery can take place after an acute attack of bulbar poliomyelitis has subsided. This is not due to repair of the grey matter itself but to the disappearance of oedema. Grey cells which have been destroyed cannot recover or be replaced and the muscle fibres connected with the lower motor neurone fibres suffer total atrophy. The possibility of response to speech and voice therapy is wholly dependent upon the quantity of muscular tissue preserved.

Since the widespread use of anti-polio vaccines the disease is now controlled and it is a rare cause of nasal speech in children. The seasonal epidemics which were frequent only a few years ago and produced each year a number of nasal dysphonias in the speech clinics are now fortunately a thing of the past. In the underdeveloped countries poliomyelitis is still a hazard and especially for workers from the developed countries who were not immunised as children before the discovery of an effective vaccine.

CEREBELLAR LESIONS

Cerebellar Dysarthria

Lesions involving the cerebellum give rise to decrease in muscle tone and disorders in co-ordination and balance (ataxia). 'The smooth, sweeping, continuous movements of the normal individual are dissociated into their constituent parts' (Berry and Eisenson, 1962). Movements are exaggerated and may overshoot their mark. The co-ordination necessary for modulation in phonation is so clumsy and slow that speech seems jerky and slurred. The rhythmic disturbance in speech may be so pronounced that one can identify the changeover from one muscle group to another. The most conspicuous symptoms of ataxia according to Grewel (1957a) are slurred and slow speech (bradylalia or bradyarthria) and hesitation or cluttering, besides failure in modulation and inconsistent pitch. Peacher (1950) states that rhythm and phonation are more impaired than articulation. Speech is slow, drawling, monotonous, with a tendency to staccato and scanning. Vowels may be nasalised and bilabial consonants explosive. Speech may be only slightly affected or so clumsy and slurred that it is unintelligible.

Disseminated sclerosis (multiple sclerosis) may give rise to many symptoms of neurological lesion, but commonly causes ataxic dysarthria. Sudden exacerbations and remissions of the disease are to be expected and speech therapy can be helpful at certain stages of this progressive disease. A primary attack in the twenties may not be followed by a secondary for 10 or 20 years. Speech practice must, in the initial stages of recovery, be moderate and muscular tension and fatigue avoided during treatment, since rest seems important in recovery.

In Friedrich's ataxia and hereditary cerebellar ataxia, the ataxic speech movements produce unstable high pitch and abnormalities in speech melodic patterns. Nasality is a characteristic symptom. Breathing patterns are also abnormal and the voice disorder gross. An inspiratory laugh is often a peculiar phenomenon

CRANIAL TRAUMA

Speech and voice disorders after severe cranial trauma are seen in increasing frequency in patients involved in traffic accidents (Kremer *et al.*, 1947). Recovery from a long coma may be followed by complete lack of speech (akinetic mutism). Aphasia may exist, and a differential diagnosis between aphasia and the akinetic mutism (anarthria) owing to lesions in the central grey matter has to be made. Speech when it returns is slow, monotonous, nasal and blurred. Laughing may be characterised by a hollow and nasal tone. There is frequently some limb involvement associated with brain damage. The patient when recovering consciousness is exceedingly disorientated, restless and noisy and must be kept quiet, and stimulation must be avoided as much as possible. Speech demands should not be made upon the patient until some degree of emotional control has returned. Visits from the speech therapist during the period of mutism, however, are valuable and reassuring. The therapist can talk quietly, promising to help with speech when the patient is well enough, recounting news without expecting answers and gradually forming a relationship in which voice and speech therapy may subsequently prosper besides currently alleviating the despair and suffering experienced at this time.

St. Onge and Calvert (1959) emphasise the value of this good relationship with patients recovering from brain stem damage due to trauma. Hostility may develop towards those in attendance and resemble paranoid symptoms. In the cases they described, the patients did not include the speech pathologist in their resentment, which permitted continued help with voice and speech and personality adjustment. These authors stress the psychological shock of awaking from coma to a nightmarish existence of helplessness and handicap, with amnesia for the traumatic incident which caused this condition. We have encountered antagonism to any form of testing which puts pressure on the patient; this should not be attempted until the patient is able to co-operate.

PERIPHERAL NERVE PALSIES

Damage to the cranial nerves may also be caused by neuritis or trauma.

In facial (Bell's) palsy due to neuritis in the 7th cranial nerve, one side of the face is paralysed. The muscles may in time recover entirely especially in younger adults but not so well after late middle age. The muscles may be severely flaccid and speech be muffled by the lips on the affected side which are pulled askew by the healthy muscles from the opposite side. The flaccid muscles of the cheek may also balloon out under the pressure of articulated breath and the voice lacks definition and projection. In long-standing cases a neurosurgical operation can be performed and a facio-hypoglossal anastomosis greatly improves the appearance and speech. It takes three months after the operation for the nerves to regenerate, also at first the tongue movement is weakened and the patient may become depressed. It is helpful at this stage to reassure the patient and give some tongue exercises. Later, patients learn to press the tongue-tip automatically against the teeth in order to activate the facial muscles into a smile.

A neuritis may affect the muscles of the palate after diphtheria causing severe nasal escape (page 254). The movements of the palate recover after a time in all cases.

Neuritic laryngeal nerve palsy may also follow influenza or 'Asian flu'. The voice is lost at first but recovers. Laryngeal palsy also occurs in thyroidectomy (see 'Laryngeal Palsy', Chapter 15).

SYSTEMIC DISEASE

Myasthenia gravis has been described in connection with disorders of nasal resonance (Chapter 12, page 254). The voice may be weak and tires very quickly, and there may be dysphonia and breathlessness (Friedman and Goffin, 1966). Alleviation of the illness results in improvement of voice and articulation. Speech therapy is not indicated. The problem is a medical or surgical one.

ARTERIOSCLEROSIS

The study of the voice in degenerative cerebral disease is largely neglected but may provide important diagnostic clues to the general health of the individual. The voice is such a sensitive barometer of physical and psychological states that it may give the first warning that all is not well with the body. In many middle-aged men and women referred with vocal strain or neurotic ('functional') voice disorders, high blood-pressure has been confirmed, and slight signs of upper motor neurone involvement have explained the vocal weakness or so-called aesthenic voice.

The voice of individuals after stroke and accompanying aphasia have been studied very little. The soft monotonous and mumbling speech of senile patients is difficult to understand. It is often taken to be due to emotional difficulties but appears to be, in many cases, a neurological symptom. The 'broken accent' or dysprosody in residual expressive aphasia has been described in one patient by Monrad-Krohn (1947). The phenomenon is rare but probably not so exceptional as the paucity of literature on the subject indicates. So much attention is paid to the syntactical and phonemic errors in dysphasia that the voice and its message is neglected. We have met several patients with residual expressive aphasia and dysprosody but each presenting very dissimilar features of broken accent. This is an interesting field of aphasology meriting more exact neurological and phonic study. It is sometimes difficult to distinguish, for example, between a severe amnesia and dysphasia in brain-injured patients, but an indication comes from the voice. In amnesia the voice is normally inflected. In the case of jargon aphasia accompanying receptive aphasia, speech is often expressively inflected and similar to the conversational jargon of the two-year-old. Dysprosody occurring in the relatively fluent speech of a resolving expressive aphasia is thought to be due to a dysarthria or dyspraxia and may remain, as in Monrad Krohn's patient, the only persisting symptom of the original lesion.

DYSARTHROPHONIA IN CEREBRAL PALSY

The neurological picture in most cases of children suffering from considerable brain damage is exceedingly complex. The damage follows no set pattern. Every child differs regarding the particular individual involvement of the nervous system as Peacher (1949 and 1950); Grewel (1960); Ingram and Barn (1961), and many others emphasise. Baf and Ingram (1955) have drawn attention to the dire need for a system of classification which may provide a common plan for diagnosis and treatment and so resolve the utter confusion which exists over the comparative advantages of rival methods of treatment and claims made by physiotherapists, speech therapists and educationists. Grewel (1960) has attempted to describe the speech symptoms of 'encephalopathy'. Ingram (1960) and Grewel (1960) stress the common occurrence of mental defect, language disorders, spatial constructive, and temporo-spatial disorders, besides directional (left-right) difficulties. Hearing disorders in athetoid children have been emphasised by Fisch and Bach (1961). Developmental aphasia, dyslexia and dysgraphia are common. Strauss and Lehtinen (1947) and later Strauss and Kephart (1955) gave impetus to research in America into the profound emotional and educational problems arising out of the disabilities in sensory organisation experienced by brain-injured children. In England research has lagged behind but the generous endowment of university research centres by the parents' organisation of the Spastics' Society has in the past decade opened up a new and hopeful era in the history of cerebral palsy in this country.

Besides the articulation and language disorders encountered, the voice is often seriously impaired. Rutherford (1944) conducted a comparative study of rate, force, pitch, rhythm and quality in the speech of children handicapped by cerebral palsy. He compared the speech of normal, spastic and athetoid children in order to define more clearly the differences between them. By 'speech' he specifically states that he refers to production of speech and the attributes of voice, recognising their inseparable dualism. The speech of 48 athetoid and 74 spastic children was rated on a three-point scale for pitch, loudness, rate and rhythm. He came to the conclusion that there was no such thing as 'characteristic' athetoid or spastic speech. The speech of both groups showed similar and divergent symptoms. Generally speaking, however, the athetoids had more loud, low-pitched, monotonous and breathy voices. Rutherford also noted that the speech attributes examined (rate, rhythm, loudness, pitch, breathiness) were correlated with control of the breathing apparatus. Differences between mobility of the speech musculature and breath control are based upon the neuro-physiological impairment and should determine differential therapy for the two groups of athetoid and spastic.

Byrne (1959) evaluated the speech of 37 athetoids and 37 spastics with normal hearing who were judged educable by a psychologist. The spastics were found to be considerably better at accurate production of vowels and diphthongs than the athetoids. Both groups were considerably more proficient in the area of voice than in that of consonant articulation. Although the differences between spastic and athetoid groups for consonants and vowels were not statistically significant, the spastics had higher or mean scores on all sub-tests.

Ataxic disorders are described in cerebral palsied children by Ingram and Barn (1961), who emphasise the associated speech dysrhythmia and pitch disorders. Speech is described as being divided into irregular segments, resembling cluttering, and it has a tendency to accelerate on a high pitch, then slow down on a falling pitch.

SUGGESTED LINES OF TREATMENT IN DYSARTHROPHONIAS OF
CEREBRAL PALSY

Treatment of dysarthrophonia in children must differ radically from that for the adult with established conditioned speech co-ordinations. The adult knows what he did to speak before his illness and what he must do now; his intellectual concepts of utterance remain largely unimpaired and he has the memory of old patterns against which to match the new. The child, however, has to learn from the beginning and by imitating what he hears he must learn to accommodate to his motor disorders. He will need guidance in the achievement of movements which will only partly approximate normality. The physiotherapist and speech therapist need to work together, literally side by side, establishing relaxation, the best posture and the respiratory co-ordination and controlled movements which form the basis of voice work. But how often is this ideal of physiotherapy and speech therapy and the team approach stressed in teaching, and how often is it neglected in practice? The cerebral-palsied child requires assessment by neurologist and psychologist, psychiatrist, paediatrician and otologist, whose explanations and advice need always to be available and give direction to the practical work of physiotherapist, speech therapist and teacher. Too often ortho-education is practised by the expert in isolation struggling in ignorance to do his best for the child.

Levitt (1962) in her realistic and practical little book on physiotherapy in cerebral palsy advocates combining the best techniques from all the seemingly conflicting methods of physical treatment for cerebral palsy, most of which have value in some but not all conditions. She believes it is wrong to impose the aim of normalcy on children with incurable lesions. The aim is adequate function with as good a pattern of movement as is possible for each individual child. Levitt's remarks are as valid for speech and voice as for locomotion and posture. Insisting upon normality imposes anxiety on all concerned and introduces harmful emotional factors into the educational picture owing to discouragement due to failure and extreme frustration. Ingram (1960) also comments against the dangers of speech therapy with these children. The child must receive encouragement and experience success. Guidance must be given in the acquisition of new speech skills and help provided in the passage from one developmental mile-stone to the next when each particular child is physiologically ready to take the next step. Thus co-ordination of expiration with phonation of vowels, with inflexion and rhythm must precede babbling of syllables as is the way in the normal development of infant vocalisation (Grewel, 1959). It is important to encourage cooing and babbling early, in the first year, though articulate speech always develops late in these children. Byrne (1959) found that in the three main stages of speech development the cerebral-palsied child was much later than the normal child. On an average the first word did not appear until 15 months, two-word sentences until 3 years and three-word sentences until 6 years 6 months. She also noted that sounds were acquired in the following order:

[w, b, j, m, d, n, h, g, p, k, tʃ, f, v, ŋ, ð, z, dʒ, l, ʃ, s, r, θ, ŋ].

This would appear to provide a guide from which consonants may be selected for babble syllables. She also noted that consonants were mostly used at the beginning of words; fewer were used in the medial position and very few in the final position. This matches the obvious and increasing difficulty in organising a complex sequence of articulatory increments when co-ordination is severely impaired. In speech work, omission of medial and final consonants should be accepted as they are probably impossible until the age of 5 or 6 when dysarthria may moderate, and consonant blends should not be attempted till later. The child using initial consonants only and a well-inflected and flowing voice may be sufficiently articulate to be intelligible. Intelligible communication and not perfect articulation is the primary goal. Consonants may be taught in isolation and the auditory and kinaesthetic training involved will ensure inclusion of consonants in speech when neuro-physiological maturation allows. It is a grave mistake in our opinion to stress consonant articulation at the expense of sacrificing the melodic features of speech.

Snidecor (1948) describing the speech correctionist in the cere-bral palsy team, stresses the need for relaxation as the cornerstone to all speech work. He advocates a reclining position for the child and the development of flowing vocalisation—bilabial syllables for the athetoid and prolonged vowels for the spastic. Simple nonsense syllables are recommended in place of tongue exercises. 'Easy does it' is the basis throughout.

The Bobath (1953) method based on reflex inhibition for

eliciting speech has also been described by Marland (1953) and
Mysak (1959a). Desensitisation of the oral zone is recommended.
Secondly, facilitation of phonation follows with the child in a
supine position with flexed abducted knees, with shoulders fixed
on the therapist's arm and head falling back. Voicing is elicited
by vibrating the chest with the therapist's other hand while the
therapist vocalises the desired sound for the child to imitate.
After a period, vocalisation follows. Efficient respiratory patterns
must be developed. Facilitated babbling along the lines of motokinaesthetic speech training first described by Young and Hawk
(1955) may be introduced.

Reverse breathing and inspiratory phonation are corrected by
some physiotherapists by rolling the child over on his back,
giving support to the neck and shoulder on the therapist's arm
as he goes over and bringing the knees up on to the chest. Expiration takes place as the diaphragm ascends under the tensed and
compressed abdominal muscles. Inspiration takes place as the
child lies flat on his back while the therapist moves his legs into
the bent knee position and straightens them, synchronising
movements with expiration and inspiration. Vocalising on the
expiratory phase of the cycle follows. Then in a resting position,
back, head and neck supported by cushions, the therapists' hands
on chest guiding the respiratory movements, vocalisation may
also be elicited. Imitation of cooing or vowel glides and babbling
with different rhythmic patterns should follow. Even though
speech and language and the symbolic use of these sounds may be
greatly retarded the inherited and reflex urge of the infant to
vocalise should be capitalised. The normal infant cries as a reflex
reaction to hunger and discomfort, later he uses voice to demand
attention to his needs, but it must not be forgotten that he also
uses voice in gurgles, coos and song to express happiness and well-
being and make social contact even before he babbles. Even deaf
children express their inherited vocal patterns in this way. Just as
it is important that the genetic inheritance should be fostered and
not allowed to atrophy in the first year of the deaf baby, so it
should be fostered in the cerebral-palsied child until such time as
neuromuscular and intellectual development allow the raw
materials of speech to be used to full advantage in communication.
Grewel (1959) says, 'The value of the sentence melody behaviour
in the infant cannot be overestimated in the later use of language.
It is a fact of primary importance that children make use of
sentence melodies, long before the use of real language is possible'.

Palmer (1947) advising upon the age at which speech training (articulation) should commence, says that a degree of motor control must be achieved first. The usual signs are control of the muscles holding the head erect and development of sucking, swallowing and chewing reflexes out of which articulate speech may evolve. Froeschels' chewing methods are advocated (page 172). Evans (1947) advises as little effort as possible in speech. Fothergill and Harrington (1949), in discussing the stretch reflex of spastic muscles, describe the 'ballistic' movements of normal articulation and believe that drills for exercising and loosening up the tongue, lips and jaws must set off the stretch reflex. Articulatory movements should be 'vowel-like', and controlled slow movements are necessary within the threshold of the stretch reflex. In the athetoid the reverse policy may be necessary and Palmer (1949) advocates repetitive movements of the mandible, lips and tongue to loosen up the muscles.

If the child is deaf, and this possibility should always be investigated in the routine examination of hearing and comprehension for speech, the educational difficulties are greatly increased. The speech therapist will in this case need the help and advice of a teacher of the deaf who may take over treatment altogether. Both teacher of the deaf and speech therapist may, however, collaborate and the speech therapist can undoubtedly contribute her specialised knowledge and skill in obtaining voice and speech improvement.

Co-ordination, rhythm and inflexion in speech and voice may be assisted in musical activities such as tapping, clapping, singing and reciting to a musical accompaniment. This is advocated by most remedial teachers as described by Alvin (1961). These rhythmic exercises develop the necessary stress, inflexion and flow of voice which are such features of intelligible expression. Levitt (1962) stresses the benefit of group treatment in speech and singing activities, which is greatly enjoyed by the children and often achieves more than individual treatment.

A concept of treatment very foreign to western ideas has emerged from Budapest and the institute for movement therapy established by Professor Peto (Cotton, 1965). Children are admitted to a residential school where they are taught by 'conductors' in which the role of mother, teacher, physio-, occupational and speech therapists and teacher are incorporated in one person. The method is based on the concept of 'rhythmical intention' and the child is encouraged to perform active movements by himself unaided and guided by the child's own speech and cortical control of movement. The method is based on the teaching of Luria (1961, 1963). A simple example of the principle involved is that a small child told to squeeze a bulb in his hand cannot do so and initiate the movement unless he says 'go-go'. Play activity we know stimulates speech and vocalisation (Greene, 1967a). Conductor therapy may probably succeed, not so much by reason of its basic principles as by the extreme consistency of method, avoiding the conflicting aims and instructions in at least the British idea of a 'team approach'. In this, each individual expert attached to a team takes over the child for treatment separately for physical exercise, speech or lessons, one after the other and, deplorable as it is, often working alone and along his own lines. Moreover each expert advises the mother according to the best of his ability. The prospect, of course, is happier if the child is in a residential school but in the vitally important early years he is, of course, at home.

This brings us to the absolute need of the mother's co-operation which at every stage of treatment is vital to the achievement of any progress. The mother must perforce be regarded as the most important member of the rehabilitation team. The child's difficulties must be explained, the reasons for the treatment given, and not only adequately demonstrated to her but the special aim of specific exercises described. The mother must not set the goal too high nor too low. Being the parent of a physically and possibly mentally handicapped child is no easy task. The mother bears the brunt of the educational difficulties involved but the father's help and support, especially in keeping up his wife's morale, is essential. Mothers tend to reject or to develop an over-protective attitude towards the child in a desperate attempt to make up to him for all those things of which he will remain deprived, and for which she consciously or unconsciously may feel to blame. She needs guidance, education and encouragement every bit as much as the child. She has to learn not to do too much, not to over-protect, to hold back when it is so much easier to help, yet to help when necessary and not allow failure to destroy confidence. The brain-injured child, more than the normal child, needs the security of a loving, accepting and harmonious home in which to develop his limited potentialities.

15   Laryngeal palsy

In this section we shall not discuss laryngeal paralysis due to lesions in the upper motor neurone, which were described in connection with dysarthophonia, but lesions in the lower motor neurone tract. These may occur either at the point of origin in the medulla oblongata (bulb), causing the bulbar syndrome (Chapter 13), or in the peripheral pathways to the laryngeal muscles. The nervous lesions may be either bilateral or unilateral. The muscles affected are rendered flaccid at first and are later subject to varying degrees of atrophy and fibrosis. These factors influencing the paralysed laryngeal muscles are of some importance in determining the eventual position adopted by the affected vocal fold after a period of time.

The Vagus (10th cranial nerve) which supplies all the muscles of the larynx has an interesting course which must be known if damage to the nerve pathways at different levels is to be understood in terms of laryngeal paralysis. Some of the fibres originate in the medulla in the nucleus ambiguus while others originate at a higher level. Fibres from the upper section of the nucleus ambiguus join the glosso-pharyngeal nerve (9th cranial) and those from the inferior portion join the accessory cranial nerve (11th cranial) (Gray, 1949). These nerves, the 9th, 10th and 11th cranial nerves, are so intimately connected in the medulla that all the muscles supplied by them are frequently involved either equally or progressively in lesions of the medulla oblongata. For this reason Walshe (1952) groups them together in pathological conditions affecting the nucleus ambiguus in what he terms the 'glossopharyngeal-accessorius complex'. Nuclear lesions of the vagus may be associated, therefore, with paralysis of the palate, pharynx, tongue and larynx (Bosma, 1953).

The vagus forms a flat cord from its many united filaments and leaves the skull through the jugular foramen and passes vertically down the neck within the carotid sheath. The superior laryngeal nerve branches off from the vagus at the ganglion nodosum (or inferior ganglion) below the level of the jugular foramen and subdivides into the internal and external superior laryngeal nerves. The internal branch of the superior laryngeal nerve consists of both sensory and secreto-motor fibres. The external branch of the superior laryngeal nerve provides the motor supply to the crico-thyroid muscle.

The left and right recurrent laryngeal nerves supply the rest of the muscles of the larynx. They differ significantly with regard

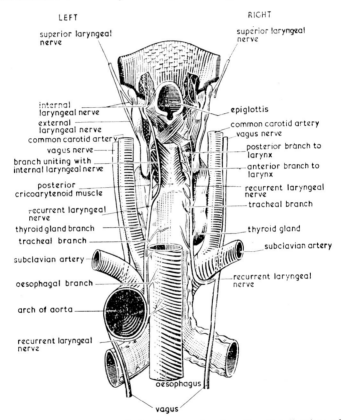

LEFT   RIGHT

superior laryngeal nerve

superior laryngeal nerve

internal laryngeal nerve
external laryngeal nerve
common carotid artery
vagus nerve
branch uniting with internal laryngeal nerve
posterior cricoarytenoid muscle
recurrent laryngeal nerve
thyroid gland branch
tracheal branch
subclavian artery
oesophagal branch
arch of aorta
recurrent laryngeal nerve

epiglottis
common carotid artery
vagus nerve
posterior branch to larynx
anterior branch to larynx
recurrent laryngeal nerve
tracheal branch
thyroid gland
subclavian artery
recurrent laryngeal nerve

oesophagus
vagus

Fig. 37   Posterior view of the larynx showing the distribution of the left and right laryngeal nerves

to their origin and pathway (Fig. 37). The right recurrent laryngeal nerve arises from the main trunk of the vagus in front of the subclavian artery and the left recurrent laryngeal nerve arises from the vagus at the arch of the aorta round which it winds before ascending to the larynx. On account of its more extensive course the left recurrent nerve is more liable to injury than the right, and is especially open to pressure from aortic aneurysm. The left vocal cord is found to be affected twice as frequently as the right in laryngeal palsy according to St. Clair-Thomson and Negus (1955).

The recurrent laryngeal nerves on both sides ascend the groove between the trachea and oesophagus for a variable distance in different individuals and then divide into anterior and posterior branches before entering the larynx behind the cricothyroid articulation. The recurrent laryngeal nerves are especially vulnerable in the operation of thyroidectomy below the level of their entry into the larynx.

On account of the distribution of the superior and recurrent laryngeal nerves it is important to remember that in order to produce a total paralysis of the larynx on one side, the lesion must occur at, or above, the level of the ganglion nodosum before the superior laryngeal nerve branches off from the vagus. This means that in lesions involving the recurrent laryngeal nerves the cricothyroid muscle will be spared. Nuclear lesions of the vagus already described in connection with bulbar palsies are caused by a variety of pathological conditions (Walshe, 1952): disseminated sclerosis, medullary tumours, encephalitis lethargica, tabes dorsalis, focal thrombosis and chronic bulbar palsy. Poliomyelitis (Bosma, 1953) is also a possible cause of a lesion since it confines itself to focal infection of motor nerve cells in the brain-stem and spinal cord. Damage to the nucleus ambiguus may result in complete laryngeal paralysis as it involves both superior and recurrent laryngeal nerves.

The consequences of peripheral damage to the recurrent laryngeal nerves have long been recognised. The following quaint account of the crude experiments of Andreas Vesalius is to be found in his *De Corporis Humani Fabrica*, 1943 (Taylor, 1949), and is of historical interest. In order to demonstrate the connection between the voice and the recurrent nerves, Vesalius chose to carry out dissection of a living sow because this animal could be relied upon to squeal continuously. Having described how by a long incision in the neck he exposed the wind-pipe by division of the muscles, he continues: 'Then I observe the recurrent nerves also attached to the wind-pipe, and these I sometimes compress by ligatures and sometimes sever; this I do first on one side so that when the nerve is compressed or severed it may be clearly observed that half the voice is lost, and that when both nerves are damaged the voice is completely lost, and that if I loosen the ligature it returns'.

This, an early account of the effect of this experiment upon the voice, is not entirely accurate, of course.

Peripheral damage to the recurrent nerves may be caused by tumours in the neck or in the apex of the lungs by enlarged bronchial glands, lung tumour, aortic aneurysm, mitral stenosis and enlarged left auricle. Patients may be referred with functional voice disorder when suffering from heart trouble and it must be remembered that there may be a real vocal weakness due to pressure on the laryngeal nerve.

External injuries from gunshot wounds or blows sustained in car accidents may also cause laryngeal palsy.

Enlargement of the thyroid gland and penetration into the retro-oesophageal and tracheal areas can create pressure on the laryngeal nerve and thus impair function of the muscles. This is of rare occurrence. Sonninen (1960) reports only one such case of laryngeal palsy pre-operatively due to compression in a series of 131 patients. Thyrotoxicosis itself does not produce palsy, though it may change the voice.

Peripheral neuritis and a temporary palsy may be caused by toxic conditions which prevent conveyance of nervous impulses to the muscles. A complete paralysis fixes the cord in the para-median position in these cases. The condition is usually unilateral, and complete recovery is to be expected once the toxaemia subsides. Lead poisoning is a toxic condition causing laryngeal neuritis. Commonly cited examples of systemic disease causing neuritis and vocal fold paralysis are diphtheria and typhoid (Musgrove, 1952). Virus infections such as measles and pertussis (whooping cough) and influenza also cause nerve neuritis. Acute localised inflammation in herpes zoster (shingles) can also reduce nervous efficiency. Jasienska and Kuzniarz (1964) described a case of a 50-year-old man with herpes zoster in the head and hemiplegia of palate, pharynx and larynx.

CHILDHOOD VOCAL PALSIES

Vocal palsies in children are not uncommon. Cavanagh (1955) reviewed the available literature on the subject and reported upon her personal examination of 107 children. Thirty-seven of these children had laryngeal paralysis, most were unilateral but 10 were bilateral, some were congenital and others acquired. A wide degree of variation in improvement of the airway and recovery of vocal fold movement was noted. Of interest are her observations on those children with unilateral paralysis in which the healthy fold was seen to abduct 3 to 5 times to one abduction of the recovering fold. In several babies with congenital laryngeal stridor, one arytenoid was placed further forward than the other while the aryepiglottic fold on the affected side was usually rolled towards the mid-line and seemed shortened. We ourselves examined a 7-year-old boy with this condition which was accompanied by a unilateral palatal palsy on the opposite side to that of the affected fold. He had an inspiratory stridor on effort and when speaking.

Van Thal (1962) reported upon an interesting case of familial laryngeal palsy with four generations of aphonia in the same family. This report appears to be unique in the literature on the subject of congenital laryngeal palsy.

THE BEHAVIOUR OF THE LARYNGEAL MUSCLES IN LARYNGEAL PALSY: SEMON'S LAW

In 1881 the laryngologist Felix Semon propounded his famous clinical observations by which he endeavoured to explain the anatomical reasons for the various well-recognised but little-understood types of laryngeal paralyses known to clinical laryngology, and the fact that in some cases of paralysis the vocal fold was initially close to the mid-line and later took up a position more laterally. In his clinical remarks Semon commented upon 'the proclivity of the abductor fibres of the recurrent laryngeal nerve to become affected sooner than the abductor fibres, or even exclusively in cases of undoubted central or peripheral injury or disease of the roots or trunks of the pneumogastric, spinal accessory or recurrent nerves'. By 'central' Semon made it quite clear that he referred to nuclear and not supranuclear lesions (Musgrove, 1952). The validity of these observations was accepted so completely that they came to be known as Semon's Law. Sir Felix Semon, like Sir Victor Negus today, was the greatest authority on the larynx in his time and so was able to expound opinions which nobody dared to question. It is charming to know that he treated Gladstone (who addressed Queen Victoria always like a public meeting) for hoarseness, and prescribed vocal rest (Hutzinga, 1966).

Negus (1931) put forward his explanation in support of Semon's law which he based on his study of the comparative anatomy of the larynx in animals, birds and fishes, and evolutionary development. He postulated that the abductor fibres are affected first in laryngeal paralysis because they are of later evolutionary development than the adductors. The 'sphincteric' group of muscles (adductors), because of their vital and protective function in prevention of foreign bodies entering the larynx and lungs, were thought to be of earlier origin phylogenetically than the abductor group, and therefore less easily disturbed than the abductor muscles. This is Negus's phylogenetic theory, now considered old-fashioned.

If the hypothesis incorporated in Semon's Law is correct, it follows that in organic lesions involving the vagus the abductor muscles will be paralysed before the adductor and, moreover, paralysis of the adductor muscles cannot occur alone but only in association with the abductor muscles. An adductor paralysis occurring in isolation will always be of non-organic origin and psychogenic by nature (i.e. hysterical). In such a paralysis, abduction of the folds is unaffected and the abductor movement is observable in deep inspiration, while the function of adduction is preserved in coughing.

Semon's Law, though providing a simple diagnostic rule in clinical practice which is generally found to be sound, never explained all the bizarre positions assumed by the folds in paralysis. As the numbers of exceptional cases following thyroidectomy increased, the infallibility of Semon's Law came to be questioned, especially in America and this promoted a number of research projects and reports (King and Gregg, 1948; Morrison, 1952; Stroud and Zwiefach, 1956).

Capps in his Semon Lecture (1958) gives a comprehensive historical survey of the facts and theories put forward in this controversy since Semon made his original observations. He concludes that Semon's observation concerning the greater vulnerability of the abductor fibres represents an undisputed clinical observation which signifies either an *incipient* sign of a progressive lesion or a *terminal* sign of a subsidiary paralysis. He avoids linking type of paralysis with actual site of lesion and speech therapists are advised to follow his example.

Arnold (1957) has also reviewed the literature and gives an extensive bibliography. He concludes that the majority of authors favour Grossman's concept (1897) to the effect that the median position of the vocal cord indicates complete recurrent paralysis while an intermediary position of the cord is interpreted as a combination of paralysis from both superior and recurrent laryngeal nerves.

Faaborg-Anderson and Nykøbing (1965) came to a similar conclusion from an up-to-date and scientific electromyographic investigation of patients suffering from laryngeal palsy. They state that a lesion of the recurrent laryngeal nerve without paresis of the crico-thyroid muscles is associated with *paramedian* position of the vocal cord. A lesion of the recurrent laryngeal nerve plus superior laryngeal nerve results in paresis of the cricothyroid and complete paralysis producing an *intermediate* position of the vocal cord. These authors stress the importance of the cricothyroid muscle for positioning of the vocal cord. When it is involved the vocal process of the arytenoid cartilage is in a lower position on the paralysed side than that on the

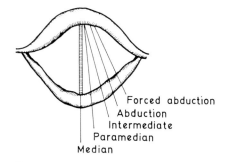

Forced abduction
Abduction
Intermediate
Paramedian
Median

FIG. 38   Vocal cord palsies: lines of orientation

healthy side, despite the fact that the transverse arytenoid muscle is supplied by both left and right recurrent laryngeal nerve branches. The transverse arytenoid of course assists in adduction only; the posterior cricoarytenoid braces the arytenoid back and when paralysed the arytenoid will be pulled and tilted forward by the cricothyroid. On the other hand in total paralysis of one side the transverse arytenoid muscle on account of its double innervation from both recurrent nerves does not atrophy and may, therefore, be responsible for the final position of the cord (Kirchner, 1966). Furthermore, atrophy and shrinkage of muscle tissues and replacement by fibrous tissue in thyroarytenoid and cricoarytenoid muscles could explain the rare case of a vocal cord, originally paralysed in the mid-line, gradually returning to a more abducted position.

The view today of vocal-cord paralysis is that the position of the vocal cord is not subject to any fixed neurological laws, evolutionary or otherwise, but is determined entirely by the interaction of a combination of neuropathological and anatomical factors (Hiroto *et al.*, 1968). Millar (1969) advocates discarding the concepts of adductor and abductor paralysis altogether. Millar favours simple reference to the position of the vocal cord as seen and whether it lies in the paramedian or intermediate position. This information is what actually concerns the speech pathologist in rehabilitation, but possible changes of position and the terminal result in long term treatment must be understood and reasonable predictions concerning voice improvement formed. The foregoing neuro-pathological review is therefore not an interesting academic exercise but needs to be related to the anatomical and neurological study of the larynx by the student in training.

In summary the factors influencing position of the vocal cords and listed clearly by Capps (1958) are as follows:

(a) continued tensor action of the unparalysed cricothyroid muscle
(b) the plane of the cricoarytenoid joint
(c) the comparative dead weight and pull of the abductor and adductor musculature
(d) the eventual degree of fibrosis of the atrophied musculature
(e) continued adductor action of the interarytenoideus muscle on the unaffected side in unilateral paralysis.

DYSPHONIA IN LARYNGEAL PALSY

The degree of slackness in the paralysed cord, the relative levels of the cords when approximated and the distance from the mid-line at which the affected cord is stabilised, account for a wide variety of dysphonic symptoms among patients all referred to the speech therapist for treatment of one condition—'vocal cord paralysis'. There may be aphonia, a breathy voice with little true voice, a harsh voice with abrupt pitch changes or a relatively good voice but an inability to raise vocal volume without cracking and total inability to manage pitch changes in singing. The prognosis is virtually unpredictable. Some patients recover a normal voice quickly, others do not do so for from six months to a year, despite the paralysed cord shifting towards the mid-line slightly and the healthy cord approximating with it soon after the trauma. Roy, Gardiner and Niblock (1956) comment on the fact that the voice may greatly exceed expectations and unilateral paralysis even go unsuspected after thyroidectomy, so normal may be the voice.

Another important factor which should also be taken into account when treating laryngeal nerve paralysis is that of the degree of damage which may have been sustained by the nerve fibres. This may be complete and irrevocable, or partial and temporary. If the nerve is cut through, no recovery of movement in the muscle concerned is possible. Anastomosis between the severed nerve endings seldom, if ever, takes place despite popular belief, according to Morrison (1952).

Doyle, Brummett and Everts (1967) reported two cases of bilateral abductor paralysis after thyroidectomy in which there was partial recovery of cord function after nerve repair. The nerve will regenerate if the severed ends are sutured in time. These authors advocate immediate exploration when a post-operative abductor paralysis develops. If delayed, the nerve is difficult to find and end-plate degeneration will have occurred and any hope of nerve regeneration is thus lost.

The lower motor neurone type of lesion produced when the nerve is severed results at first in a flaccid paralysis and this is followed by atrophy, fibrosis and contracture of the muscle involved as already described.

Temporary damage to the nerve may be caused by stretching or bruising when the thyroid gland is removed by digital manipulation. In some cases the nerve is caught up when the thyroid artery is ligatured. A nerve is incapable of conveying nervous impulses to the muscle it supplies until it has reverted to normal and this may take weeks or even many months (Harpman, 1952).

The six classic positions assumed by the vocal cords in health and disease as listed by Negus (St. Clair-Thomson *et al.*, 1955):

1. *Median* (adductor, phonatory and mid-line are synonymous with median). The cord adopts a position in the mid-line.

2. *Glottic Chink*

   The cords are adducted but slack allowing minimal separation during respiration.

3. *Paramedian*

   The cord lies slightly to the side of the mid-line and if both are paralysed they are separated posteriorly by a distance of 3·5 or 4 mm.

4. *Cadaveric*

   The cord lies in a position which is between paramedian and gentle abduction. The cord is slack and in the same position as it assumes in the cadaver, hence the name.

5. *Gentle Abduction*

The cord is abducted further than in the cadaveric position, but not fully. This is the position in quiet respiration.

6. *Full Abduction*

The cord is abducted to its fullest limit and the position occurs in forced inspiration when the maximal air-way is necessary.

EIGHT TYPES OF LARYNGEAL PARALYSIS

1. *Unilateral Abductor Paralysis*

The abductor muscle (criocoarytenoid posterior) is paralysed; the affected cord lies in the median position, with the arytenoid tilted forward. The obstruction is sufficient to cause dyspnoea and in phonation the healthy cord approximates with its fellow, the arytenoid passing in front of that on the paralysed side. The voice is hoarse at first but recovers quickly. The singing voice will, however, be impaired.

2. *Bilateral Abductor Paralysis*

Both cords lie in the median position and this condition provides the most serious of the paralyses which may afflict the patient. 'Prognosis is at best uncertain and at worst disastrous' according to Musgrove (1952). The cords assume the glottic chink position and can separate as much as 1 mm. Phonation is possible and the voice strong but difficulty in breathing is extreme and there is pronounced stridor. During sleep breathing is so noisy that it has been described as a respiratory howl. There is considerable danger from asphyxia if the patient should choke or contract an infection of the respiratory tract.

A tracheotomy operation can be performed and a cannula inserted in the tracheal opening, through which the individual can breathe in comfort. By covering the orifice of the cannula air can be directed past the cords and a strong voice is obtained when speaking. If a flap-valve cannula (speaking tube) is used there is no need for digital closure of its orifice.

3. *Complete Unilateral Recurrent Paralysis*

This is the most common type of paralysis and accounts for 90 per cent of all vocal cord palsies, according to King and Gregg (1948). The adductors and abductors are paralysed but the cord does not lie in the cadaveric position for it is maintained in the paramedian by the action of the cricothyroid muscle. When paralysis has been established for some length of time the cord may move over to the mid-line. The transverse arytenoid being innervated from both sides retains some ability to contract,

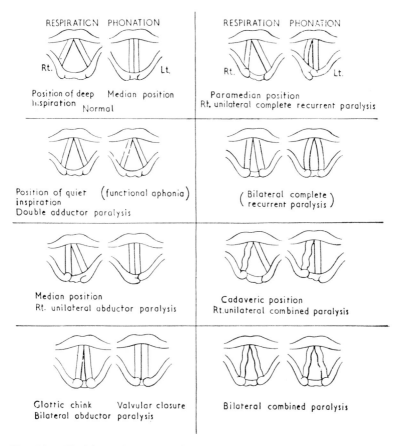

FIG. 39   Positions of the cords in various types of paralysis after Negus (St. Clair-Thomson *et al.*, 1955)

though this is much reduced. It can assist the cricothyroid in shifting the cord towards the mid-line.

The healthy cord continues to adduct normally and is even able to pass over the mid-line and compensate for the deficiency of movement in its fellow. The voice is at first hoarse and breathy but gradually reverts to normal.

4. Complete Bilateral Paralysis

Both cords lie in the paramedian position and the voice is lost. At first the cords are flaccid but in time fibrosis and contracture takes place. The pharyngeal muscles in all probability participate in the excessive effort to approximate the cords and obtain an audible whisper when speaking, Clerf and Baltzell (1952) believe.

After some months, and as much as a year in some cases, the cords approximate and lie in the median position and the patient suffers all the sequelae of a bilateral abductor paralysis and requires similar surgical treatment: arytenoidectomy and lateralisation of the cord by the Woodman operation (page 330).

5. Unilateral Superior Laryngeal Nerve Paralysis

This is a comparatively rare type of palsy on account of the short course followed by the superior laryngeal nerve. The criocothyroid alone is affected. The unopposed pull of the thyro-arytenoid and posterior cricoarytenoid muscles produces slackening along the edge of the cord and the voice is rendered hoarse and rough. In some cases only slight breathiness and lack of pitch change is evident but no visible signs of paralysis. Electromyographic investigation may reveal impaired muscle action. Such cases may be referred to the speech therapist with the incorrect diagnosis of 'functional' disorder of non-organic origin whereas a paresis exists.

6. Bilateral Superior Laryngeal Nerve Paralysis

The cricothyroid on both sides is paralysed. The voice is hoarse, drops in pitch and lacks inflexion.

7. Combined Unilateral Paralysis

A lesion of both recurrent and superior laryngeal nerves produces total paralysis of the cord which lies in the cadaveric position. Aphonia results but with the development of compensatory movement in the healthy cord the voice may recover; recovery of movement of the injured fold or change in position is not to be anticipated.

8. Combined Bilateral Paralysis

The paralysis of both cords is complete. Permanent aphonia exists and there is no means of alleviating the condition.

THYROTOXICOSIS AND THYROIDECTOMY

The thyroid gland is situated in the lower part of the neck opposite the fifth, sixth and seventh cervical vertebrae and first thoracic vertebra. It consists of two lobes joined by an isthmus which crosses the second and third rings of the trachea. The apices of the lobes reach up to the larynx and are in contact with the inferior constrictor of the pharynx and posterior portion of the crico-thyroid muscle. In this area, therefore, the lobes of the gland are in close relation to the recurrent laryngeal nerves before these enter the larynx via the articulation of the cricoid and thyroid cartilages. In the hands of a skilled surgeon severance of the nerves rarely occurs especially as the gland is gently prized away from the larynx by the fingers before surgical removal of any part of it. Holl-Allen (1967) in 1,200 consecutive cases of thyroidectomy reported 1·08 per cent unilateral vocal cord palsies.

Thyrotoxicosis

The thyroid gland, which is controlled by the anterior pituitary gland, is concerned with the maintenance of the metabolism of the body by discharging thyroxine into the blood. The regulation of all life functions, as Arnold (1962) points out, is dependent upon the hypothalamic-pituitary-thyroid-adrenal system. Disturbance of the thyroid will upset the whole chemical and emotional balance of the body. When the normal secretion of thyroxine is diminished (hypothyroidism), cretinism results in infants and myxoedema in adults. When the secretion of thyroxine is increased (hyperthyroidism) the individual suffers from thyrotoxicosis; or if associated with protrusion of the eyeballs it is called ex-ophthalmic goitre, commonly known as Graves' disease. The gland may be visibly and palpably enlarged, but not necessarily so.

Graves' disease is characterised by well-recognised symptoms: tachycardia (abnormally rapid pulse); a warm moist skin and increase in perspiration; diarrhoea; and a big appetite, but with loss of weight on account of increased body metabolism. There is also a pronounced nervousness, and excitability associated with the physical condition (Wittkower and Mandelbrote, 1955). Women are prone to fits of weeping. There are menstrual changes in both hyper- and hypothyroidism.

Sometimes the illness can be arrested by medication. Treatment by X-ray is no longer a popular procedure and thyroidectomy is the most common treatment. Most of the gland is removed in the operation but a sufficient part must be left to prevent myxoedema (page 236). Thyroid disorder is far more common in women than in men. Of 1,000 patients who underwent thyroidectomy reported upon by Lange (1953) only 90 were men. (Five of these cases suffered from temporary laryngeal paralysis, and three suffered permanent injury.)

Goitre is the lay term given to any enlargement of the thyroid gland. Endemic goitre is due to a deficiency of iodine in the drinking water which prevents the blood from assimilating iodine which the thyroid gland must extract in order to manufacture the hormone thyroxine. Endemic goitre may be corrected by minute doses of iodine. Enlargement of the gland may also be due to the growth of an adenoma of the thyroid. Malignant tumour of the thyroid gland is fortunately very rare. In all cases of toxicosis and enlargement of the gland there is the possibility of pressure symptoms: discomfort and difficulty in swallowing may be present, also voice changes may occur due either to pressure on the recurrent laryngeal or changes in the vocal cords as a result of interference with the circulation.

Sonninen (1960) has given a valuable analysis of the symptoms presented by 131 patients before undergoing thyroidectomy. He classified these cases according to the symptoms of toxicosis and tracheal compression present. The table shown below gives his case analysis. Cases having neither toxicosis nor compression are separated from the others.

Group	Certain	Uncertain	Total
1. Compression	22	18	40
2. Toxicosis	23		23
3. Toxicosis and compression	17	39	56
4. No toxicosis, no compression	12		12
			131

The two most important groups are 1 and 2. Laryngeal symptoms occurred mainly in the compression group. This group included cases so slight that they normally tend to be excluded by clinicians. The importance to the speech pathologist of Sonninen's account is that it confirms the opinion that compression from the goitre may be so slight that it may go undetected and be present without signs of toxicosis from the blood analysis, yet produce vocal change which is attributed to functional disorders. Sonninen judged weakness of the voice in shouting to be a symptom of laryngeal asthenia due to compression, a test which would not normally be carried out nor thought sufficiently positive and valid by the average medical specialist.

The tracheal compression symptoms listed by Sonninen are well known to every speech pathologist. They include constant desire to clear the throat, sensations of pressure and pain; paraesthesia; difficulty in swallowing; lowered pitch of the speaking voice; lack of volume; difficulty in singing on a high pitch and uncertainty of pitch. The compression cases may show slight reddening and swelling of the folds, which explains the desire to clear the throat and the discomfort felt. In treatment of many dysphonic middle-aged women diagnosed as 'functional' (psychogenic) cases of voice disorder, it has been impossible to avoid noting the great similarity in their complaints of vocal weakness and discomfort in the throat, besides generalised signs of debility pointing to thyroid disorder. Endocrine imbalance during the climacteric may cause extreme fatigue and muscular weakness, besides changes in the mucous membrane covering the vocal folds. Perello (1962) has emphasised this well-known connection between functional voice disorders and endocrine imbalance in his paper on premenstrual dysphonia.

It may be difficult to persuade medical experts to reconsider diagnosis of functional dysphonia in the case of climacteric neurosis or depression and to consider the possibility of compression from the thyroid gland when there are no signs of thyrotoxicosis in the blood analysis. The experienced speech pathologist, by means of careful observation and assessment of vocal symptoms and emotional balance, may be able to distinguish the real neurotic from the organic case. On the other hand, one must not minimise the undoubted possibility of neurotic pseudo-hyperthyroidism where organic treatment is of no use. The vague complaints put forward by some patients may be a sign of laryngeal neurosis described by Arnold (1962) or really organic as described by Sonninen (1960). Wittkower and Mandelbrote (1955) say: 'The thyroid hormone is primarily a stimulator of cell metabolism and as such it promotes intellectual activity and performance and increases sensitivity and alertness'. It is especially active in adolescence and accounts for the heightened emotional reactions, vitality and growth of intellectual interests at this time. Over-excretion has profound psychological effects upon the individual and the clinical picture of thyrotoxicosis so often closely resembles an anxiety state that diagnosis is extremely difficult. Here we see the psychosomatic 'servo-system' of the body at its most complex. Thyrotoxicosis can be precipitated by shock and it is to be remembered that hysterical aphonia and dysphonia develop frequently after shock or periods of ill health and overwork and mental strain. Thyrotoxicosis can in some cases be cured by rest and the relaxation of a holiday. The families of thyrotoxic patients tend to show nervous traits and over-reaction to the trials and tribulations of life. Wittkower (1955) found disturbed interpersonal relationships between all thyrotoxic patients and their mothers.

LARYNGEAL PALSY AND VOICE THERAPY AFTER THYROIDECTOMY

Wittkower (1955), writing as a psychiatrist, emphasised the need of continued support after thyroidectomy. Treatment of the diseased organ alone is only a temporary expedient in the management of the most disturbed patients. In addition it is necessary to have an appreciation of the patient's personal problems and of the close relationship these problems have on the metabolic disturbances of thyrotoxicosis, which in turn aggravate the emotional disorder present. A long history of personality maladjustment is generally an indication that even thyroidectomy and restoration of normal basal metabolism will not improve the psyche.

The psychological aspect of speech therapy following thyroidectomy resulting in voice impairment is of great importance. Patients suffer considerable depression and complain of excessive fatigue for some time and appear to be unduly concerned with perhaps a slight vocal weakness. They need moral support and sympathy until their body chemistry settles down, and the family's co-operation is needed to provide help and relief from anxieties as far as possible. It is often very reassuring to the nervous patient to have his symptoms explained rationally on the basis of a temporary continuing endocrine disturbance, and to avoid too much emphasis upon the psychological and environmental difficulties which may exaggerate their importance.

A policeman of 59 years who had a particularly strong and resonant voice which was a great asset in his profession, could send mischievous children, as he said, 'scuttling like rabbits into their holes' when he called down the street. He suffered a unilateral paralysis of the vocal fold after thyroidectomy and developed severe depression and anxiety. He could not sit in a room and listen to people talking when he returned home and had to escape into the garden. He had nervous attacks and felt suddenly and unaccountably anxious with tachycardia and sweating and felt ashamed of this. Reassurance that such symptoms were due to temporary endocrine imbalance was helpful. His voice, which had been weak and rough and disappointing considering the degree of compensation achieved by the healthy fold, now quickly improved and his speaking voice became normal.

Hysterical aphonia may undoubtedly follow thyroidectomy especially if the voice is weak after operation. A female patient whose voice was husky for a few days but quite normal when she left hospital, suddenly became aphonic while talking to her mother-in-law. Subsequently her voice alternated between aphonia and falsetto, and she invariably became aphonic when her daughters were 'difficult'. Another patient who was making good progress towards recovery of voice after total unilateral paralysis persisted in losing her voice unaccountably for short periods. Then one day she reported that she had fallen off a kerb and the jolt had restored her voice for good.

Because of the marked emotional lability and anxiety of these patients the speech therapist must be fully aware of the possibility of functional disorder hampering vocal recovery. We have had several patients under treatment for vocal cord palsy dysphonia in whom a great discrepancy between voice production in vocal exercises and spontaneous speech developed. Such a discrepancy is of considerable diagnostic significance. In the two case histories outlined below there was repressed deep resentment directed at the surgeon who had ruined the voice which, unexpressed verbally, was unresolved and caused an unconscious desire to retain the injured voice and demonstrate how badly treated the patient had been. Although litigation was contemplated it was not taken up.

Mr F., aged 27 years, underwent a sub-total thyroid lobectomy in order to have removed a long-standing nodule and old haematoma. He was hoarse after operation but his voice was improving when he left hospital. However, when examined three months later he was complaining of vocal weakness and hoarseness and was found to have a vocal cord paralysis. The cord was fixed only slightly lateral to the mid-line and the healthy cord compensated well and the laryngologist did not understand why the voice was so poor. He was referred for speech therapy. The voice produced had a double note or broke pitch. He complained he could not make himself heard on the factory floor where it was noisy and he had to give instructions. He was a 'storage consultant'. He was able to obtain a normal voice in vowel sounds but forced his voice when speaking. It was felt that there was a strong psychological element interfering with voice production. He was given an amplifier to use, which he liked.

During the next few weeks the following details were divulged gradually as at first he was far from communicative, politely agreeing to everything we said. He was a Belgian married to a physiotherapist and he obviously felt his education and job were much inferior to hers and envied her training and hospital status. He complained about the excessive taxation of his salary and talked of returning home and getting his firm to post him to England and so avoid taxation. He was sorry he had ever had the operation and he certainly would not have agreed if he had known he would have his voice damaged.

The therapist arranged to see Mr F.'s wife and asked her opinion and whether her husband felt very resentful towards the surgeon. She said, 'Oh, yes, it's surprising how many of his friends have told him he should sue the hospital'. She said also she would have 'another go at him' for being so unreasonable. There was never any question of not having the operation since the long-standing adenoma had suddenly haemhorrhaged and he had developed pressure symptoms and obstruction of the air-way. This information was not in the medical notes and was news to us. On his next visit Mr F. was using a deep husky voice but after some discussion of his wife's visit and being challenged with his un-reasonable attitude regarding the operation, coupled with an explanation that the cord was probably paralysed before removal of the adenoma, he seemed happier and his voice improved. He attended once more and this time his voice was normal, strong and well inflected although the slight unilateral abductor paralysis remained.

Mr H., aged 47, had a large nodular goitre removed one year previously. It extended into the chest and behind the trachea and was causing symptoms of stridor and breathlessness. In the operation the left recurrent laryngeal nerve was unavoidably damaged with a resultant vocal cord palsy. The patient was sent to a speech therapist who treated him for ten months after which she felt he was not making progress and that there was a functional basis to the pronounced dysphonia. He asked the surgeon to refer her for treatment to our hospital department and he was seen by one of our laryngologists first who reported that the left vocal cord was immobile in the paramedian position, but the right vocal cord compensated well and he was able to produce a good voice. However, the voice was weaker than to be expected with these laryngeal findings and the impression was that dysphonia was by now largely psychogenic.

When we examined the patient he was exceedingly talkative and communicative, although he said he did not speak much at work or at home, on account of his weak and broken voice. He was obviously tense and anxious and stated that after 23 years of never a cross word at home and very happy marriage he was now an impossible person to live with: irritable and impatient and constantly losing his temper with his wife and two boys. He was afraid of losing his job and was sure he would not get a promotion (but did). He was a marine-paint salesman and was most successful in selling huge quantities of paint to shipowners. He was perfectly able to obtain a good clear voice on vowel sounds but insisted this was useless as he was totally unable to maintain the voice in speech, and produced habitually a spastic type of dysphonia. He had a fine voice before the operation and used to love singing opera as he washed up with his wife; now he was a freak and was driven mad by people asking him what was wrong with his voice.

It was a very long time before we were able to get to the bottom of this man's mental attitude towards his voice disorder. He gradually began to be less anxious and admitted that his voice improved sometimes at home and was even normal when talking to himself or singing in his van driving to and from the docks. Then during one visit he quite suddenly began to talk about his operation. He had been very ill with pneumonia some years before and when he went into hospital for thyroidectomy the first time he had a severe cold and he was sent home, being told that he could not be operated upon as he might develop pneumonia. The second time he was admitted he had a cold and though he pointed out that he might get pneumonia they took no notice and operated. He was sure he was going to die and when he regained consciousness he was not surprised to learn he had pneumonia, and was on the danger list. When he got better he felt that it was all the surgeon's fault that he had ruined his voice. After discharge from hospital his throat felt sore and painful and then one day he felt and saw a piece of tubing coming through the skin (presumably a drainage tube). He went to the hospital and was seen by a registrar who examined his throat, whipped out the tube with forceps, said 'Oh, that's nothing, nothing wrong there', and hustled him out of the clinic without any apology or explanation. This apparently was the final insult added to the injury which produced a smouldering resentment. He contemplated suing the surgeon for damages and his friends advised him to do so, but he did not see the use, it would not bring his voice back. Soon after making a clean breast of it, his voice came back quite suddenly one weekend and he spent hours ringing up all his friends on Sunday and the speech clinic on Monday morning. When he came to see us he was annoyed that his voice was not so good and showed some tension and pitch breaks; he attributed this to his hatred of hospitals, saying his heart always sank as he crossed the threshold. The following week he telephoned to say that as his voice was now normal all the time and it only weakened when he came to see us, he thought (if we did not mind) he would not come any more for treatment. We agreed happily to this arrangement and he was discharged ten weeks after his first visit.

VOCAL RECOVERY FOLLOWING VOCAL PALSY

Many patients suffering from slight vocal weakness after thyroidectomy will need help in voice production which either assists in the recovery of the muscles or possibly, in a sectional paralysis, allows other parts of the same muscle to compensate for partially impaired function. In cases of complete unilateral recurrent paralysis, where the affected fold is in the paramedian position, 'pushing' vocal exercises will help to shift this to the mid-line and induce also the compensatory movement of the healthy fold (pages **178** and **331**). The voice remains breathy for some time owing to escape of 'wild air' and lacks power, but may eventually become normal. When both folds lie in the paramedian position similar treatment should be given. Either fold may recover from paralysis but if this is not so, and both eventually assume the mid-line position, then it will be necessary to obtain the same surgical treatment as described below for bilateral abductor paralysis.

TEFLON INJECTION INTO PARALYSED CORD

Arnold (1962a) described experiments with tantalum injected directly into paralysed vocal cords in rehabilitation of dysphonia under local anaesthetic. In 1964, Arnold reported further experiences with intrachordal teflon injection and indicated criteria for selection of cases suitable for this form of treatment and listed contra-indications. The chief indication is unilateral vocal cord paralysis when the cord is fixed in the paramedian or intermediate position and its level is below that of the healthy cord. A greater gap between paralysed and healthy cord cannot be compensated for by the foreign bulk of teflon—the anterior two-thirds of the vocal cords may approximate and the vocal processes toe inwards, but not the arytenoids (Rubin, 1965). Rubin describing some pitfalls of treatment of dysphonias by intrachordal injection of synthetics says that voices that are weak or tire easily benefit the most. All surgeons recommend postponement of teflon injection till after six months waiting period in the hope of spontaneous recovery. Goff (1969) calculates that at the time of writing over 500 patients in the USA have received teflon injection for vocal-cord paralysis. All reports agree that the vocal results are excellent, both immediate and dramatic. Only a little discomfort and laryngitis may be felt for a few days after the injection. Phonation time, singing range, intensity and coughing all improve. Von Leden, Yanagihara and Werner-Kukuk (1967) evaluated vocal-cord movement from ultra-high-speed motion pictures. Their aerodynamic and acoustic studies showed marked improvement in all physiologic and acoustic parameters after teflon injection of the cord.

In Britain the use of teflon treatment has not been practised to any great extent. Siegler (1967) carried out the procedure with satisfactory results in Liverpool. British surgeons are cautious and conservative and the possible risk of malignancy developing from introduction of synthetics into the body has held them back. Teflon, a substance used for lining non-stick saucepans, is a highly neutral and non-reactive substance, and apparently safe. Lewy (1966) found no evidence that it is cancerogenic when examining microscopic section of the larynx eighteen months after injection. Kirchner, Teledo and Stroboda (1966) found teflon to be stable and inert in their experiments with dogs.

In 1969, however, a case of cancer of the vocal cord after teflon injection was reported and the federal drug agency of the

USA froze all further issue of the material pending further investigation and research. So there the matter stands.

BILATERAL ABDUCTOR PARALYSIS AND ARYTENOIDECTOMY

Réthi (1963) in 1928 first described an operation for the alleviation of the distressing condition of bilateral abductor paralysis. King (1953) first described his surgical technique, which was later simplified and improved by De Graaf Woodman (1946), and the procedure is now generally known as the Woodman operation.

An incision is made along the anterior border of the sterno-mastoid muscle and the arytenoid cartilage is exposed, dis-articulated and all but the vocal process is removed. The vocal process and fibres of the thyroarytenoid muscle are then pulled laterally and sutured to the inferior cornu of the thyroid. The cord is thus fixed in a position of abduction and the cord of the opposite side may be able eventually to pass over the mid-line and approximate with it. The ideal glottic aperture is 5 mm. If less, the air-way is inadequate. If greater, the voice will be hoarse or lost (King, 1953). Sometimes the original lateralised position of the vocal cord alters during healing and is shifted by formation of scar tissue. Woodman (1953) reported the answers to a question-naire from 90 surgeons on 521 cases of arytenoidectomy via the open approach (Woodman, 1948). The percentage of failure in providing an adequate air-way, which is the primary purpose of the operation was 9 per cent when no previous surgery had been attempted. The resulting post-operative voice was reported as adequate in 75 per cent of cases, good to excellent in 20 per cent and poor in 5 per cent.

A direct approach to arytenoidectomy by means of a Lynch-suspension apparatus and electro-cautery, which minimises bleeding and scarring, has been advocated by Thornell (Edwards, 1952).

A degree of recovery from abductor paralysis is possible up to 6 and even 12 months. Arytenoidectomy is therefore postponed for this period. Possibility of shrinkage in the bulk of the cord and replacement by fibrous tissue and shift from the mid-line to a paramedian position must be given a chance (Kirchner, 1966).

Anxiety and tension may cause an aggravation of breathing obstruction in talking and on effort. Patients sometimes develop a habit of talking on ingoing as well as outgoing breath. Training in relaxation and diaphragmatic breathing can help. Frail and old patients unable to withstand surgery will not be subjected to arytenoidectomy but a tracheostomy can be performed if breathing is difficult, and a flap valve cannula permits air to pass through the larynx and voice to be produced satisfactorily.

Speech therapy is necessary for the improvement of voice after arytenoidectomy and should be based upon approved methods of voice production. Relaxation and central breathing assume more than usual importance on account of the need that generally exists for the practice of forceful phonation exercises to increase adduction of the folds (Woodman and Pollack, 1950, and Pollack, 1952). Energetic use of the arms assists in the reflex sphincteric closure of the glottis which accompanies the need for fixation of the thorax and voice-restoring exercises may be based on this mechanism.

The strength of voice ultimately attained depends upon the post-operative result, the width of the glottic aperture and the nature of the paralysis. In bilateral total recurrent paralysis, difficulty in adduction is aggravated by contracture and fibrosis so that adduction over the mid-line will be impossible for the unoperated cord. The voice will be hoarse and never normal. In abductor paralysis, the folds being capable of adduction, there is no reason why compensatory movement should not be obtained by the unfixed cord, and voice become almost normal.

If the voice never recovers sufficiently to be audible under occupational conditions, amplification may be obtained by wearing a throat microphone or using a pocket amplifier and hand microphone. Telephones which amplify the voice are obtainable. The use of an amplifier in the early stages of treatment when at work or under any circumstances in which a patient has difficulty in making himself heard, may reduce anxiety and fatigue.

EXERCISES TO OBTAIN BETTER ADDUCTION OF FOLDS

The following exercises are recommended for patients who have undergone the Woodman operation, and those suffering from total unilateral paralysis of one fold where 'compensation' by the healthy fold is needed.

1. Laugh or cough and endeavour to prolong the spasmodic phonation thus achieved into a protracted vowel.
2. Swallow and phonate [i:] as recommended by Pollack.
3. Link the fingers, lift arms to level of clavicle and pull against each other phonating on [i:].

4. Push hands against a table and phonate.
5. Sitting in a chair push down strongly with hands grasping the seat on either side.

Froeschels (1948a), who appears to have been the originator of these exercises, stresses that the push must be perfectly synchronised with phonation, voicing being attempted simultaneously with the maximum reflex sphincteric action of the glottis. Moolenaar-Bijl (1956) recommends fast repetition of syllables with [f] and [s], and without pushing, as 'a useful basic laryngeal gymnastic'. Later on, the sustaining of a vowel and practice of vowel glides will stimulate the suppleness of the voice. Van Thal (1961) recommends strongly articulated syllables preceded by plosives following production of voice after pushing exercises. The vowel [u] is the most propitious and syllables [bu bu].

These exercises should be practised at frequent intervals during the day, but for short periods only. Care must be taken not to strain the throat and produce inflammation and soreness similar to that following vocal strain. In those cases of vocal-fold paralysis treated by us, however, it has not generally been found necessary to have recourse to forcing exercises. Voice has developed through use of the hard attack and the simple instruction to breathe deeply and voice loudly. Marland (1952) also reports good results in cases of vocal-fold paralysis without forcing exercises.

Difficulty in maintaining voice throughout phrases is encountered at first; a few words may be voiced and then speech deteriorates into a whisper. The length of phonation may be increased by the methods below.

1. Singing vowel sounds, or humming and feeling the vibrations in the larynx with the finger tips.
2. Phonating a succession of vowels in a staccato string, attempting a glottal plosive before each.
3. Counting or reciting the alphabet.
4. Speaking phrases of gradually increasing length, for instance: a blue sky; a bright blue sky; a bright blue clear sky; etc.

The most common fault is the tendency to speak on the ingoing breath (Woodman and Pollack, 1950). This must be discouraged since approximation of the folds on inspiration naturally obstructs the air passage and reduces the amount of inspired air which, in turn, reduces the amount available for voice. Thus a ruse which temporarily serves to prolong the voicing of a phrase defeats its own ends in the long run. When a glottic chink persists despite all training in adduction of the folds, the voice remains hoarse but audible. Breath is wasted in phonation and the patient must learn to replenish the breath supply at more frequent intervals than is customary when in possession of a normal larynx. At first there is a persistent tendency to carry on speech with very little breath, which produces tension and undermines good breathing patterns, but constant attention to breathing technique will correct this in time.

LARYNGEAL PALSY AFTER THYROIDECTOMY

Case Reports

Mrs B., aged 52. Bilateral vocal-fold paralysis four months previously. Both folds immobile, the right in cadaveric and the left in paramedian position. Right fold congested but the left normal. Respiration stridulous. Voice raucous, obtained by use of ventricular bands and pharyngeal muscles. Patient very tense and nervous. Breathing was quite remarkable and executed with an extraordinary degree of muscular effort. The sternomastoid muscles stood out like ropes and the lower lip and jaw were thrust forward in the inspiratory effort. Although the position of the folds provided a perfectly adequate air-way, such was the tension that an inspiratory stridor was audible with each breath. This unhappy state of affairs had come about as a result of the patient having been instructed in hospital by a physiotherapist to utilise the upper portion of her chest in breathing. She was able to maintain voice only for a few minutes at a time, and reading aloud to her children was rendered impossible by breathlessness.

Relaxation and instruction in diaphragmatic breathing in the first treatment dispelled the stridor immediately, and then vocalisation was attempted upon a sigh. A weak but unmistakable vocal note was thus produced and convinced the patient of the need for reducing tension and allayed her fear that relaxation would result in loss of voice. Treatment continued for three months during which the voice improved steadily and became well inflected, and a pitch range of an octave was achieved. The greatest difficulty encountered was that of establishing relaxation and central breathing in this patient, who was of an extremely excitable and talkative nature.

Six weeks after commencement of speech therapy another laryngoscopic examination showed that the right fold was still in the cadaveric position but no longer congested. The left fold, although lying in the paramedian position at rest, was moving across the mid-line in phonation and making contact with its partner.

In this case partial recovery from paralysis after thyroidectomy must have taken place before speech therapy had commenced, otherwise voice could not have been achieved instantaneously nor would ventricular band voice have been possible. Excessive tension, however, had prevented the discovery that vocal fold phonation was possible.

Mrs X., aged 64 years. Dysphonia following thyroidectomy three months previously. The right fold paralysed in paramedian position, left fold freely mobile and compensating well, despite the fact that it had been paralysed before the operation.

The patient's voice was weak and grating, giving evidence of inco-ordination, and it faded readily, especially when she was tired or upset. Breathing was shallow, and there was considerable pharyngeal tension, with inspiration audible though not stridulous.

Relaxation and breathing exercises, followed by simple vocalisation exercises, produced a good clear voice and an octave range after three treatments. The patient, a German Jewess, as a result of her tragic experience in wartime Germany and the postponement of thyroidectomy long after it was necessary, was extremely nervous and anxious. She was housekeeper to an exacting gentleman who alarmed her considerably, and should he complain of a dish set before him she lost her voice for a day. She complained of a lump in the throat and choking sensations, also pains in the head, neck and shoulders, and was convinced she had cancer. She had had arthritis in the past and an X-ray photograph showed narrowing of the spaces between several of the cervical vertebrae (see globus hystericus, page 181). A further laryngoscopic examination at this time (four months after thyroidectomy) showed that the right fold and arytenoid had now become fixed in an over-adducted position past the mid-line. The air-way was still adequate and the left fold being freely mobile was approximating well with the right fold.

The throat sensations were naturally attributed to the patient's nervous condition and she was assured that her fears and pains lacked foundation, without this, however, making them any the less real to herself. Since the patient was moving into her own house and an improvement in her domestic affairs promised alleviation of her apparently hysterical symptoms, speech therapy was discontinued for two months. When seen again her voice had deteriorated and she complained of feeling very ill and tired and declared with conviction that her throat grew more uncomfortable every day, and that her voice also came and went.

A thorough X-ray examination was now carried out and this revealed the presence of an adenoma behind the oesophagus and trachea causing their forward displacement. The growth was removed successfully with immediate improvement in voice and alleviation of the pain and discomfort and 'hysterical' symptoms.

It is always a temptation to attribute psychological causation to the aches and pains complained of by those of highly nervous temperament, especially when they tend to lurid descriptive details. But an unshakeable conviction of discomfort must always be subject to a thorough physical examination before a diagnosis of hysterical symptoms can be made, as this case very clearly illustrates.

Mrs M., aged **65** years. Aphonia following Woodman operation. She had undergone thyroidectomy twelve years previously. She had no voice afterwards though this gradually improved, but as it did so difficulty in breathing increased and 4 years later a tracheotomy had to be performed. Her voice remained good. Prior to performance of the Woodman operation on the right fold, examination of the larynx showed a bilateral abductor paralysis with a glottic chink on inspiration. The voice was fairly good.

The result of the operation was disappointing, the glottic aperture exceeding **5** mm. Recovery from the operation was slow owing to the development of pneumonia. Speech therapy was started two months after the operation. The patient was tense and upper thoracic breathing was so deeply ingrained that great difficulty in establishing central breathing was experienced. A very hoarse and breathy voice was obtained after three months speech treatment and the left fold when inspected was seen to be moving, but not meeting, the fixed fold. A holiday now resulted in deterioration of the voice as a result of an increase in tension and loss of ground gained in breathing technique. A further examination showed that the ventricular bands as well as the vocal folds were being used in phonation. Emphasis upon relaxation and breathing again brought an improvement in voice. This patient, after a year's treatment, can now obtain sometimes as many as ten words on the same breath, but the voice is very hoarse although a range of four or five notes is possible. It is adequate for normal purposes and is produced without effort; in fact she often states that the less force she puts into speech, the better her voice becomes. The attempt to achieve greater vocal volume by forcing is, however, often irresistible. There has always been a marked inclination to speak on inspired air and this has been hard to eradicate. Lapses still occur even in the clinic.

Forcing exercises were at no time used in treatment for fear of developing excess ventricular band movement. The co-operation of this patient has been excellent but her age, health and anxious temperament have not been factors operating in her favour. The wide glottic aperture might have been of less significance had not twelve years elapsed between thyroidectomy and arytenoidectomy. In the circumstances it is perhaps surprising that this patient obtained any serviceable voice at all.

PERIPHERAL NEURITIS OF THE LARYNX

Paralysis of the larynx as a result of laryngeal neuritis may follow any acute toxic infection, such as diphtheria, typhoid, whooping-cough, measles and influenza, but it is an occurrence of considerable rarity except in the case of influenza. The toxic neuritis prevents the conveyance of nervous impulses to the laryngeal muscles; a complete paralysis fixes the fold in the paramedian position. The condition is generally unilateral. The neuritis is fortunately almost exclusively of a temporary nature and permanent paralysis due to toxic invasion is practically unknown, although the unexplained paralyses of the larynx which do occur may be attributed to such infection (Clerf, 1950). In the great majority of cases, however, laryngeal neuritis disappears after several weeks at most. During the period of recovery, anxiety over the loss of voice while straining to overcome aphonia or hoarseness may give rise to all pernicious accompaniments of vocal strain, and eventually it is these circumstances which generally convey the patient to the laryngologist and subsequently to the speech clinic.

Treatment of such cases consists in reassurance concerning the temporary nature of the vocal disorder, and the correction of tension and shallow breathing. The possibility of functional complications in the organic disorder must not be overlooked. The use of forcing exercises to restore mobility to the affected fold should not be necessary since mobility returns naturally as the neuritis subsides, but this may take up to three months or even six, and a small percentage do not recover (Siegler, 1967). Indeed the use of force in phonation may aggravate inflammation and positively delay recovery.

The general health of the patient is an important factor in the restoration of vocal health. He is generally found to be in a state of debility after his illness, but the severity of the illness is often due to over-tiredness as a result of anxiety or overwork and consequent lowered resistance to infection. Such precautions as a tonic, attention to diet, and insistence upon a sensible programme of work and play will help to rid the system of the toxic effects of illness, but a holiday, if it can be arranged, is the best curative measure of all.

Case Reports

Mr T., aged **56** years, referred with a diagnosis of paralysis of the right fold following severe tonsillitis and pharyngitis two months previously. There was slight evidence of return of mobility to the fold, which was immobilised in a paramedian position.

The patient had become aphonic two weeks after the onset of flu, just as his throat was getting better. His voice had grown slightly stronger during the following six weeks but was still severely hoarse and his throat ached after the day's work, which involved much telephoning and conversation. He had been working under pressure for the past **18** months, had failed to take a summer holiday and was feeling 'worn out' before his illness. Although an apparently tranquil individual he confessed to having been very anxious about his voice because a near relative had lately died of cancer of the throat. His voice, he said, had improved considerably following the laryngologist's examination and diagnosis which had relieved this anxiety.

Breathing and vowel exercises produced an immediate strengthening of the voice but it continued to tire for some weeks towards the end of the day. This patient was then prevailed upon to take a fortnight's holiday from which he returned sound in body and voice and ready for discharge from the speech clinic.

Mr P., aged **47** years, referred with a diagnosis of paralysis of the left fold lying in paramedian position following influenza and laryngitis two months earlier. The affected fold still showed slight inflammation. He was using ventricular bands and pharyngeal musculature for phonation and his voice was high and strident.

When examined by the speech therapist he was found to be

excessively tense and in a very nervous condition. His breathing engaged the use of the upper thoracic region almost entirely, and such was the tension in the throat that the voice was harsh in the extreme and no vocal fold vibration could be heard. It transpired that the patient had been unemployed before his illness and had fallen into debt. His wife and children had also been ill with severe influenza and this had added to his anxieties.

Treatment consisted very largely in relaxation and reassurance. Vocal fold phonation was soon achieved in exercises as the neuritis dispersed but he reverted to ventricular band voice production the moment conversation was resumed. Recovery of normal voice came quite suddenly and coincided with re-employment.

This is yet another example of the conversion of organic vocal disorder into hysterical disorder following traumatic occurrences in the individual's life.

LARYNGEAL PARALYSIS AS THE RESULT OF EXTERNAL TRAUMA

Permanent damage to the laryngeal nerves as a result of a blow is an infrequent occurrence. More commonly bruising and internal bleeding is followed by temporary swelling and immobilisation of the folds. The throat is painful, there is difficulty in swallowing and perhaps in breathing, and the degree of vocal disorder reflects the severity of the laryngeal condition. Apparent paralysis of the folds is more often due to local swelling than actual damage to the laryngeal nerves. Of six cases suffering from haematoma of the larynx following external trauma described by Putney (1952) all made a total recovery, even in three patients in whom fixation of a fold had existed. An irreversible paralysis due to a nervous lesion, however, is by no means impossible nor improbable expecially in wartime (Harmer, 1919).

Vocal rest should be prescribed until the swelling of throat and larynx has subsided. The voice recovers in most cases as the vocal folds revert to their natural condition and speech therapy will not be necessary, except in those cases in which a functional disorder develops from the original trauma and is perhaps aggravated by faulty voice production. Treatment will also be necessary in those few cases in which permanent paralysis remains.

Case Reports

Mr N., aged 24 years, referred with a diagnosis of vocal weakness following an accident 4 months previously. Movement of the folds normal. No inflammation.

The patient had lost his voice after a car accident in which he had been struck on the larynx by the steering wheel. His voice recovered but he began to be troubled by a constant feeling of tiredness in the throat. He was an inveterate talker and the temporary muscular weakness following trauma to the crico-thyroid muscle may have produced a slight vocal strain. He had no pronounced bad habits of voice production and the voice was not abnormal. The difficulty was felt to be mainly functional, although he responded well to the reassurance provided by an ordinary course of voice production.

Mrs O., aged 35 years, referred with a diagnosis of left unilateral total recurrent laryngeal nerve paralysis, the result of a car accident 5 months previously. The right fold was moving well.

The patient had been driving when the accident occurred, had been concussed and had several cuts on the head. She had a pain in her Adam's apple for 2 or 3 days following the accident, but no dysphagia. Her voice was hoarse when she regained consciousness but had grown stronger in the interval that elapsed before speech treatment was commenced. On examination her voice was asthenic, breathy and deep, breathing was shallow and there was some generalised tension. The patient felt a considerable degree of guilt concerning the accident in which she had jeopardised the lives of the other occupants of the car; she also had acute matrimonial difficulties and a difficult mother to contend with. A strong functional element in the dysphonia prevented the recovery of normal voice. She invariably lost her voice at home when upset and her voice always improved greatly during treatment but regressed during the week. She could not be induced to practise vocal exercises at home. Vocal exercises introducing force were found not to produce such good results as the vocalisation of vowels when relaxed, but employing strong breath pressure. Good results were obtained when Barany boxes were used as recommended by Labarraque (1952). When the instruments were held to the ears, the patient's voice grew stronger in reading, though not entirely normal; as she endeavoured to hear herself she automatically raised the volume of voice. The boxes were then removed abruptly so that she might hear the vocal improvement which she endeavoured to maintain as she continued to read.

She was eventually discharged after 8 months' treatment. Her speaking voice was still rather deep and husky but she stated that it was normal and had always had this characteristic. She was unable to achieve more than a range of six notes when singing. The right fold obtained good compensation with the paralysed left fold.

This patient turned up at St. Bartholomew's Hospital 15 years later and was astonished to be reminded that we had met before at her other hospital. She had been free from dysphonia during the interval but was now complaining of dysphonia after the death of her husband whom she had actually deserted some time before his death; she was now suffering from bereavement guilt and depression, from which she quickly recovered with the help of discussion.

TUBERCULOSIS OF THE LARYNX WITH MYOPATHIC PARESIS AND
ULCERATION

Although inflammation of the vocal folds is commonly due to
vocal abuse and the chronic irritation set up by excessive friction
between their opposing surfaces, it must not be forgotten that
inflammation may be caused by pathological infection. Tuberculosis
of the larynx (phthisis laryngea) is such a condition. The infection
in the vast majority of cases is a secondary complication of
pulmonary infection, the tubercle being implanted by sputum
coughed up from the lungs. It may develop as a secondary site of
infection from lupus in the nose. There has been a dramatic
decrease in the incidence of laryngeal tuberculosis in the last
thirty years due to the early diagnosis and treatment of pulmonary
tuberculosis by antibiotics and the condition is now one of great
rarity. But it may still occur in old age. Smurthwaite (1919)
states that in the early stages of infiltration an adductor paralysis
(myopathic paresis) may appear before any positive signs of
inflammation are visible and this may possibly be diagnosed
incorrectly as an hysterical disorder. If infection progresses,
ulceration of the folds can develop. Complete vocal rest is essential
and resting of the voice must be strictly observed. Scarring and
irregularity of the folds may occur during healing with resultant
impairment of the voice dependent upon the degree and site of
the damage. If webbing of the folds develops, division of the web
and skin grafting may be necessary, as described in St. Clair-
Thomson et al. (1955). The possibility of such severe complications
is now unlikely since the use of antibiotics, at least in the developed
countries with good medical services.

Speech therapy may be necessary after cure of the disease.
Slight thickening of the mucous membrane may remain along the
length of the folds or in the posterior region. The voice always
has a characteristic deep, husky and rather hollow tone (Guthrie,
1952). We have treated two female patients with this condition.
One was referred soon after cure of tuberculosis and had developed

considerable anxiety over her health and economic situation besides tension in attempting to obtain a louder voice. She responded well to relaxation, breathing exercises, hearing training and raising the vocal pitch. The other patient had recovered from tuberculosis some years previously and had not been anxious about her impaired voice until domestic difficulties produced a functional aphonia. Vocal exercises and discussion of her difficulties brought the voice back. She said it improved in clarity and strength during treatment and was better than it had been since her tubercular illness. In neither of these cases did the huskiness and 'veiling' of the voice disappear entirely, since permanent changes and thickening of the vocal membrane had taken place.

SYPHILITIC INFLAMMATION AND ULCERATION OF THE LARYNX

Syphilis of the larynx may occur as a congenital infection or as an acquired condition, secondary to primary infection. The disease may be manifest by acute inflammation of the larynx with a timilar involvement of the pharynx and, in advanced stages of the disease, ulceration occurs. The symptom of hoarseness is a prominent feature of syphilitic laryngitis, the voice is strong, of a peculiar rough quality and generally causes no discomfort (Guthrie, 1952). In the early stages the intractable laryngitis and pharyngitis can be mistaken quite easily for a simple catarrhal infection. In very advanced stages, the formation of syphilomata may resemble cancerous tumours. Accurate diagnosis depends upon a positive Wasserman reaction being obtained from a test of the patient's serum, but in a small proportion of cases in the tertiary stages of syphilis a positive reaction is not obtained.

Scarring of the vocal cords following ulceration is generally severe and may cause stenosis of the larynx and breathing difficulty (dyspnoea). Treatment must obviously be directed to the cure of the disease, and only after this has been achieved and the laryngeal symptoms alleviated can any attempt at improvement of the voice be undertaken. The patient may now be helped to make the best use of his voice. Prognosis is unfavourable unless cicatricial tissue is minimal or can be removed surgically, so that the vocal cords present even edges in adduction.

RHEUMATIC LARYNGEAL ARTHRITIS

Laryngeal arthritis involving the cricoarytenoid joints is another condition of considerable rarity which may cause aphonia or dysphonia according to the degree of immobility imposed upon the folds. In the early stages of invasion of the larynx by the disease there is acute local inflammation and extraordinary pain attendant upon phonation. Great difficulty is experienced in moving the folds and there is pronounced hoarseness. The principle treatment is medical, directed at alleviating the arthritic disease which is widespread throughout the individual's system before the larynx becomes involved. Cortisone treatment is often prescribed. In the past it was thought advisable to rest the voice while inflammation was acute (Ellis, 1952). Nowadays it is considered advisable to exercise the voice and keep the criocoarytenoid joints mobile. Local short-wave diathermy may relieve the pain, which is acute, and improve vocal-fold movement. Severity of symptoms vary and a flare-up of arthritic episode is often linked with respiratory infection and subsides spontaneously (Wolman, Darke and Young, 1965). Sometimes arthritis subsides without leaving permanent changes in the cricoarytenoid joints, apart from some stiffness and resultant sluggishness in vocal-fold adduction, which resolves in time. At this stage vocal exercises can be helpful.

In a small proportion of cases, however, total fusion of the cricoarytenoid joint (ankylosis) takes place, in which case there is no chance of recovery. The position of the fold in ankylosis of the arytenoid joint resembles that of an abductor paralysis of the recurrent laryngeal nerve with the fold fixed in the paramedian position. Rarely it is held in a position of extreme abduction by the fibrous bands which form through arthritic changes in the arytenoid joint. Should compensation by the opposite fold be impossible, a stronger voice may be obtained after a 'reverse King operation' has been performed and the fold transplanted to the median position (Morrisson, 1948) (page 330). The most common form of laryngeal arthritis is, however, bilateral with both folds immobilised in the mid-line. If there is difficulty in breathing a tracheotomy will be performed. If the condition is not alleviated by medication and both folds remain permanently fixed in the mid-line, a Woodman operation can be performed (Woodman, 1948). It is doubtful whether speech therapy will help the voice post-operatively since the fold not operated upon remains immobile. Operation may not be feasible if the patient is aged and frail. A tracheotomy and use of a flap-valve type of tracheotomy tube will be the preferred choice of the medical adviser with such cases.

When rheumatic laryngeal arthritis resolves before occurrence of ankylosis of the joints, the folds sometimes remain sluggish in movement and the voice is hoarse or breathy. This condition can be improved by speech therapy. A female patient's voice was severely hoarse following a brief attack of arthritis of the larynx which rendered adduction of the folds difficult; she quickly developed a normal voice through the practice of vocal exercises. Movement of the folds was stimulated by attempting their rapid abduction and adduction in quick succession. The patient was instructed to drink in a cold gulp of air to obtain full abduction, and then to shout a vowel sound to promote full adduction. Relaxation and diaphragmatic breathing exercises are, of course, necessary preliminaries to such vocal exercises.

CONGENITAL STRUCTURAL ABNORMALITIES OF THE LARYNX

Congenital abnormalities causing stenosis of the larynx are mainly a matter of theoretical interest to the speech therapist since the condition in most cases is alleviated in infancy or early childhood.

Arnold (1958) in discussing 'dysplastic dysphonia' and congenital cases of hoarseness, describes various abnormalities found in adult larynges which may be familial and associated with hoarseness in childhood. Laryngeal anomalies may also occur in conjunction with other bodily deformities. Possible laryngeal anomalies producing hoarseness are: sulcus of a vocal fold described earlier (page 128); one fold placed higher than the other; one fold broader than the other; and one ventricle may be larger than the other. The arytenoids may pass one in front of the other upon adduction. Differences in the size of the wings of the thyroid cartilage or an abnormal shape to the epiglottis may be present. A 7-year-old boy referred to us for examination, whose voice had been severely hoarse from birth and lacked inflexion, had also an inspiratory stridor upon exertion. When speaking rapidly he frequently spoke upon an inspiratory breath. Laryngoscopic examination showed the left arytenoid fixed in a forward position and slightly lateral to the mid-line with bowing of the fold. This was associated with unilateral paresis of the palate. Adenoidectomy when performed did not produce nasal speech as was feared might be the case and was the reason for a speech therapist's assessment before operation.

A child may be born with a membranous web across the anterior portion of the folds. The web may be quite small and cause no inconvenience, or may extend back into the glottis joining nearly the whole length of the folds and causing serious obstruction.

Symptoms of hoarseness, dyspnoea and stridor are dependent upon the severity of the obstruction. In male children the existence of a congenital web may not be detected until adolescence when failure of the voice to break leads to a laryngoscopic investigation (*see* under disorders of pitch, page 220).

Simple division of the web surgically may not be satisfactory because the folds being active organs do not heal easily on account of the friction between their surfaces. Fibrosis may occur, or the raw edges adhere as they heal and the web thus reform. There are two methods for dealing with the problem.

An acrylic plate can be inserted between the folds after their division and left in place for a period of two or three months until the folds have healed (Hall, 1954). Alternatively the raw surfaces of the folds after division may be covered by a Thiersch skin-graft, which is held in position by an acrylic mould until the graft is established and the larynx healed (St. Clair-Thomson, 1955). In either case a laryngofissure operation (page 361) must be performed in order to gain access to the larynx.

The voice after operation depends naturally upon the contour of the folds, but is generally rather deep and hoarse. Speech therapy should be tried and some improvement in the voice may be gained.

Another possible congenital deformity of the larynx concerns the epiglottis. In place of the usual flattened structure, it is folded in such a way that its lateral edges almost approximate (Wilson, 1952). The aryepiglottic folds offer considerable resistance to the air stream in inspiration and cause a vibratory stridor which is always present, but grows alarmingly louder upon exertion and especially when the infant cries, when it is said to resemble a crowing cock. There is no serious cyanosis but dyspnoea may be present. The child, however, remains comparatively healthy. The condition requires no treatment and there are no symptoms by the third year.

ACQUIRED LARYNGEAL STENOSIS

Stenosis of the larynx may follow accidental scalding, inhalation of smoke and flames in a fire, or swallowing acid. Webs can form in healing and present the same difficulties in surgical management as congenital webs described above.

Gun-shot and stab wounds and blows on the larynx in boxing and especially in car accidents are relatively common. The thyroid and cricoid cartilages may be fractured and the vocal cords torn and arytenoids dislocated (Harris and Ainsworth, 1965). Hollinger, Schild and Maurizi (1968) advocate early repair as soon as the patient is well enough, to avoid chronic laryngeal stenosis. Shumrick (1967) states the case for wearing of seat belts with shoulder harness to prevent laryngeal trauma in car crashes. In laryngeal fractures a tracheotomy should be performed early and stabilisation of the cartilage fragments achieved by endolaryngeal stenting in order to prevent webbing and preserve the airway and voice. The danger is that in concentrating upon treatment of multiple bodily and head injuries, perhaps in a general or neurosurgical unit, the condition of the larynx and problems of air-way and phonation be left too late. After tracheotomy and breathing have been dealt with in an emergency situation the laryngologist needs to be consulted (Duff, 1968).

Speech therapy will be necessary when the larynx has healed and must be adapted to the laryngological report. Vocal-cord palsies are the most common residual disorder. Fracture of the larynx need not occur to produce paralysis of the vocal cords. A patient who had been hit on the larynx by a cricket ball in Jamaica sustained severe bruising but had little breathing difficulty, and was found to suffer from a complete paralysis of one cord which did not recover. He was aphonic at first and then the voice gradually returned as compensation by the healthy cord was obtained.

In motor-car accidents it is well to remember that litigation and claims for damage are often in progress. In this case, if the patient can claim for loss of voice and damage to his career, this will be taken into account in settlement of compensation. Full potential vocal recovery may not be achieved until the law courts have settled the case. Another factor is the long time it takes for a serious laryngeal injury to recover and function to be restored. The voice may go on improving over the period of a year or more. Sometimes delayed shock and anxiety produce aphonia or dysphonia out of proportion to the injury and the psychological trauma needs treatment.

CHRONIC HYPERPLASTIC LARYNGITIS

Kleinsasser (1968) describes the absolute confusion of terms and conditions associated with the collective term 'chronic laryngitis' and remarks that every laryngologist has a different concept of the clinical picture presented by such terms as pachydermia, keratosis, leukoplakia, polyp, papilloma, etc. We have already run into this difficulty in discussing contact ulcers and pachydermia (page 136). It is with some trepidation, therefore, that we embark upon chronic hyperplastic laryngitis, but since it is now treated surgically and voice therapy is generally required subsequently, it seems necessary to include the condition under inflammatory conditions of the larynx to distinguish it quite clearly from chronic laryngitis due to vocal abuse which is not treated surgically.

'Chronic hyperplastic laryngitis' is characterised by a diffuse inflammatory process that extends over a wide area of the laryngeal mucosa—although it is usually most highly developed on the cords—and eventually leads to epithelial hyperplasia (Kleinsasser, 1968). The condition, unlike acute and chronic laryngitis does not heal when infection or irritants are removed and it is a potentially pre-cancerous condition. Kleinsasser recommends stripping of the cords (decortication) and removal of the thickened epithelium since it arrests the disease and achieves voice improvement. It may also prevent malignancy developing, although it is too early yet to be sure of this being the case as patients have not been followed up for long enough periods.

It is necessary to remove all possible irritants to the larynx including vocal abuse (Shaw and Friedmann, 1964). This develops as a result of the hoarseness and phonation difficulty secondary to inflammation, of course. Most patients have been or are heavy cigarette smokers and they must be warned against the dangers of smoking and advised to stop. Any dust, heat or fumes which may be encountered at work must be avoided, and if necessary other occupation found.

Post-operatively voice rest is recommended but if the patient must talk then Kleinsasser says a normal tone of voice is less harmful than whispering. Only when the vocal cords have fully healed and re-epithelized—usually after 3–4 weeks—is speech therapy prescribed if necessary. It is remarkable how much voice improvement can be achieved in a short time if the patient is co-operative and carries out instructions for better voice production. In the cases we have treated the voice has improved but never recovered normal quality.

Illustrative case history of Hypertrophic laryngitis

Mr L., aged 50, had, even in his teens, a hoarse rough voice which he may have cultivated in order to sound 'tough' in a Cockney manual workers' environment. Ten years before seeing us he had laryngitis and lost his voice and was examined by a laryngologist who advised him to change his job of coalman as his 'tubes were congested with coal dust'. He recovered his voice and changed his job to that of a floor-cleaning specialist, using mechanical polishers and scrapers. He had no trouble for nine years, when he suddenly became very hoarse. His doctor prescribed linctus and inhalations and he had a month off sick but the voice deteriorated to a whisper. He was then seen by our laryngologist who prescribed further treatment for laryngitis and advised Mr L. to stop smoking, which he did. The cords were mobile but the larynx was red and ulcerated and the edges of the vocal cords were roughened and irregular. Medical treatment did not produce any improvement, so on account of the possibility of malignancy and need for biopsy, a direct microlaryngoscopy and micro-surgical stripping of the right cord was performed. Two weeks later the right cord presented a healthy 'satin' appearance but the left cord was oedematous and red posteriorly. There was a tendency to phonate with the false cords. Three weeks later the voice was worse and the left cord more inflamed and 'plicae ventricularis' more pronounced. The patient on account of developing vocal abuse was referred for speech therapy and also stripping of the left cord was prescribed and carried out two weeks later.

Mr L. was told not to speak for a week and subsequently to rest the voice as much as possible and speech therapy was not recommenced until two weeks later, when both vocal cords were reported to be looking thick and slightly red. Although the patient had a harsh, grating dysphonia similar to that of contact ulcers he declared his voice was back to how it always had been and this was corroborated by his wife. His breathing appeared not to be at fault but air flow was constricted by over-adduction of the vocal cords and ventricular bands. He attempted to shout all the time. He had a hearing loss in one ear and this was thought to be a contributory factor and a hearing aid was ordered. He was extremely tense and had a habit of clenching his fists and flexing his biceps. When asked about this he said that when a coalman and needing to lift 2-hundredweight sacks of coal he used to walk round with a hard rubber ball in each hand, flexing the muscles of arms and shoulders to strengthen them. He prided himself on being very fit and physically strong. He was super-ficially cheerful and carefree but looked a worrier.

Speech therapy was arranged three times a week for a month,

then reduced to twice a week and eventually once a week as the voice improved. Considerable time was spent on hearing training and the production of smooth, clear vowel sounds in the tenor range, which after a time he could achieve perfectly. At first this voice sounded affected and artificial to him and he needed convincing that it was acceptable and pleasing by playing back recordings of good and bad voice. The difficulty was to obtain a carry-over into spontaneous speech and eradicate his habitual forced, hoarse voice production. He was given an amplifier to use at home and in the clinic used it for speaking, which automatically caused him to reduce his vocal volume. He then switched the instrument off and was instructed to carry on quietly, with no more effort than before. If he raised his voice, the instrument was again switched on.

Mr L. is now using a very much smoother and easier voice but it was two and a half months before there was any appreciable improvement and his voice has remained slightly 'veiled' or husky. His larynx looks healthy and it is hoped that the hypertrophic laryngitis is now cured and will not prove to have been a pre-cancerous condition.

VOCAL-CORD POLYPS

True vocal-cord polyps represent the most common condition needing surgery and not all patients require speech therapy. Kleinsasser (1968) in a series of 100 cases reports 67 men and 33 women; 36 per cent of the patients between 20 and 40 years; 55 per cent between 41 and 60 years. The oldest patient referred was 71 years and the youngest 6 years. The cause of polyps is obscure and although they sometimes appear to follow an increase in voice exertion and therefore to be related to vocal abuse, this is not at all certain. Neither do polyps appear to be associated with irritants. They are larger than vocal nodules and there are different types: a soft 'gelatinous' type develops inside an oedematous sac and a fibrous type may consist of vascularised and hyalinised connective tissue. The gelatinous polyp occurs typically about 3 mm behind the anterior commissure on the under surface of one cord and sometimes both. The fibrous polyp occurs on the middle of the vocal cord and on the upper surface. Polyps may be tiny or almost occlude the glottis. Colour photos of three-dimensional magnified images of the larynx are shown in Kleinsasser's book (1969) and illustrate beautifully the different types, sites and shapes of polyps encountered.

The voice is often affected but surgery is always carried out, even in the event of a very small polyp, as it is difficult to distinguish by appearance alone from a malignant neoplasm (Brodnitz, 1953). The voice improves immediately after surgery but should not be used for a week, by which time it should have recovered fully. Should this not be the case, speech therapy is prescribed. The larynx is such a sensitive zone, both from sensory and psychological angles that any discomfort and surgical interference generally provokes aggravated sensations and anxieties. Reassurance and exercises to improve the tone of the vocal folds and adduction in phonation as a general rule are needed, rather than a comprehensive rehabilitation programme. This is especially the case in elderly patients who are not great voice users but need to be heard by deaf relatives and enjoy chatting in the local pub or old peoples' club. This may constitute the highlight of their lives and hoarseness may cause real hardship.

PAPILLOMATA OF THE LARYNX

Papillomata are benign neoplasms consisting of fibrous stalks of areolar connective tissue covered with a very much thickened stratified squamous epithelium which grow in the larynx. It is now generally accepted that they are caused by a virus (Dekelbaum, 1965, and Rabbett, 1965). They are essentially a disease of childhood, may start as early as in the second year and are potentially dangerous to the child on account of obstruction in breathing. Rabbett (1965) says that 'papillomatosis of the larynx is one of the most frustrating diseases in the field of otolaryngology. Although inherently a benign disease, its rapid recurrence after removal and its extremely prolonged course, make it a trying experience for the physician and a dangerous, debilitating disease for the afflicted patient'.

The papillomata do not invade the muscular tissue of the folds and can therefore be plucked off quite easily. They proliferate like warts or bunches of minute grapes. Rabbett (1965) points to the fact that they tend to increase and multiply after respiratory infections but antibiotics favourably control bacterial infection and restore the larynx to health quickly. This is of importance as it renders the laryngeal mucosa less susceptible to invasion by the virus.

Repeated surgical removal seems the most satisfactory, safe and effective treatment, when all things are considered including the long-term effects of other forms of treatment. It is largely a question of playing for time: recurrence may be delayed some years and in any event the disease is generally self-limiting and at puberty the papillomata may vanish like the Cheshire cat, never, it is to be hoped, to be seen again, whether in boys or girls, there is little sex difference. Dekelbaum (1965) reviewing 67 cases treated between 1928–1962 believes the disease is increasing in incidence.

There appears to be in some female patients a connection with hormonal changes when recurrence coincides with puberty, pregnancy and menopause. Since papillomata regress at puberty in both male and female subjects treatment in childhood is largely palliative and there is a strong case for playing a waiting game and not taking strong action.

Birrell (1954) for this reason states that the only satisfactory palliative treatment in the case of multiple papillomata on the folds is tracheotomy to relieve dyspnoea. An incision is made well below the level of the cricoid cartilage and the child is fitted with a tracheal cannula through which he can breathe in comfort. This may have to be worn for years until the laryngeal condition improves. The child must be kept under frequent observation since there is a possibility of papillomata spreading into the trachea and causing obstruction of the airway at a lower level than the larynx. Tracheotomy is not an agreeable condition for a child, however.

Hollinger (1959) advocates forceps removal without anaesthesia at frequent intervals. He mentions the case of one child from whom he removed nodular masses 134 times in the course of four years. The advantages of avoiding tracheotomy are the prevention of respiratory infections and bronchitis to which a child with a tracheotomy is subject. The nature and extent of papillomatous formations must influence the choice of surgical treatment in individual cases. The temperament of the child and mother must also be taken into account. Some children obviously cannot tolerate forceps removal at frequent intervals.

Thermal cautery has been tried and is initially successful but there is a danger of scarring the vocal cords. Radiotherapy has been used successfully in so far as papillomata are dispersed but there is a proved connection between radiotherapy and early laryngeal cancer (Rabbett, 1965; Vermeuling, 1966). A new treatment is the use of ultrasonic waves of great concentration directed carefully at the site of the papillomata (Jenkins, 1967). Ultrasound is known to have a deleterious effect on viruses. It is not known what the ultimate effects will be in terms of damage to nerve tissue, growth and later development of malignancy. Evaluation will not be possible for many years and until the children treated have passed through puberty and become middle-aged.

Morres, Wentges and Brinkman (1966) described a child of 20 months who suddenly became aphonic and papillomata were discovered. Ultrasonic therapy failed but a cryogenic cannula filled with liquid nitrogen as is used in Parkinson surgery, and the tip applied to the papillomata was successful with no recurrence 2 years later.

Hollinger *et al.* (1968) give interesting figures in their report of 174 patients suffering from papillomata over a 15-year period:

77 patients under 13 years of whom 38 were male and 39 female. 97 patients over 13 years of whom 64 were male and 33 female. In 5 of the 33 female patients the condition disappeared during pregnancy but recurred afterwards.

Disappearance of papillomata during puberty, pregnancy and menopause in studies such as these has drawn attention to a connection between hormones and growth of papillomata as mentioned above.

Language develops normally in children suffering from papillomata of the larynx. Though the voice may be severely impaired and perhaps whispering only is possible for several years, the voice should recover when once the growths disperse, although this is by no means certain when a substitute voice has been used for many years.

An Indian child of 9 years, who had undergone polypectomy frequently, when we examined her had developed a strong buccal whisper in speaking and was unable to produce any laryngeal phonation. Air was vibrated orally by vigorous movements of the tongue, and air appeared to be pocketed in the cheeks and pharynx in a manner similar to that acquired by some laryngectomised patients. This buccal whisper is described by Bateman and Negus (1954). Although this child could breathe through her larynx after the repeated surgical removal of papillomata she could not be persuaded to vibrate air in the larynx or speak on a laryngeal whisper. She was flown home soon afterwards but it is unlikely that this child would ever speak normally without special training in co-ordinating expiration with phonation.

Brodnitz (1959) has described the case of a boy with a damaged larynx who developed voice by vibrating air in the hypopharynx by movements of the base of the tongue, sometimes described as 'frog speech'. After reconstructive surgery had rendered phonation possible all conventional methods of voice production failed. Use of a stethoscope by the boy and placing the diaphragm alternately against the larynx of the phonating therapist and then his own larynx produced good results with the help of 'vibrating-tactile sensations'.

Curry (1949b) describes an interesting case of a 16-year-old girl who had suffered from laryngeal papillomata since early childhood and had no voice all her life but began to develop voice following successful surgery. Some months later when re-examined she suffered from continuous abrupt voice breaks, the voice shifting from a hoarse chest voice to an unpleasant rasping falsetto. The larynx presented a normal appearance, however. The results of voice therapy, if any, are not reported in this case.

The voice should develop normally as the papillomata disappear as long as the vocal cords have not been damaged by plucking the growths off during childhood. This is now less likely if the Kleinsasser microsurgical technique is used. It is possible that psychological disturbance may arise out of a child being constantly under surgical treatment or, if wearing a tracheotomy tube, from being different from his fellows. This is by no means certain and one boy we knew, at least, far from being upset by his affliction, was able to compensate for it and gain much kudos from his enviable accomplishment of being able to blow smoke out of his neck.

In cases in which tracheotomy has existed for many years, upper thoracic breathing habits often develop and breathing exercises may be necessary. Failure to use the vocal muscles adequately on account of papillomatous obstruction may produce an asthenic dysphonia when once the laryngeal condition is normal. Training in voice production will be necessary if this happens. Special emphasis will have to be given to hearing training since the patient, never having produced a normal voice, will lack the necessary auditory control of the vocal muscles. Dysphonia persists as a result of habit rather than of actual muscular inadequacy in most cases and the voice disorder may be aggravated by emotional difficulties as already mentioned.

Papillomata which recur in adult life are much less troublesome than in childhood since when removed they may be cured or not recur for many years. After stripping the cords of multiple papillomata voice therapy may be necessary, depending upon the degree of deterioration of the voice and the length of time dysphonia has existed before operation.

Case History

Joan at the age of 4 years began to develop a husky voice and slowly increasing noisy breathing. At 6 years she was found to have papillomata of the vocal cords, which were removed surgically. At 7 years she was operated on again and tonsils and adenoids were removed. At 8, 9 and 10 years papillomata were removed and twice at 12 years and finally at 14 years. After each operation the voice recovered fully but immediately after operation she suffered from dysphonia for some weeks. On the last occasion this persisted rather longer than usual although the vocal cords looked entirely normal. She was a shy adolescent at this time and a short course of speech therapy improved the volume of voice and increased confidence.

Mrs G., aged 50, came to our department for surgical removal of papillomata. She had first developed papillomata of the larynx at age 5 in India but was not operated upon and they dispersed while she was at school in England. She returned to India at age 18 and a year later papillomata returned but she did not have them removed. The voice was husky and there was no difficulty in breathing. She returned to England and had no more trouble until aged 28 when she had a recurrence associated with pregnancies and had surgical removal of papillomata twice with a year's interval between. She had a hysterectomy at age 38 and no more trouble until a recurrence at age 48 when she was living in Africa. Breathing became so difficult that she eventually had to return home for treatment. Her larynx at this time was congested with papillomata clustering like bunches of tiny grapes over the vocal cords. Her voice was breathy and only a squeak was possible now and then. She was placed on vocal rest after surgical removal of the growths and when seen 2 weeks later had no voice at all. There remained one or two papillomatous remnants which prevented full adduction of the vocal cords. A month later when Mrs G. was able to free herself from family commitments, she had the remnants removed, after which the larynx was pronounced healthy. It was expected that once the vocal cords were presenting normal surfaces and capable of normal excursions the voice would return. This was not the case and for approximately 4 months her voice remained hoarse and breathy but a high-pitched note could be produced with tension. During this period she returned to Africa but wrote to say that her voice had returned suddenly while singing carols in church at Christmas. The delay in voice recovery may have been due to persisting pre-operative habits of phonation; certainly it was no psychological problem as she was an exceptionally happy, extrovert and stable person. The extensive surgical interference with the laryngeal mucosa in plucking off the papillomata was more probably responsible for delay in return of normal voice dependent upon reintegration of the mechano-receptor reflex laryngeal system.

This patient has now returned to England for permanent residence and her voice is almost normal although a couple of papillomata have returned. These are not to be removed as they are causing no inconvenience and the patient is convinced that the red lateralite dust to which she was exposed in India and Africa implanted a virus in her larynx which may disperse with residence here.

Mr J., aged **54**, first had a papillomata removed from vocal cord at age **24** years. Eighteen years later he had difficulty in swallowing and felt pain and was referred to the ENT department suffering from 'globus hystericus' by his general practitioner. He was found to have some swelling on the anterior section of the left ventricular band. This was the cause of the feeling of a lump in the throat. No surgery was indicated. His voice was husky at this time, but the swelling disappeared and his voice improved. Eight years later at age **50** he had papillomata removed from the cords and again a year later. His voice was hoarse after this but fairly strong. Four years later his voice faded and he was put on vocal rest, his vocal cords looked 'glazed' (laryngis sicca) and did not approximate adequately posteriorly. The laryngologist thought the trouble was part nervous and part vocal strain and referred him for speech therapy.

Mr J.'s voice at this time was hoarse and harsh. He was an assistant manager in an insurance firm in an office block surrounded by noisy streets congested with traffic. He had to telephone, interview and dictate letters all day. He was tense and anxious and smoked 10–15 cigarettes a day. He was happily married with two children, had no domestic or financial worries and enjoyed his work. Speech therapy did not produce any improvement in voice and the speech therapist felt the trouble was organic and asked for another laryngoscopic examination. This time a more experienced laryngologist detected thickening of both vocal cords anteriorly over the first third and separation of the cords in the middle third, with normal apposition in the arytenoid region. The patient was admitted for a scrape and biopsy and a month later when re-examined the vocal cords looked healthy. There was no sign of further papillomata but the voice remained bad and the false cords looked thick. Speech therapy continued for two months: in exercises he was able to produce high notes better than low but there was no improvement in speaking voice and he had another check with the ENT specialist. There was again thickening of the left cord in the anterior third. It was decided to discontinue speech therapy, although the specialist was convinced that the cause of the laryngeal symptoms was vocal abuse with a functional basis. Mr J. has continued to have laryngoscopy checks every 3 months. Four months after we saw him last he had a further papillomata removed from the anterior region of the cord. Two years later he developed a keratotic plaque in the anterior commissure and contact ulcer posteriorly which were treated by surgery and vocal rest. Since that time and elapse of three years he has had no further organic signs but his dysphonia has remained severe.

LARYNGEAL CYSTS

Cysts of the vocal cords occur rather rarely but are especially common on the false vocal cords in persons over 50 or 60 years of age (Kleinsasser, 1968). Almost all are retention cysts on the false cords and develop secondary to degenerative processes in the ductal system of the mucous gland network. They may be multi-focal and bilateral. They may hang from the inlet to the ventricle of Morgagni and obstruct the air-way or may be situated deep in the false cord but are not painful. Surgical treatment presents no problems. The cysts have to be opened up and drained and mucosa sutured thereafter. Lymphatic cysts also occur on the free edges of the aryepiglottic folds and epiglottis but generally are so small that they need not be removed.

Although the removal of cysts on the false vocal cords and ventricle should not disturb the voice, we have had a number of such cases referred for speech therapy and dysphonia afterwards. One woman of 45 developed, besides hoarseness, an anxiety state after the fright of a rather sudden enlargement of a cyst which obstructed breathing. She began to have difficulty with breathing after discharge from hospital on exertion, and then an inspiratory stridor developed in speech. She was given relaxation and deep-breathing exercises and was treated as a case of anxiety state since there was no impairment of the vocal cord movements. Delay in being admitted to hospital for surgery and further delay subsequently in obtaining speech therapy upset her. Another woman of 70 developed a severely deep and broken voice after removal of a cyst situated in the false cord. Although the larynx presented an entirely normal appearance it was some months before vocal rehabilitation restored a normal voice. In this case there were no anxiety symptoms and, in fact, the patient, a very active and young 70, was impatient with therapy but her husband did not like her changed voice, which had been a very pleasing and musical one.

17   Laryngeal car-
cinoma: partial and
total laryngectomy
and pseudo-voice

Carcinoma of the larynx is rare under 30 years and is mainly a
disease of middle and old age. Early cases are often related to
papillomata treated by radiotherapy in childhood (Rabbett, 1965;
Vermeuling, 1966). One of the youngest patients reported in the
literature developed a fibrosarcoma of the larynx at age fifteen
and underwent a total laryngectomy fifteen months later after
recurrence of the growth which had been initially arrested by
radiotherapy (Garfield-Davies, 1969).

Malignancy occurs in the larynx more frequently in men than
in women approximately in the ratio of seven to one (Jackson,
1945). Women are prone to gynaecological cancer. If the individual
is fated to contract this frequently lethal disease, he may derive
considerable consolation from the fact that the prognosis for
intrinsic cancer of the larynx is better than for any other site
in the body.

Primary cancer may spread by direct penetration into the
surrounding tissue and there is always a danger of recurrence
near the original site of a primary growth which has been removed
surgically. It is often impossible to excise all the affected cells if
the growth is not well encapsulated, even though wide-field
surgery is carried out. A more serious risk of secondary cancer
arises with involvement of the lymphatic glands since cancer
may now occur widely throughout the body by lymphatic metastasis. As there are practically no lymphatic vessels in the vocal
folds, lymphatic metastasis will only occur when considerable
invasion of the larynx has taken place.

Direct extension of the tumour in the early stages is confined to
the membranous and muscular tissues of the larynx and limited
by its cartilaginous structures, and is therefore of low malignancy.
A tumour is generally not painful in its initial stages and gives no
danger signal of its existence, penetrating deep into body tissues
before it is finally detected. Laryngeal tumour, however, produces
immediate symptoms of hoarseness followed by discomfort,
obstruction, and an irritating cough if allowed to progress. If

358

symptoms of hoarseness are investigated immediately and within a few weeks of inception, diagnosis may be made in time to save life, or at least prolong it for several years. In many cases permanent cure is effected by radiotherapy.

Surgery aspires to the cure of cancer by total excision of the growth, and radiotherapy at the destruction or arrest of active growth and stimulation of fibrous tissue formation. Radiotherapy may be given as an alternative to surgery or ancillary to it at any stage in treatment (Negus, 1950).

The development of cobalt-ray therapy has improved the chances of cure by radiotherapy (Lederman and Daly, 1965; Shaw, 1966a), although Lenz, Okrainetz and Berne (1959) were of the opinion that there is not much difference in long-term results from cobalt- and X-ray therapy. One of the main advantages to the patient is that irradiation burns are less severe and much less discomfort is felt during treatment.

Early cancer of a vocal cord when full movement is retained should be treated with radiotherapy as the first line of attack, with surgery left in reserve if necessary. Surgery is used as a first procedure in cases that are too advanced when first seen. Surgery is also necessary when radiotherapy fails and when a recurrence of malignancy recurs and this can be at any time within a period of a few months or several years. The voice may be hoarse during X-ray treatment and the throat dry but the voice normally recovers fully. Vocal abuse may cause laryngitis rather readily subsequently and then speech therapy is of value.

Differences of opinion now exist not so much as regards radiotherapy versus surgery in primary cancer of the larynx but as regards the extent of surgery advisable and the degree of safety precautions necessary. There are considerable differences in attitude observable among British and American surgeons—the former being usually more conservative (Shaw, 1966). In Britain it is the convention to perform a total laryngectomy when radiation has failed but there is no reason why partial laryngectomy should not be done if stage one (primary) carcinoma is present (Shaw, 1966). A cordectomy (laryngofissure) can be carried out if the recurrence involves the same cord to a similar and minimal extent. A simple laryngectomy on the other hand may be considered safer in the long run especially if there is some extension of laryngeal malignancy observable.

Block dissection (radical neck dissection) will be necessary if metastatic lymph nodes have to be removed.

PHARYNGO-LARYNGECTOMY

Hypopharyngeal, post-cricoid and cervical oesophageal cancer do not respond to radiotherapy and are more difficult and less rewarding to surgeon and speech therapist (Greene, 1967).

OESOPHAGO-PHARYNGO-LARYNGECTOMY

Extensive involvement of larynx, pharynx and oesophagus necessitates removal of these structures and surgical reconstruction

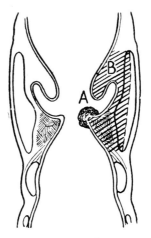

FIG. 40   Coronal view of larynx, showing extent of excision in partial
             laryngectomy with removal of true and false cords

of the oesophagus is now advocated, using part of the stomach or free colonic grafts.

Kirsch (1962) reports that five-year cures occur in 80 per cent of patients who undergo laryngofissure and 60 per cent of those undergoing laryngectomy, but that these figures relate to selected cases. When the cervical glands are affected the outlook is less sanguine. Pharyngo-laryngectomy and radical neck dissection may have just as good results as simple laryngectomy as far as longevity is concerned if combined with irradiation therapy. Some individuals in the laryngofissure and laryngectomy categories live to normal old age and eventually die from other causes. Guthrie (1966) reported a case of a man who underwent laryngectomy at 35 years and was still alive 42 years later. Usually, the outlook is more optimistic for the aged than for the young because carcinoma tends to be more ebullient in youth than in old age when the general rate of cell replacement is slowed down.

PARTIAL LARYNGECTOMY (LARYNGOFISSURE OR CORDECTOMY)

Laryngofissure means cleft of the larynx and is actually only descriptive of the vertical and medial incision made through the anterior angle of the thyroid cartilage in order to gain access to the interior larynx. Partial laryngectomy is a more accurate term. Thyrotomy and thyrochondrotomy are synonyms for the same operation.

Partial laryngectomy is performed only in cases of well-localised tumour situated on the extreme outer edge of the cord. In some cases the vocal cord alone may be excised in one piece with a surrounding margin of 1 cm of healthy tissue (Jackson and Jackson, 1945). In the majority of cases, however, it is considered safer to remove both the vocal cord and the ventricular band and the thyroid ala of the affected side with it. The larynx is left lined with the external perichondrium which heals more readily than if stripped cartilage is left exposed, and also the wound heals with the formation of a fibrous band of cicatricial tissue. Thus in the place of the thyroarytenoid muscle a substitute vocal cord conveniently forms. In time the healthy cord may pass over the mid-line to meet the adventitious cord and a serviceable voice be acquired.

The formation of granulomas on the healing surfaces may interfere with phonation at first and if these do not disperse of their own accord in the course of two or three months they may be removed by direct laryngoscopy. Granulation occurs in approximately 30 per cent of cases undergoing partial laryngectomy, according to Jackson *et al.* (1945). The speech pathologist needs to know that this is not a case of local recurrence of tumour, in order to reinforce the reassurances given by the surgeon in charge, and allay the patient's anxiety.

Sessions, Maness and McSwain (1965) reviewed the literature and 40 cases of laryngofissure performed between 1938 and 1963, on 34 males and 6 females. They draw attention to the fact that the resultant voice is dependent upon the position of the substitute cicatricial cord. The voice is strong if the healthy cord does not have to pass over the mid-line. The voice depends on the degree of approximation achieved between cicatricial and true cords. Eighteen patients in this series had good voices and eighteen only fair voices (4 were not followed up).

Figi (1953) described hemilaryngectomy and skin graft in reconstruction of one vocal cord.

Conley (1962) devised a single-stage operation after partial laryngectomy and removal of both cords, whereby regional flaps are transposed to form imitation vocal cords. Brodnitz and Conley (1967) described the vocal rehabilitation necessary after this procedure. The voice is deep but strong. In speech treatment, gentle pushing exercises with great circumspection are advised.

The operation of laryngofissure is far less traumatic than that of laryngectomy: the patient retains a normal air-way and, though hoarse, has an acceptable voice from the outset. For these reasons in America partial laryngectomy is performed when feasible, keeping in reserve total laryngectomy for if carcinoma recurs and without any greater hazard to the patient. Pressman and Bailey (1968) have related surgery to recently gained knowledge concerning embryonic development of the larynx and anatomy and the spread of cancer and its escape routes via the submucosal lymphatic compartments. The embryologic development of the larynx into two halves and the significance of superficial and deep lymph routes are of prime importance in the new surgical techniques being employed. Whereas a superficial tumour in the mucosa of the larynx may freely travel across the anterior commissure and invade the other half of the larynx, the deeper structures and lymph routes do not readily communicate with each other. The interior of the larynx being divided as it were into a number of compartments anatomically segregated from each other, allows a wide variety of surgical procedures. These may be vertical, horizontal and frontolateral procedures, besides supraglottic horizontal procedures combined with radical neck dissection for removal of involved nodes (Shaw, 1966). All methods preserve the air-way and the voice to a greater or lesser extent. With supraglottic procedures the vocal cords are not involved and the patient's voice will remain unimpaired despite possible difficulties in swallowing.

SPEECH THERAPY FOLLOWING LARYNGOFISSURE

Speech therapy plays an important role in vocal rehabilitation after standard laryngofissure without reconstructive-cord surgery. The substitute cord on the excised side does not project so far into the larynx as the normal cord and is also quite immobile; the healthy cord of the opposite side must be trained to pass over the mid-line and compensate for the deficiency of its fellow much in the same way as in the case of a total unilateral vocal cord palsy. Forcing exercises (pages 178 and 331) are generally recommended but often equally good results may be obtained, without the danger of building up laryngeal and pharyngeal tension, if the patient is merely encouraged to fill up his lungs and raise the volume of his voice. It may assist to press the wings of the thyroid cartilage between thumb and finger to emphasise tactile and kinaesthetic cues. Relaxation and correct diaphragmatic breathing are vital preliminaries to the vocal exercises since there is considerable air wastage. The practice of strong vowel sounds with hard attack is carried out to eliminate breathiness.

The voice may become comparatively good but is never quite normal and is generally rather deep and hoarse. Because of the amount of breath wasted in phonation and the precipitate emptying of the lungs, there is always a strong tendency to continue speech in a forced whisper, involving much tension, in an attempt to achieve the old and habitual length of phrase despite inadequate breath pressure. The patient must be taught first to increase his usual breath capacity and then to obtain better control over expiration. When approximation of adventitious cord and vocal cord is poor, there is sometimes a tendency to attempt vocalisation on inspiration. The patient must learn to inspire more frequently than was his former custom and to use shorter phrases. A contact throat transducer for increasing volume can be used very successfully when voice is inadequate, or a hand microphone with amplifier.

Some improvement in tone can be obtained by the usual vocal exercises. Increase in inflexion may also be achieved by practising scales and variously inflected phrases, and even the singing of well-known tunes. Many patients thus acquire surprisingly serviceable voices in a very short time. On the whole the vocal results with the elderly are disappointing. Levin (1962a) makes the following observations on wide experience: 'Following healing, repeated observation on these patients indicates that there is partial or complete replacement of the removed fold by a scar tissue band. Since approximation is only partial or non-existent, the voice is very harsh and seriously impaired. The outgoing air cannot be interrupted properly. There are extraneous harsh noises as a result of the more or less continuous flow of air'. The exceptional case of a reasonably pleasing voice can occur, however.

Case Report

A male patient of 59 years had an extraordinarily strong voice after laryngofissure, and this appeared to be not so much the result of speech therapy as the fact that he had a well-formed adventitious cord and a naturally well-produced voice before the operation. He was a physically fit and athletic person, a keen swimmer, an ardent cyclist, and regularly touched his toes twenty times night and morning while taking deep health-giving breaths. He was a singularly happy individual and begrudged every moment spent in the hospital away from his engine. Unlike most small boys, he fulfilled his early ambition to be an engine driver and had the good sense to remain faithful to his first love for thirty years.

LARYNGECTOMY

Carcinoma which does not respond to radiotherapy or which recurs after radiotherapy, necessitates, sooner or later (depending

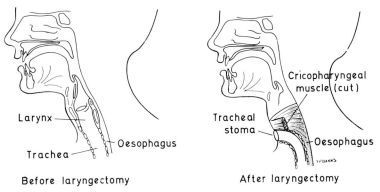

Before laryngectomy   After laryngectomy

Fig. 41   Respiratory tract before and after laryngectomy

upon the surgical considerations described above) a total laryngectomy. If the tumour is causing dyspnoea a tracheotomy may be performed before the main operation but generally this is done at the same time, but precedes laryngectomy. The new air-way assures freedom from breathing complications as far as possible and gives the surgeon freedom of action in the laryngeal field above.

Wilson (1952) states that as little interference with the inferior constrictor of the pharynx as possible is desirable consistent with removal of the tumour. This muscle, when detached from the cricoid cartilage, forms the cricopharyngeal sphincter at the top of the oesophagus and becomes the vibrator for production of oesophageal voice. Levin (1962) says that an effort should be made to create an ample hypopharyngeal pouch without constrictions because upper oesophageal stenosis is a serious handicap in acquisition of pseudo-voice.

Many excellent X-ray cine-radiographic studies have been carried out in recent years and the configuration and function of the pseudo-glottis and hypopharynx examined during the speech of laryngectomised patients. Robe, Moore, Andrews and Hollinger (1956), also Di Carlo, Amster and Herer (1955) and Vrtička and Svoboda (1963) investigated the relation of type of operation performed and the speech result, but did not find evidence to support any particular surgical technique. Slight deviations from the usual technique appear not to influence the functional result. Though theoretically surgical techniques may be devised to obtain a favourable anatomical and physiological result the imponderables of site of tumour and the formation of scar tissue which are individual to each patient are factors beyond control. Mason (1950) states categorically that the precise nature of the pseudo-glottis cannot be predicted and varies with each individual. There is no question, however, that the shape of the hypopharynx and pseudo-glottis is important for the acquisition of good speech. Though it may vary quite widely there are certain irregularities which operate against good functional control over the vicarious 'lung', 'glottis' and 'resonator', which have been emphasised by Hodson, and Oswald (1958), Damsté (1958) and Vrtička and Svoboda (1963).

Preservation of the hyoid bone has been advocated, and Vrtička and Svoboda report that an intact hyoid bone was found much more frequently in their good speakers. They point out that preservation of the hyoid often signifies preservation of the strap muscles whose importance for facilitating aspiration of air into the oesophagus for production of pseudo-voice was emphasised as early as 1922 by Seeman. Bateman and Negus (1954) state that the site of the pseudo-glottis must be expected to vary since it is produced in a muscular tube scarred by operation. However, Vrtička and Svoboda reviewing their 100 cases do not agree with Negus, Hodson nor Damsté. In most of their cases the crico-pharyngeal sphincter was found to be situated at the normal level between the 5th and 6th cervical vertebrae. There was, however, great variability in size and shape of the hypopharynx defined as that part of the pharyngeal tube immediately above the narrowly constricted area of the cricopharyngeal sphincter. Four basic forms were distinguishable: conic, cylindrical, triangular and irregular. In good speakers the conic type prevailed while the irregular type was mostly found in poor speakers. It seems that though surgical technique is not related directly to speech proficiency the final form of the reconstructed pharyngeal tube after healing certainly is. Narrowing at some point in the crico-pharyngeal area is necessary to act as a vibrator but constriction by scarring impedes dilation of the hypopharynx and prevents easy intake and ejection of air from the oesophagus. Moreover, a normal contour to the throat which denotes a pharyngeal cavity above the new vibrator is necessary for resonance of the sub-stitute voice.

Block dissection of metastatic nodes is often necessary and a further complication to laryngectomy, because the throat will be flattened and tighter as more tissue has been removed. If a fistula forms, which is often the case, further scarring and cica-tricial tissue may form. The tongue may be weakened by unilateral dissection of the hypoglossal nerve, and 'drop shoulder' follow unavoidable section of the spinal accessory nerve. The latter is painful and physiotherapy should be given (Levin, 1962a; Hunt, 1964). Despite these complications most patients acquire reason-able oesophageal voice but not so easily as after a simple laryn-gectomy (Smith, Rise and Gralnek, 1966). Putney (1958) did not find type of neck incision, method of pharyngeal closure or amount of cervical tissue excised had any appreciable effect on voice. In our own experience it is difficulties in healing of a fistula which contribute mostly to difficulties in producing speech. The other important factor which only time will eradicate is the unavoidable inflammatory reaction to modern radiotherapy. In the days before cobalt therapy the skin ulceration and the redness and peeling of the neck of a patient brought the muscular condition well to the forefront. With cobalt therapy the patient only feels some soreness and dryness of the mouth but fibrosis and a board-like induration occurs (Harrison, 1964). The speech pathologist should include in her examination and assessment *feeling* the patient's throat for hardness and also anaesthetic areas. The irradiated skin, of course, is ischemic (anaemic) and has a poor blood supply and it is this which causes difficulties in healing. A well-vascularised pedicle of normal, non-irradiated skin has often to be brought up to cover a fistula. This operation, which involves a specialised surgical training, is most successfully performed by a plastic surgeon.

PHARYNGOLARYNGECTOMY

Carcinoma in the hypo-pharynx, post-cricoid and cervical oesophagus necessitates surgical removal of the larynx, pharynx and variable amounts of the oesophagus. In addition most cases will need also a unilateral or bilateral block dissection. Repair presents many problems and sacrifice of the cricopharyngeal sphincter means that voice production will be difficult, and though patients may obtain a whisper or a little voice it lacks volume and is very tiring to sustain. Dornhurst and Negus (1954) state that in very favourable circumstances the voice may be as strong and as fluent as that of the patient who has undergone simple laryngectomy. Such cases are very rare in our experience.

In repair of the cervical oesophagus a single-stage operation and Thiersch graft round a Portex tube may be used in reconstruction and was first described by Negus. This procedure is fraught with difficulties (Harrison, 1964). Stenosis of pharynx and oesophagus may occur and difficulties in swallowing, the patient having to be admitted to hospital for bougienage and stretching of the reconstructed tube under anaesthetic. Plastic reconstruction of pharynx and oesophagus is possible from thoracic flaps but this multiple-stage operation necessitates long hospitalisation and in view of the fact that recurrence is anticipated within 2–3 years it is not generally considered worth while. Recently I met a Canadian patient who had had this treatment and not only did he have a throat of normal appearance but an excellent and fluent voice. Stuart (1966) because of the difficulties of reconstruction and hazards of operation, and of the short life expectancy, advocates insertion of a plastic tube prosthesis. Patients who have a tube prosthesis obtain characteristic hollow and sometimes quite strong voice with great ease and without speech instruction.

THE ASAI TECHNIQUE

Surgeons are constantly endeavouring to improve and explore ways and means of providing patients with better voice after laryngectomy. Dr Asai of the University of Kobe, Japan, has devised a technique which is carried out in three stages after laryngectomy. The first is carried out at the end of an ordinary wide-field laryngectomy and the next two follow at intervals of a month or so later. A tube of skin is constructed in the throat above the tracheal stoma and opening into it and running up to the base of the tongue and opening into the pharynx. Miller (1967, and 1968) is the exponent of the Asai technique in America. Voices are reported excellent with a wide range of pitch and tonal quality. No learning has to take place—the patient places a finger over the tracheal stoma, driving the air up the dermal tube and thus producing voice which is less deep than oesophageal voice, while phrases as long as those of a normal speaker on one breath can be produced. Some patients have to exert digital pressure on the neck at the level of the internal pharyngeal opening to obtain sufficient constriction to air flow for voice production. Others have to close the pharyngeal stoma with the hand when swallowing fluids. A film with sound track was shown in London at the Royal Society of Medicine by Miller (1970) and certainly the speech of the patients was good, but not better than good speakers having a simple laryngectomy. The Asai technique can be performed on patients who have had a laryngectomy some time before and this conversion technique promises to be successful. Such complicated operations are possible only with normal healthy tissue and in Britain where radiotherapy has generally preceded laryngectomy not many patients would be suitable for the multiple stage surgery.

OESOPHAGO-PHARYNGO-LARYNGECTOMY

Extensive involvement of the oesophagus besides larynx and pharynx presents even greater difficulties than those already described in connection with pharyngolaryngectomy. Stomach and free colonic grafts are now advocated in reconstruction of the oesophagus, the colonic transplant being the most popular. (Harrison, 1964; Lall and Evison, 1966; Fairman and John, 1966; Hobbs and Mullard, 1966.) The operation is hazardous and even if the patient survives the prognosis is poor. Fairman and John report 19 survivals from the operation and immediate complications. Harrison (1964) remarks gravely that the surgeon has 'both moral and technical responsibilities' and quotes Gardham: 'How often by prolonging life do we really add to its sum of happiness and how often do we prolong the quantity of life at the expense of its quality?' The speech pathologist must often times be thankful that these ethical responsibilities are not hers but on the other hand she must be aware of them in order to maintain perspective and plan the rehabilitation programme. It is unwise to call in a good laryngectomised patient to demonstrate how a colon transplant patient will speak after operation. It is wiser and kinder to explain that the voice will be weak but whispering will be possible and to speak encouragingly of amplifiers and vibrators. Some of these patients she will never treat and others she may be able to provide with a vibrator. A few patients, however, do develop good colonic voice. Lall and Evison (1966) report on the performance of 4 patients; one developed excellent speech and one reasonable voice and X-ray showed narrowing of the transplant while the diaphragm obtained air fluctuation. One patient showed no narrowing of the reconstructed oesophagus and had only a strong whisper. The last patient was unable to shift air in the tube transplant and so obtain a whisper. We have had a couple of patients who produced very serviceable voice before they died.

LIFE AFTER LARYNGECTOMY

Bateman and Negus (1954) reassure that 'laryngectomy at the present day is not an upsetting or painful operation; healing is usually secure in ten days, when normal swallowing should be resumed' (after removal of the nasal feeding tube inserted immediately after operation). In some cases who have had X-ray therapy a section of the wound obstinately refuses to mend, but a plastic operation can be performed to close a neck fistula and this is generally entirely successful.

In normal conditions healing is rapid and the development of septic conditions is prevented by the administration of antibiotic drugs. If no complications arise the patient is feeling well and cheerful within 10–14 days after the operation and will be found ambling round the ward already trying out his legs and sometimes his new voice.

The most common and troublesome post-operative complication is bronchitis induced by the aspiration of secretion into the bronchi during operation. The patient is distressed by the difficulty in breathing and becomes exhausted by the effort to cough up mucus. A Moure's cannula is inserted in the tracheal opening at first; this cannula consists of two tubes fitting one within the other. The outer tube is left in position until the wound is healed, but the inner tube can be removed, cleaned and sterilised frequently by the nurse in charge. Special suction apparatus is also used to extract mucus from the cannula while in position. This provides temporary relief for the patient and prevents the formation in the bronchial tubes of plugs of mucus which can endanger life through asphyxiation. The acute catarrhal condition is generally only temporary and use of the suction apparatus will not long be necessary. Although the glottis is usually considered a necessary part of the mechanism of coughing, the laryngectomised patient is perfectly able to cough efficiently using the abdominal muscles and diaphragm for increasing intrathoracic pressure. The alveoli offer considerable resistance to sudden pressure, and the air in them is trapped and not immediately expelled. The maintenance of thoracic pressure is difficult for prolonged fixation of the thorax to meet the needs of manual work, but even so, many patients have been able to continue in their employment as porters and dockers. If the patient has a drop shoulder, of course, lifting weights will not be possible and even turning the wheel of a heavy vehicle such as a brick lorry will be too much.

Persistent post-laryngectomy bronchial catarrh may hold up the patient's recovery and his discharge from hospital for several weeks. Breathing exercises may be prescribed by the surgeon in charge, also postural drainage of the lungs, which is undertaken by the physiotherapist. If this is the case and the speech therapist wishes to give instruction in breathing for speech, contact should be made with the physiotherapist in order to avoid possible conflict of exercises and instructions. If the breathing technique taught by the physiotherapist is different from that of the speech therapist, and it may be, then the latter must explain that her instructions relate exclusively to the breathing patterns necessary for speech and not the bronchial condition.

It is important that the patient should be rid of the bronchial infection early for, quite apart from the considerations of health, it renders the acquisition of oesophageal voice difficult on account of the interference with breathing for speech. Patients with bronchial congestion cannot produce oesophageal voice. Bronchitis frequently develops with a cold in the laryngectomised patient. Inspired air-borne bacteria are deposited in the chest and cause infection there instead of in the upper respiratory tract. The nasal mucosa on the other hand remains remarkably healthy and the pseudo-stratified squamous epithelium with which it is lined is replaced in the course of time by ciliated columnar epithelium (Dixon, Hoer and McCall, 1949). Head colds are few. Loss of smell is often noticed, due to inability to inhale through the nose and stimulate the olfactory nerve endings. The sense of taste is also impaired, since we scent most flavours. Smoking, using the buccinator muscles, can be enjoyed for the flavour and does no harm or less so than formerly as the smoke is not inhaled. Swimming is no longer possible. A plastic stoma apron or bib can be worn in the shower.

A small shield consisting of a wire lattice may be worn over the tracheal stoma and suspended by tapes round the neck and covered by clean white gauze or a bib. The shield prevents the discomfort of gauze and clothing being sucked into the orifice upon inspiration. One female patient wore a silver filigree buckle on a chain, which looked attractive. The gauze acts as a filter preventing the inspiration of dust and smoke particles, especially necessary in industrial centres and in foggy weather. Since the gauze is warmed and moistened by respiration it partly replaces the lost function of the upper respiratory passages. Cold air in winter may promote coughing: the bib also gives protection to clothing from mucus in coughing. Medical bibs or aprons can be bought from surgical suppliers but they are thick, hot and unattractive. Buchanan's Laryngectomy protector is supplied by Thackray Limited, Park Street, Leeds, England. Many patients wear home-made aprons of a machine-stitched nylon gauze envelope containing a thin sheet of foam rubber or simply white cotton surgical gauze. All types of bib need to be washed frequently and kept scrupulously clean. Care must be taken to use a plain soap and to rinse thoroughly as scented soaps and detergents may be irritant and make the patient cough and even develop an allergy over a period of time. The foam rubber may also disintegrate and dust or particles be inhaled if a bib is used too long.

The tracheal tube can be discarded when the surgeon in charge gives permission or a tracheal stoma button can be worn to keep the stoma patent (Lauder, 1968). Ability to produce voice may be improved when the tracheal tube is removed.

Some male patients prefer to wear a white silk scarf instead of collar and tie but on an office worker, for example, more formal dress looks more usual and is preferable. Women can wear a lace fichu, a high-necked blouse, or a chiffon scarf with a rope of pearls and thus perfectly conceal all visible evidence of their disability. Some patients, strangely enough, do not appear to be sensitive about their appearance or perhaps wish to obtain sympathy by drawing attention to the disability by not covering the stoma in any way. If this is the case the speech therapist must advise on the proper management of dress on the lines above. The aesthetic management of the stoma and tracheal airway problems are of great importance. The audience reaction to the patient is conducive or otherwise to communication. Patients often complain that people look away, avoid them or do not want to know them. Even friends and relations may be distressed unnecessarily by the appearance of the patient and yet not know how to tell him tactfully about conspicuous mannerisms and hesitate to suggest covering the 'blow-hole' adequately and tastefully (see case history of Mrs R., page 420, in this connection).

The most difficult and unacceptable aspect for the laryngectomee to tolerate, if a normally sensitive individual, is the tracheal opening and airway and in some this takes precedence in importance over loss of voice. It is particularly difficult to cope with coughed-up mucus discreetly and excessive coughing may be an affliction for many weeks after leaving hospital.

Whereas blowing the nose and wiping the mouth with a handkerchief are socially permissible, wiping mucus from the stoma and attacking the problem under a blouse or shirt or bib is another thing altogether. Embarrassment may at first prevent a patient from leaving the house and this may contribute substantially to his depression. Meeting other patients in a group, whether in a class or lost-chord club, is very helpful. Moral support is derived from other sufferers with the same troubles and individuals who have had the same difficulties and found ways of overcoming them.

Violent coughing can render a patient incontinent. One patient with a persistent irritating cough could not go back to work for 18 months for this reason despite acquiring excellent speech very early.

PSYCHOLOGY OF THE LARYNGECTOMEE

In hospitals with ear, nose and throat departments fully organised to deal with cancer patients, a patient who is informed that he must have a laryngectomy operation receives tremendous support from all the staff. He will know his surgeon, radiologist and radiotherapists and the nursing staff and especially the ward sister and feel 'at home' long before he actually has to have the operation, if he has had early radiotherapy. The nature of the laryngectomy operation is explained to the patient and family by the surgeon, the nursing sister explains nursing and feeding problems and the speech therapist explains how speech will be achieved. Although not all surgeons agree on the necessity of a laryngectomee with good speech visiting a patient before operation, most do, and all speech therapists are anxious to provide this facility. There can be nothing more reassuring to a terrified patient than to meet somebody who has not only come through the operation but is alive and well, at work, speaking, and leading a normal life.

The moral support given before operation continues after it and must be maintained until the patient is fully rehabilitated. The natural depression and anxiety which precedes operation and depression which may follow it are normal and understandable and it is often a bad sign when a patient is unnaturally euphoric after operation while in hospital. Often he relapses and goes into a prolonged state of misery when he gets home. By and large the laryngectomee adapts extraordinarily well to the disaster and exhibits great courage and willpower. But a mature approach of this nature 'represents a tremendous emotional and physiological victory and should be recognised by physician and family' (Barton, 1965).

The patient confronted with laryngectomy has to adjust to sudden physical changes in himself which will have widespread repercussions in every aspect of daily life. He will be overcome by anxieties about eating, breathing, speaking and co-habitation. How can he cough? How can he blow his nose or smell? What are the implications of loss of voice as regards his work? Horror may be felt over the necessity to breathe through a hole in the neck and fears concerning loss of sexual attractiveness and desirability arise in both men and women. The surgeon will do his utmost to allay the patient's fears and those of his family, explaining the results of the operation and answering questions. The speech pathologist if introduced to the patient before operation may assist with further reassurance. In this we are in accord with Oswald (1949), Di Carlo (1955), Damsté (1958), Fontaine and Mitchell (1960) and Levin (1962a).

The patient will be greatly comforted if he can meet and speak with a proficient oesophageal speaker. The laryngectomised, 'cured', and successfully rehabilitated individual is able to demonstrate more convincingly than any other that life may go on with enjoyment and without too great inconvenience. He is able to describe from actual experience what laryngectomy means in terms of physical discomfort and personal, social and economic difficulties.

The speech pathologist by keeping in touch with the patient before and after operation pays out a life-line on to which he can hold and the strength of which even the therapist may not fully realise. A patient of Mitchell (Fontaine and Mitchell, 1960) who produced voice very early after operation and developed extraordinarily natural speech described to me, several years afterwards, his abiding gratitude to this therapist. On hearing he was admitted to hospital on Saturday afternoon for operation on Monday, she spent most of the weekend tracking down a good oesophageal speaker in the rural district and introducing him to the patient, besides making several visits meanwhile to explain cheerfully and amusingly the difficulties arising out of so many patients being on summer holiday with no bus or train services available on Sunday.

The importance of the larynx in communication, and of the voice as a means of expressing feelings and personality, has been stressed sufficiently in preceding chapters for the shock sustained by a patient from amputation of so vital an organ not to be underestimated. Many writers have stressed depression in relation to the hindrance it provides in acquiring serviceable speech and in getting back to work. Every speech therapist should be fully aware of the social and family background of the laryngectomee and of his emotional state. A careful case history before operation should be taken. This provides a good basis for forming a real supportive relationship with the patient.

Kallen (1934) refers to the acute depression which often interferes with speech progress. Fontaine and Mitchell (1960) have stressed the emotional and sexual difficulties which may arise after laryngectomy. They emphasise the need for co-operation between almoner (medical social worker) and speech therapist in the alleviation of anxiety, and obtaining adjustment of interpersonal relationships within the family of the patient before voice can be expected to develop. Heaver and Arnold (1962) emphasise the same point and write as psychiatrist and laryngologist 'co-ordinately' as follows:

'A pathologic reactive depression is the usual sequela to the doctor's dictum that the larynx is cancerous, that it must be removed at once, and that natural speech no longer will be possible. Fright, anxiety, insomnia, confusion, self-pity, fear of death, and suicidal impulses pervade and devitalise the patient's psychic energy. It also should be remembered that a depression occasionally masquerades as euphoria'. This is often evident in our experience when the patient is in hospital, depression overcoming him when he returns home. For this reason the above authors advocate the use of an artificial larynx until oesophageal voice is mastered. This is an unconventional procedure and many speech pathologists especially in Britain question its wisdom, preferring to recommend mechanical aids only as a last resort.

Barton (1965) in examining the adjustment of 50 patients to

total laryngectomy, among whom there were 5 suicides, and 50 patients to partial laryngectomy is concerned that evaluation of the individual's adjustment to the disease and operation should be of primary concern to the surgeon in charge. He emphasises that many patients are mentally ill before the operation and are overwhelmed by the catastrophe. Inability to speak and express fears causes acute anxiety. Failure to try fully to speak is a danger signal. Of major importance is the understanding and forbearance of spouse and family. Sleeping together, Barton says, is a haunting experience; coughing of the patient may alarm the partner who becomes over-tired and over-wrought. Instability in a patient in the past is an indication for extra care and vigilance in rehabilitation and psychotherapy may be advisable.

Murphy, Bisna and Ogura (1964) reviewed 24 laryngectomised patients, 4 of whom were judged to be suffering from depression, 3 of whom had not returned to work. They are not interested in the technicalities of diagnosis by experts and whether depression is reactive, endogenous, psychotic or neurotic. Whether depression antedates surgery is fortuitous, and whether depression is a reaction to surgery is not germane since they believe the general symptoms, course, treatment and final outcome are the same. Depression in the absence of other psychiatric illness is readily treatable with gratifying results. These authors describe depression as a sustained mood of dejection, sadness and joylessness, accompanied by insomnia, undue fatigue, anorexia, disinterest, social withdrawal, crying spells, feelings of hopelessness, impaired concentration, indecisiveness, neglect of personal cleanliness or grooming, and either a passive wish for death or thoughts of suicide. Many of these symptoms are normal in the circumstances after laryngectomy and resolve themselves spontaneously. It is a cluster of symptoms Murphy *et al.* (1964) emphasise, persisting for months which characterise real depression and which need psychotherapy, discussion and support, combined with anti-depressant drug therapy, and if necessary electroconvulsant therapy.

Murphy *et al.* (1964) examined their group of patients for the following: age, education, employment history, marital relations, over-indulgence in alcohol, psychiatric history, estimated importance of speech in patients usual employment. None of these factors or group of factors were predicative of the patient's final adjustment, mastery of oesophageal speech and return to work.

In fact the belief of many workers in the area of rehabilitation of the laryngectomised is that psychological factors are more important than any others in determining whether the patient will speak with voice or not. Diedrich and Youngstrom (1966) say that personality, motivation and family environment are all important to success and it is these factors which militate against achievement and account for their estimated one-third of all laryngectomees who fail to learn to speak. These authors believe psychological adjustment is not given enough attention. The operation is, after all, an amputation and marked deformation of the body. Women find it harder to accept the deeper voice and regret the loss of a beautiful voice. The husband of one of our patients left her because, he said, he could not bear her loss of voice. Many patients deplore the fact that they cannot enjoy a good laugh and feel their sense of humour is reduced accordingly.

OESOPHAGEAL PSEUDO-VOCAL MECHANISM

The most skilful laryngectomised speakers acquire extraordinarily natural and fluent speech so that strangers may think the speaker is suffering from a cold or laryngitis and have no idea that he has no larynx. It is now proved beyond any shadow of doubt that pseudo-voice is produced by expelling air from the cervical oesophagus and vibration of the cricopharyngeal muscle. This is always called oesophageal voice, but why is a mystery since logically it should be called cricopharyngeal voice. Purists insist that one should not speak of voice but pseudo-voice but this seems to me too precious. A considerable amount of prejudice and misconception still attaches to the production of oesophageal speech. The term 'pharyngeal voice' is used by those who believe that air is vibrated exclusively in the pharynx. Some go to the opposite extreme, and not believing in the charging of the cervical oesophagus by other means, think that air is swallowed and teach this as the best method for obtaining air intake. The fact that some patients cannot possibly produce voice or do not want to do so is insufficiently recognised. Therapists assume a patient must be psychologically disturbed if he does not learn to use oesophageal voice, viz. Diedrich and Youngstrom (1966) above. Electronic aids, vibrators and amplifiers are still regarded with distaste and disapproval by speech therapists and surgeons, and patients are denied the undoubted solace of these instruments.

It seems therefore, that despite the many excellent American publications now available to students on the subject of teaching laryngectomees to speak, a historical survey leading up to present-day knowledge and treatment based on sound physiological principles will still not come amiss. However, the student is strongly recommended to read and study carefully the scientific research summarised in *Speech Rehabilitation of the Laryngectomised* by J. C. Snidecor and others (1968) and the more practical clinical account by D. M. Diedrich and K. A. Youngstrom of *Alaryngeal Speech* (1966).

The acquisition of oesophageal voice is no new discovery and long before speech pathologists were at hand to rehabilitate these patients they learned to speak on their own initiative. Dr S. Solis Cohen (Bateman and Negus, 1954) reported in 1895 the case of a patient who taught himself to speak. In those days, of course, few individuals survived long enough to do so. The cricopharyngeal sphincter, described by Killian as early as 1908, is composed of the lowest fibres of the inferior constrictor and, when these are freed from the cricoid plate, they lie as bands just beneath the mucosa and circular muscle layer of the oesophagus and form the vibrator of the substitute glottis (Morrison, 1931) (Fig. 41). The walls of the oesophagus are highly elastic and capable of considerable expansion in accommodation of the food bolus, and of air adventitiously after laryngectomy. The oesophageal sphincter (cricopharyngeal muscle) is relatively atonic after operation. This and the upper portion of the oesophagus are composed of striated muscle innervated by the recurrent laryngeal nerve and voluntary relaxation and tension of the sphincter can be acquired in oesophageal voice production (Levin, 1962a). Should scar tissue impair the elasticity of the sphincter it is unlikely that speech will be good. At best it will be explosive and staccato, since swallowing air into the stomach will be unavoidable and it can only be forced up by belching. Adequate speech cannot develop without the use of oesophageal muscle, or vibration of air by its passage through a narrow lumen of the reconstructed oesophageal pharyngeal tract in the case of pharyngolaryngectomy.

The early teaching of voice without a larynx consisted simply in instructing the patient to swallow air and belch it forth. The patient was aided perhaps in the acquisition of this skill by beer or aerated drinks or sometimes a solution of bicarbonate of soda (Oswald, 1949). The voice had the unmistakable quality of belching and was also laboured, the patient having to pause and swallow before each phrase of two or three words was uttered. In the course of time, however, it became apparent that the whole method of voice production underwent a radical change as greater proficiency in voice production developed. The patient apparently ceased to swallow air but somehow seemed to manage to vibrate it in his throat and 'higher up' by almost imperceptible pharyngeal and lingual movements. This 'pharyngeal voice' was thought to be produced entirely in the pharynx. The tone was less deep and considerably more natural and speech more fluent than when the 'oesophageal' voice, dependent upon air swallowing, was used.

An interesting description of how it feels to produce this so-called 'pharyngeal' speech has been given by Sawkins (1949), Miss Oswald's highly accomplished laryngectomised speaker. He states that a vibrating column of air is passed backwards and forwards between the pharynx and mouth. The back of the tongue with the tip in position for the articulation of [n] performs a piston-like movement and sets the air column in motion between the approximated muscular tissues. The back of the tongue, pharynx and the pillars of the fauces, he believed, acted as 'substitute folds' causing the vibration of air and therefore voice. This belief, was of course, quite erroneous.

In actual fact the pharyngeal cavity does not participate in the production of the fundamental oesophageal note, though it acts as a resonator for it. We knew one patient who used the pharynx exclusively to vibrate air in the production of voice. This patient, referred by us in despair to Miss Oswald, is the case S.K. described in the monograph by Hodson and Oswald (1958). Lateral X-ray motion photography showed no expansion of the oesophagus during speech, the cricopharyngeal sphincter remaining tightly closed, but pulsations of the pharynx took place. His voice was bizarre and ugly, resembling the quacking voice of Walt Disney's Donald Duck. It had no resemblance to oesophageal speech. Damsté (1958) has described a similar case in which there was an inability to take air into the oesophagus and the sphincter remained tightly closed. Possibly the pillars of the fauces act as vibrators in these patients and account for the characteristic squawking 'voice'.

In his patient, Damsté obtained relaxation of the cricopharyngeal sphincter by stretching it artificially. The patient swallowed the thickest oesophageal catheter (weighted by bird shot!) periodically, until he mastered voluntary relaxation of the oesophageal sphincter. The early recordings of this patient's pharyngeal speech resembled exactly the speech of S.K. The recordings and the patient himself, now speaking with serviceable oesophageal speech, were kindly demonstrated to me by Mrs Moolenaar-Bijl and Dr Damsté in their Gröningen Clinic in 1957, and testified to the success of Damsté's method of obtaining artificially the mechanical relaxation of the cricopharyngeal sphincter. Oswald's case S.K. never acquired pleasing speech.

Seeman (1959) claims to have been the first to determine by lateral radiography that the oesophagus acts as a vicarious or substitute 'lung' and the oesophageal sphincter as a pseudo-glottis. In 1922 he published his report, which is unfortunately in Czech. Seeman, as cited in Kallen's review of research (1934) drew attention to the fact that: 'The cervical and upper portions of the oesophagus contain transverse striated muscle fibres, the muscles of the lower part are smooth. As the recurrent laryngeal nerve gives off branches some of which (the so-called rami oeso-phagei nervi recurrentis) are distributed to the oesophagus, the phenomenon associated with phonation is probably the result of an irradiation to the musculature of the oesophagus of the nerve impulses attending phonation'. Seeman sought to prove that phonatory contractions in the cervical and upper portions of the thoracic oesophagus were genuinely active and not dependent upon respiratory movements. Only in the middle and lower thoracic oesophageal sections did he observe changes in the lumen effected by thoracic movement. In skilful laryngectomised speakers it certainly seems possible that there is an irradiation to the oesophageal sphincter of the nerve impulses for normal laryngeal phonation, though this is naturally difficult to prove. In one of our most proficient speakers the cricopharyngeal bands on either side can be seen to approximate in the mid-line exactly like bulky vocal cords as he phonates during an indirect laryngo-scopic examination. Other patients with great difficulty in air-charging the oesophageus present a tight slit in the glosso-pharyngeal lumen.

Morrison published in 1931 a further report and his own valuable observations. This was followed in 1937 by Stetson's distinguished research study and his original suggestions for teaching oeso-phageal speech. He confirmed that the pseudo-glottis is formed by the oesophageal sphincter and that the valvular lips are separated as air bursts through them and then recoil and close automatically as the air pressure below them drops. This mechanism is much the same in fact as for laryngeal phonation. The cervical oesophagus (sometimes in association with the upper thoracic portion) provides a 'lung', bellows or air reservoir for speech. The intake of air and its expulsion, he maintained, was dependent upon changes in intrathoracic pressure coincidental with normal respiration for speech. Bateman and Negus (1954) explain that the sphincter in normal individuals is tightly closed in order to prevent this happening and the entry of air into the stomach during the respiratory cycle. After laryngectomy the muscle can be relaxed voluntarily to take advantage of this normal physiological process. Bosma (1953) has described the occurrence of air aspiration and expulsion in the same way in individuals suffering from paralysis of the pharynx following poliomyelitis. Stetson (1937) stated in fact that chest action for oesophageal speech is the same as for normal speech, the pulses in the oesophagus being largely produced by the original co-ordinations and chest pulses for speech. The only difference Stetson observed was that inspiration had to be executed at more frequent intervals in order to replenish the more quickly exhausted air reservoir of the oesophagus. This reservoir he thought was small and consisted of only 2·5 c.c. Snidecor and Isshiki (1965) (Isshiki, 1968) have, however, discovered that air flow is considerably higher than this and volume per syllable ranged from 5 to 16 c.c. and 27–72 c.c. per second in good speakers.

THE VICARIOUS LUNG

Air is constantly replenished during oesophageal speech in the vicarious lung in two ways. First, air is *aspirated*[1] into the oesophagus synchronously with lung inspiration. Secondly, minute quantities of air are *injected* into the oesophagus by muscular compression of air in the oral cavity (the implosive method). Injection may take place and precede speech and is achieved by closing the lips and elevating the soft palate with slight tensing of the cheeks and tongue, causing air to be compressed in the oral cavity, pressed backward into the pharynx and injected into the oesophagus. This injection phase commonly accompanies the lung inspiration which precedes speech. Alternatively the same result may be obtained by sudden closure of the articulatory organs during the normal flow of speech and enunciation of consonants, especially the plosives. Stetson substantiated that a patient uttering a series of [pup] syllables replenished oesophageal air on the last consonant of each syllable. Thus in the speech of

[1] Synonyms for 'aspirated' are 'insufflated' and 'inhaled'—the last being confusing since it is not always clear to the student whether oesophageal or lung air is being inhaled.

proficient laryngectomised speakers, the air in the substitute or vicarious 'lung' is constantly replenished, giving the possibility of uttering 15–20 syllable phrases upon one cycle of lung respiration, and before further aspiration of oesophageal air by lung inspiration is necessary. The incidence of vowels and continuants and nasal consonants which do not favour injection of air, gradually drains the vicarious lung of air.

Speech therapy in England before the second world war and immediately after was distinguished mainly by its remarkable insularity and almost complete isolation from scientific advances in other parts of the world. Neither the knowledge from the great European centres nor that from America infiltrated. This in some ways has been an advantage in that speech therapists have had to rely almost entirely upon clinical observation and empirical method in their practical field and are probably still unsurpassed as practical therapists (Van Thal, 1956). It is not surprising therefore that, lacking cine-radiographic and scientific examination techniques, the belief that good oesophageal voice was pharyngeal in origin persisted for a very long time in England and survives even to this day.

In 1949, however, Marland advocated a 'direct' method of teaching 'pharyngeal voice' after laryngectomy. She omitted swallowing technique from therapeutic method, basing much of her observation upon the very skilled patient of Miss Oswald, Mr Sawkins (1949). She taught patients to take in air by 'oral compression'. At this time Miss Oswald's interest and enthusiasm inspired a research project with Hodson at University College Hospital under the supervision of Myles Formby. Sir Victor Negus acted in an advisory capacity. Hodson thus embarked upon the very first lateral cine-radiographic studies in England of laryngectomised patients. Both good and poor speakers were carefully studied. The film was shown and patients demonstrated to an invited audience in 1952, but the work was not published until 1958. This valuable little monograph entitled *Speech recovery after total laryngectomy* (Hodson and Oswald, 1958) contains Miss Oswald's plan of treatment. Having been a student of this gifted therapist I am probably biased in my views regarding the best methods of teaching oesophageal voice, but nobody who watched her teach and heard the results could fail to acknowledge their value.

Hodson and Oswald established that the pseudo-glottis was of two types. It was formed in some cases by the muscular sphincter at the top of the oesophagus (the cricopharyngeal sphincter). In other cases it was formed by a 'narrowed segment' at the upper end of the oesophagus and varied from 4 to 8cm in length. This was composed probably of dissarranged and diffusely spread cricopharyngeal and inferior constrictor fibres after surgical intervention. In some patients the walls of the hypopharynx moved, but Hodson and Oswald concluded that these movements were related to quality of voice only and did not contribute to the fundamental note. They also observed that the air stream for sound formation in facile speakers was entirely derived from the oesophagus which 'fills with air by an inspiratory movement, mainly diaphragmatic; and from which air is driven by slow expiratory movement, again largely diaphragmatic in make-up. And that, finally, the inability of poor speakers is largely due to a failure of co-ordination of the mechanism of "sphincter" control and diaphragmatic breathing inherent in the above'. Oswald believed that the *sole means of drawing air into the oesophagus was by aspiration,* and expulsion was by increase of thoracic pressure through ascent of the diaphragm. Stetson's injection method of air intake did not enter into her treatment.

Moolenaar-Bijl (1952 and 1954) published accounts of her treatment for laryngectomised patients by injection of air into the oesophagus following the teaching of Stetson, and the use of oral pressure in articulation of the plosive consonants. She believed in complete contradiction to Oswald's view, that this is the only way in which oesophageal speakers achieve the necessary air intake and that respiration and inter-thoracic pressure play no part in the process. Her thesis was ably supported by Damsté and Van den Berg, who produced an interesting cine-radiographic film with synchronous sound in 1955. This is still shown to students and can mislead them. Captain Peters asking for a cup of coffee demonstrates unforgettably the pumping of air into the oesophagus by plosives, but the replenishment of oesophageal air by lung inhalation can be detected if one looks for it. A much more instructive black and white cine-radiographic film was made some years later by the same Dutch team in collaboration with the laryngologist Professor Hutzinga. It is entitled 'Oesophageal Speech' and is distributed in England by Philips. The film demonstrates both the injection of air during speech and aspiration of air before the act of speaking. This is referred to simply as replenishment of oesophageal air and the main purpose of the film is still to demonstrate implosion.

The division of opinion over the question of air intake is of great consequence in teaching. All research workers and experienced speech clinicians who have to rely upon their powers of observation are agreed that fluent oesophageal speech is perfectly synchronised with the normal respiratory cycle. Bateman and Negus (1954), Hodson and Oswald (1958), Robe *et al.* (1956), Di Carlo *et al.* (1955), and Vrtička and Svoboda (1961, 1963) are unanimous that oesophageal speech occurs only during lung expiration and that it is always prefaced by lung inspiration as in normal speech.

It is the relative importance of articulation, injection and inspiration for the oesophageal air supply which causes controversy, since the principles involved should logically determine teaching method. Vrtička and Svoboda (1961), reviewing a far larger group of laryngectomees than those in previous studies, describe a lowering and flattening movement of the tongue (also noted by Schlosshauer and Mockel, 1958) which coincided with oesophageal aspiration and preceded phonation in their best speakers. In their own words, 'this movement of the tongue never had the character of an air injection from the oral cavity and the hypopharynx into the oesophagus supposed by Moolenaar-Bijl; it did not even occur in patients using very quick and minute aspirations as some of the less good speakers did'. Patients, of course, tend to employ the methods taught by their instructors— those taught the inhalation method will use this means of air charge rather than another. Similarly those taught injection by plosives will rely more on this means. All patients with fluent speech use plosive injection, aspiration and various means of pushing air back with the tongue used rather like a pump. Damsté (1959) in fact described this as the glosso-pharyngeal press. A glossal press or a glossal pharyngeal press can be observed in many patients, with or without closed lips before speaking; this leads frequently to a gulping or clicking sound in the throat which has to be corrected in clinical practice.

Diedrich and Youngstrom (1966) by means of lateral radiographic studies examined tongue movements during air intake in 20 laryngectomees. During 'inhalation' the tongue never occluded the oral cavity and there was little or no movement of the dorsum of the tongue. The lips were open, there was velopharyngeal closure and the air-way from lips to pharyngooesophageal junction was patent. Injection showed two types of tongue movement: *a glossal press* consisted of contact by the tongue with alveolus, and frequently middle of the tongue contact with the hard palate, while the posterior portion moved backward but failed to touch the pharyngeal wall. The lips might be open or closed. A *glossopharyngeal press* occurred when the tip and middle of the tongue contacted alveolus and hard palate, and posterior portion of tongue moved back to make contact with pharyngeal wall, while the hypopharyngeal cavity might be completely obliterated. There was velopharyngeal closure and lips might be closed or not. They noted that these movements are different from a swallow movement, also that the quicker the air intake the better the speech—long pauses make for non-fluency.

Diedrich and Youngstrom also compared articulation in laryngectomees with normal speakers and found the latter used more lip tension. They also report that 's' and 's' blends and voiceless plosives are the easiest sounds for injecting air into the oesophagus, by which is meant presumably also the most effective.

Isshiki (1965 and 1968) with specially developed and very complicated electronic apparatus was finally able to check the differences reported in previous research findings described above in which spirometric, pneumographic and radiographic equipment was often used separately so that only one aspect of oesophageal speech was examined, perhaps, at one time. Also gross movements and not refined movements were noted and the extreme complexity of co-ordinated muscular adjustments were not appreciated. Another factor distorting the picture in many studies was that only superior speakers were chosen as research subjects. Isshiki chose six speakers of variable proficiency. Respiratory thoracic movements, volume of air charge, flow rate of air charge and voice were measured. It was found that air intake and use in conjunction with respiration and vocalisation vary greatly with individual speakers. Some speakers injected air while speaking and as they exhaled, which is what other researchers have found. All speakers apparently aspirated ('inhaled') air into the oesophagus synchronously with lung inspiration. Some speakers relied more on injection than inhalation. Negative pressure in the oesophagus during lung inhalation assists injection of air by the tongue. The more effective and larger the air intake, the better the speech. Lung expiration and speech are always synchronised. A slow and normal deep breathing movment itself did not insufflate air into the oesophagus. This is important and confirms the observation that a quick diaphragmatic pant is necessary for sucking air into the oesophagus and needs to be developed by the patient. It seems, therefore, that all the protagonists in the field are right and it is obviously unwise to confine speech therapy to teaching one method but advisable to introduce a combination of all methods, since this is actually what takes place when fluent speech is mastered. This was my own conclusion in 1964 and also that of Robe-Finkbeiner (1962) and Diedrich and Youngstrom (1966) besides others.

Varying methods of air intake are usefully taught at different times and all methods may produce the wrong results at any given stage in treatment until a balance is found. Efforts to conform, for example, to old breathing habits may result in excessive expiration from the tracheostoma. Then dissociation of voice from respiration, by emphasising injection of air, may help to remedy the fault. The experienced therapist will first help her patient to produce voice quickly by whatever means is found easiest. Failure to produce voice has most serious adverse psychological consequences, as Heaver and Arnold (1962) emphasise. Application of the basic principles related to air intake into the vicarious lung must develop along lines favourable to the patient's learning ability and his anatomical and physiological possibilities. The correction of faults and improvement of pseudo-voice will be effected by application of one principle after another so that the patient eventually obtains the necessary smooth synchrony of respiration and voice largely by his *own* method.

My personal conviction is that good diaphragmatic breathing is essential and that respiration must be co-ordinated with production of oesophageal voice, and this aim should form the basis of vocal training. I have taken over the treatment of a sufficient number of patients trained in swallowing and injection technique, with failure to progress from the 2–3 syllable phrase, to be convinced of this need. By applying local relaxation and respiration techniques an immediate increase in length of phrase and consequently of fluency can be obtained.

One need not confuse the patient by association of breathing technique with voice production immediately. Miss Oswald's plan of teaching relaxation and diaphragmatic breathing before laryngectomy was a sound one. Although believing that aspiration of air is necessary I am equally convinced that this must be combined with air injection, during the process of either strong raticulatory movements or a combined tongue and pharyngeal movement, or both, at different moments. In this respect I am not in agreement with Hodson and Oswald (1958) or Vrtička and Svoboda (1961).

The variation in methods of charging the oesophagus with air in their 100 patients is described by Vrtička and Svoboda and will be given below in order to emphasise the impossibility of generalisation over the laryngectomee's speech. These authors classified their patients according to the grades of Robe *et al.* (1956) as follows:

(*a*) No sounds produced
(*b*) Partial control: single sounds under fair control
(*c*) Simple words produced
(*d*) Combines 2–3 words
(*e*) Some sentences used
(*f*) Sentences consistently used
(*g*) Fluent, non-hesitant speech

The (*a*) group performed unco-ordinated swallowing movements by which means air was brought into the oesophagus. In groups (*b*) and (*c*) there was a tendency to more regular quiet dilation of the hypopharynx during aspiration, and the swallowing movements were absent. In groups (*d*) and (*e*) there was regular aspiratory dilation of the hypopharynx with lowering and flattening of the back of the tongue in the pre-aspiratory phase and only very exceptionally by swallowing movements. In the (*f*) group and more especially in the (*g*) group the aspirations were quite regular, easy, relatively quick and automatic.

The above categories fit into the categories quickly recognised by any experienced speech clinician in this field and neatly summarise the stages through which the laryngectomised patient may pass or linger or come to a halt in treatment. According to Vrtička and Svoboda (1963) in a further study of 75 cases with combined radiographic and phoniatric follow-through examinations, a gradual increase in functional control of expansion and contraction of the hypopharynx is evident. Speech proficiency is in fact in direct relation to the control eventually achieved over dilatability of the hypopharynx. This movement is thought by these authors to be related to quality of voice and not to injection of air into the oesophagus. As speech fluency increased the length of the air column in the oesophagus increased also, and therefore the air reservoir for voicing longer phrases.

18 Speech rehabilitation after laryngectomy

It has already been stated that the speech therapist should contact the patient before his operation and explain how he will be able to speak again. Many patients jump to the conclusion that they will be totally unable to speak. It is advisable to reassure them on this point at the outset and tell them that although without a voice at first, they will be able to whisper. We also tell them about the vibrators and amplifiers which are available but do not as a rule demonstrate them unless particularly requested.

A laryngectomee with good speech and a happy balanced out-look on life should visit the patient, if possible before the operation. The visitor needs to be carefully selected; some are tactless and may go into too great detail about the after-effects, wishing to air their knowledge and achievements, and may unintentionally frighten the patient. If no suitable visitor is available a tape-recording of a laryngectomee can be played as a second best. If the patient is to have a pharyngolaryngectomy and/or colon transplant we are far more circumspect. We do not arrange for a laryngectomised visitor to demonstrate but we assure the patient he will achieve a loud whisper quite easily and we mention vibrators and amplifiers (see page 422).

SPEECH THERAPY PROCEDURE

If an opportunity for providing instruction in relaxation and intercostal diaphragmatic breathing is presented before laryngectomy this provides an opportune beginning for the vocal rehabilitation programme. The patient in a state of tense expectancy and fear will find reassuring the opportunity for doing something immediately practical and constructive about his pending loss of larynx and voice. At the same time the inter-personal relationship established with the therapist is greatly reassuring.

The therapist should visit the patient as soon after operation as is allowed, to see how he is getting on and maintain contact, even if this is only a friendly wave from the door. When the feeding tube is removed and swallowing no longer painful, speech lessons can start. This contact after the operation is all the more necessary in case healing is delayed and the patient has to retain the nasal feeding tube for some weeks, and even months if an obstinate fistula forms. In these circumstances the patient should be encouraged to whisper, with the nasal tube in position as this maintains and develops clear articulation. It is helpful also if the tongue is paretic. Often a clear and audible whisper can be heard and this is naturally very encouraging to the individual and also much less tedious and frustrating than writing everything down. In fact we discourage written communication as far as possible. If the fistula is failing to heal, and depending upon its site and size, the surgeon should be consulted concerning the advisability of whispering and the possible danger of exaggerated articulatory movements of the tongue pulling at the wound. Much depends upon the height of the fistula in the pharyngeal wall and also the manner of speech—some excitable patients put far too much effort into whispering.

Once the patient is allowed out of bed, and is eating normally, voice production can commence and he should be allowed to join an out-patient group of laryngectomees if available, merely as a spectator.

Oswald (Hodson and Oswald, 1958) emphasised that no formal instruction apart from the preliminary relaxation and breathing technique should be given at first. She recommended that the patient should just sit and listen to other patients. Thus, relaxed and free from direct demands upon himself to produce voice, which may breed anxiety, tension and over-exertion, the patient is allowed to experiment by imitation when he feels so inclined, and may spontaneously produce voice. This is not a new concept but was advocated as early as 1926 by Hugo Stern, cited by Morrison in 1931.

If the patient in these circumstances produces oesophageal voice, treatment generally follows an easy course. Guidance in breathing technique, voice and articulation co-ordination helps nurture the seed which has germinated. Once voice is mastered the patient can speak, since there is no impairment of the organs of articulation. The naturally good speaker with a good speech sense automatically and intuitively adjusts articulation to the new circumstances. Speech must be slower, allowing time for more emphatic articulation, so that maximum benefit may be derived from injection of air into the oesophagus by compression of air in the oropharynx.

The patient who produces voice so easily proves to be rather the exception unfortunately in our experience with patients who have been treated by X-ray therapy. Many have great difficulty in mastering even the rudimentary elements of oesophageal voice and a single vowel sound. In these cases the therapist's example and demonstration of what is needed which provides a pattern to imitate is essential. Experimentation along empirical lines of teaching will be necessary. The therapist's exact diagnosis of why the patient is failing to produce voice suggests the remedy to be applied in every case. No fixed and rigid mode of instruction will meet the needs of all difficult cases, despite the ardent advocates to be found for the three different methods of air charge of the oesophagus. The first aim in teaching is the production of a sound; it does not matter how this is achieved, but achieved it must be at the earliest possible moment after the removal of the larynx and for purely psychological reasons. The thing the patient fears most is that he will never again be able to speak audibly. Failure to achieve voice after laryngectomy has the most depressing and disastrous effect upon the patient and may delay speech many months. As the period in which he fails to find his new voice gradually lengthens, the conviction that he never will do so naturally grows. He may resort more and more to the use of a buccal whisper. As this is produced by exaggerated articulation and high air pressure in the mouth and pharynx against which the cricopharyngeal sphincter is firmly closed, the chances are diminished of obtaining voluntary relaxation of the sphincter so necessary to voice production.

A warning is necessary here. Professional enthusiasm should never lead to a patient being deprived of an artificial vocal aid when he really needs one. It is not humane to insist upon acquisition of oesophageal voice when this is not possible. The decision should not be the responsibility of patient or therapist alone but arrived at in the light of clinical experience during treatment, and in collaboration with the laryngologist who can assess the surgical result. The patient's oesophogopharyngeal structure, its size, shape and dilatability should be examined ideally by cineradiographic filming. For decades lateral X-ray films have been regarded as indispensable diagnostic data when rehabilitative surgery is planned for cleft-palate patients by plastic surgery teams. The same investigative techniques should be available for laryngectomees failing to acquire oesophageal speech. The speech pathologist in the laryngological team may collaborate with laryngologist and radiologist to good effect, as the work of Oswald, Moolenaar-Bijl, Di Carlo and Snidecor fully demonstrates. However, many of us have not the advantages of working in expensively equipped research units and must rely on our own observations and the surgical and post-operative history. An indirect laryngoscopy is often most helpful and is a routine follow-up procedure in the ear, nose and throat department. The therapist can look over the surgeon's shoulder and inspect the pseudo-glottis and will soon begin to find this as useful as looking at vocal cords and spotting nodules, contact ulcers or tensor weakness in the normal larynx.

The patient who is not obviously going to achieve oesophageal voice easily should be given an artificial larynx (vibrator) to experiment with. It is now realised that this does not necessarily mean the patient will give up trying to speak using his own mechanism. On the contrary, most patients dislike the gadgets and want to learn to speak without them, but it may save frustration and the misery of not being able to talk freely at home, and in fact help a patient to relax and learn oesophageal voice more easily. Use of a vibrator requires slow clear speech and encourages practice in phrasing. Arnold and Heaver (1962), Diedrich and Youngstrom (1966) strongly advocate use of a vibrator from the outset. In some but not all patients this is advisable, in our opinion.

Lauder (1968), himself a laryngectomee and qualified speech pathologist, says, very sensibly, that there is no need to adopt an either/or attitude. For example, we can cite cases of patients who speak naturally and adequately at home but need a vibrator in the noisy surroundings at work or in telephoning. If deprivation of a vibrator means staying off work longer than is necessary once the patient is physically fit, then he should be given a vibrator. Another illustration which emphasises the need for imagination and latitude in approach by the speech therapist is the patient whose speech is adequate at work in a quiet office with little speech required but inadequate for communication with a hard-of-hearing spouse. This again justifies use of a vibrator and makes all the difference to happy home-life and readjustment post-operatively.

FACTORS IMPEDING ACQUISITION OF VOICE

The following factors can be expected to render the acquisition of oesophageal voice difficult or impossible:

(*a*) A poor post-operative result with formation of scar tissue which restricts facile dilation of the hypopharynx and crico-pharyngeal sphincter.

(*b*) Damage to the nerve supply to the pharynx and tongue by surgery producing muscular weakness, especially of the tongue, and difficulty in swallowing solids.

(*c*) Old age and frailty accompanied by lack of drive to learn.

(*d*) Deafness and inability to monitor speech.

(*e*) Low intelligence and inability to master the necessary new muscular co-ordination.

(*f*) Real distaste for oesophageal speech and preference for an artificial vocal aid.

(*g*) Previously inadequate speech.

(*h*) Unsympathetic spouse or deaf spouse.

(*i*) Depression.

If a patient therefore wants or appears to need a vibrator we let him have one on loan. The patient who has had a simple laryngectomy operation and uneventful recovery generally does not require one and begins to develop oesophageal voice sufficiently early to be confident that he is making the anticipated progress. A pocket amplifier may be more useful at this stage in the learning of oesophageal voice production and especially when practising at home (see also page 411). The amplified voice is satisfying, as is singing in the bath, and helps relaxation and speaking without effort. It helps self-monitoring of speech and assists in correction of such faults as extraneous gulping sounds and blowing from the stoma. A doctor of 60 years still in busy rural practice wrote: 'The amplifier has been a tremendous help to me as a tutor which enables me to hear just what sort of sounds I am producing. I am hoping to keep it for another month or two as I am beginning to be a bit more intelligible'. He was at that time using also a white noise vibrator successfully. He eventually learned to speak naturally, but used a pocket amplifier and hand microphone when having to speak against background noise.

Many patients who develop good oesophageal speech in time just do not find it loud enough for professional purposes. One of our patients who is a busy and gifted freelance photographer for colour magazines and supplements makes free use of an amplifier when needed and says he could not manage without, despite having excellent speech. He has evolved a means of overcoming the difficulty of dropping 'h's' by making a minute

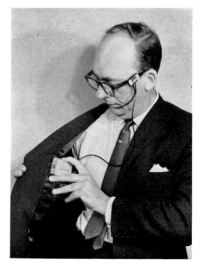

Fig. 42   Patient with S. G. Brown amplifier and Pacific head-set
microphone

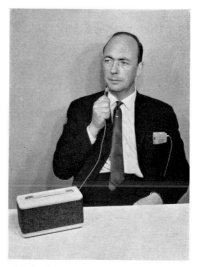

Fig. 43   Patient with S. G. Brown amplifier, hand microphone and table
loudspeaker

pause before the following vowel which he says the ear of the
listener fills in as an 'h' at the psychological level. It is certainly
most effective.

Another patient who works for a newspaper and is also a

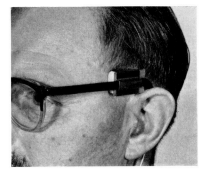

Fig. 44A S. G. Brown throat microphone worn on spectacle frame (sound source through bone conductor)

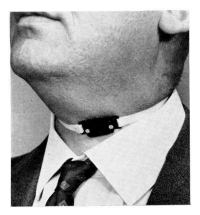

Fig. 44B S. G. Brown throat microphone

door-to-door salesman of an evening and a mason and master of his lodge, uses a pocket amplifier and speaking tube attached to a spectacle bracket. Only in this way can he be heard at the door and demonstrate his wares with free hands, and moreover perform all those mysteries a master of a lodge has to (which a woman knows nothing of). A civil servant, who had marital troubles long before his laryngectomy and was a tense anxious man, produced a tense high-pitched voice with great difficulty. He found answering queries about tax returns well-nigh impossible. He was fitted with a contact transducer on the arm of his spectacles which picked up vibrations from his temporal bone. After this his speech improved greatly in fluency, became lower in pitch and with this his anxiety and depression were alleviated. He was often able to discard his speech aid on 'good' days.

There are only certain laryngectomised patients who can use a contact transducer placed on the temporal bone in this way. It is not possible for individuals with normal anatomy and so it is no use a therapist endeavouring to test a voice aid out on herself in this way. It will not work in cases of partial laryngectomy either. The pseudo-voice has to be rather hard, tense and of relatively high pitch for vibrations to be picked up and amplified via bone conduction.

THE INTRODUCTION OF VOCAL METHODS

Since it is generally agreed and proved that the fluent laryngectomee employs both aspiration and air injection methods of air charging the oesophagus, it would seem logical to introduce him immediately to both methods and to draw attention to implosion by articulation and aspiration by diaphragmatic breathing. However, experienced clinicians in general advocate beginning with one method rather than another, or several, because it is less confusing to the patient. Vrtička and Svoboda (1961), Hodson and Oswald (1958), Di Carlo *et al.* (1955) advocate aspiration as the best teaching method to begin with. Moolenaar Bijl (1953) and Damsté (1958), also Diedrich and Youngstrom (1966), advocate the implosive method. As a rule, I find the attempt to produce pseudo-voice from syllables beginning with plosive consonants is the least difficult but I am perfectly prepared to experiment with all methods if difficulty is encountered by a patient. Belching or 'burping' may be suggested, and drinks of beer or an aerated liquid—anything, in fact, to let the patient feel and hear an air bubble going up and down in the throat. We experiment together. It is of great value if the therapist can produce the required oesophageal voice herself and this is not difficult and setting oneself the task of acquiring the skill certainly breeds humility and insight into the patient's difficulties. If this is not possible, a therapist can cheat and produce a very good imitation of an oesophageal vowel sound by drawing air in over the ventricular bands, rounding the mouth and pulling down the larynx to obtain the necessary hollow resonance. In America, of course, laryngectomee teachers are employed in many centres to teach laryngectomees Lauder. (1965) has reported on the questionnaire he carried out to obtain the views of distinguished American speech pathologists on this controversial question. Although the idea is rejected out of hand by European and British therapists, I have seen classes in progress with a laryngectomee teacher in charge in hospital clinics in America and the speech results were excellent. The laryngectomee teachers are notably far more exacting in the practice of exercises than the average speech therapist. There seems to be no valid reason why laryngectomees who have undergone an adequate teacher training course should not be used as an adjunct in the normal clinical team working under qualified speech therapists, especially in areas where there is a shortage of speech therapists.

Lauder (1968a), a laryngectomee teacher holding the ASHA certificate of clinical competence, has produced a useful and practical booklet for laryngectomees which can be recommended reading for laryngectomised patients.

1. *Air Swallowing*

If the patient has not lost the facility of 'burping' in the process of a rigid upbringing he is at an advantage since he may be able to eructate air from the oesophagus immediately. He knows the necessary kinaesthetic and tactile sensations and may readily obtain control over relaxation and dilation of the oesophageal sphincter. All small children 'break wind' naturally after meals to relieve an air-distended stomach, but this is firmly repressed by most mothers as disgusting. The small child soon loses the facility encouraged in infancy by the ritual patting and de-winding after taking the breast or bottle. Psychological inhibitions develop, associated with parental disapproval and social taboos. Many patients, especially female, never overcome their aversion for oesophageal speech for this reason. This is, of course, a strong argument against advocating air swallowing and belching as the first method of instruction.

Another objection is that air swallowed into the oesophagus travels down to stomach by peristalsis and cannot easily be voluntarily eructated. The technique aided by aerated drinks may serve a temporary purpose but since it has to be unlearned at some stage, it is wasteful of effort if another method can be readily mastered. It must be remembered that no proficient oesophageal speaker uses air swallowing for charging the vicarious lung.

2. *Injection Method*

Direct instruction in air injection is probably preferable to that of air swallowing, whether or not one has faith in co-ordinating it with lung inspiration.

Voiceless plosives and fricatives are the best to commence with, viz. [st], [sk], [sp], [skr] and [p], [t], [k] followed by vowels. It is generally far easier to obtain voice on a syllable [pa], [ta], [ka] than by the old classic procedure of endeavouring to swallow and utter a vowel. Closing of the tracheotomy tube with the finger is advocated by some therapists as an aid to injection. This I find makes patients cough.

Although it would appear logical to instruct the patient in breathing, drawing attention to the fact that he must preface speech with a quick brief inspiration, this may possibly confuse him. Some say it provides too many things to concentrate upon at once. By the time the patient has mastered the intake of air by compression of air in the mouth, however, and is able to achieve syllables successively and easily, it is generally found that expansion of the chest takes place as preliminary to speech, quite unconsciously and automatically, under the overwhelmingly strong compulsion of the old reflex and automatic speech pattern. This is why the naturally good speaker before laryngectomy is often the naturally good speaker afterwards. The possession of a good kinaesthetic sense, of responsive and brisk muscles 'tingling with kinaesthesia', and naturally good habits of breathing and articulation appear to be most important factors influencing the speech progress of laryngectomised patients with a good surgical result and healthy attitude to their disability. Tongue exercises and plosive syllable practice (page 175) may be necessary to improve clarity of speech, especially with a lingual paresis.

3. *Aspiration Method*

When an individual is tense and breathing is shallow, and the preoperative mode of speech production was poor, then proper instruction in relaxation and central breathing is essential. The slightly exaggerated and rapid descent of the diaphragm noted by Morrison is an obvious feature of the delivery of every proficient oesophageal speaker. If a patient is unable to achieve the happy co-ordination of respiratory and articulatory muscles, his speech will necessarily lack fluency and ease and he will never synchronise injection and aspiration of air into the oesophagus which is the ideal to be aimed at.

It is advisable, therefore, in such circumstances to instruct the patient in relaxation and correct breathing technique as soon as is possible, and if the patient is well enough this should start before operation. When regular speech treatment is begun relaxation and breathing exercises should form part of every lesson, but breathing exercises need not at first be taught in relation to phonation exercises. The patient may learn to produce voice by the injection method independently and later, when oesophageal voice is produced without effort, and on protracted vowels, then attention may be drawn to the intimate connection between voice and respiration. With some patients it is true that there is never any need to do so, but in the majority it is generally advisable quite early in treatment, in order to increase the air reservoir and so obtain longer phrasing and also greater volume of voice.

Di Carlo *et al.* (1955) found that abdominal expansion in breathing occurred in their poor speakers and thoracic expansion in their better speakers. Abdominal breathing is advisedly to be discouraged and the intercostal diaphragmatic method emphasised. Isshiki (1968) found that normal inspiration did not draw air into the oesophagus, therefore a quick pant-like intake is necessary. Posture is important. We have had patients who slumped in a chair improve dramatically when told to sit upright and control their diaphragmatic intercostal movement. Some patients find it easier to stand and practise phonation. Abdominal breathers need especially panting exercises for toning up the musles and developing the quick diaphragmatic inspiration so necessary for aspiration technique.

The danger of confusing the patient with 'breathing exercises' and encouraging increased blowing from the stoma is not so great as the antagonists of the aspiration method believe. The patient has in fact nothing to learn, he need only be reminded that inspiration and expiration coincide with the preparatory and active phases of speech in exactly the same way as they did before operation. There is, on the other hand, a real danger in concentrating exclusively upon injection of air. This is an unnatural process quite foreign to the reflex habit patterns of the individual, and as difficult to acquire as any other new skill demanding muscular co-ordination invariably is in adult life. It is quite common to find patients concentrating upon injection to the complete cessation of respiration. The breath is held while injection and ejection of air take place and the thorax and abdomen are held rigid. In these circumstances attention must be paid to the necessity for relaxing and co-ordinating lung respiration with injection and ejection of oesophageal air on articulation of vowels or syllables. As stated earlier, negative pressure in the thorax aids aspiration of air into the oesophagus, hence the need to synchronise exactly injection with the quick inspiration of lung air.

GROUP TREATMENT

Group treatment is unquestionably the most satisfactory medium in which to work with these patients, but may not always be possible. The great difficulty once voice is achieved is that of self-consciousness over speech which the beginner feels to be conspicuous and socially unacceptable. Women especially may dislike the deep-pitched oesophageal voice, which is more conspicuous in the female than male patient. Working in a group in a sympathetic atmosphere where everybody is in the same predicament breeds confidence, and gives the patient the courage eventually to speak freely at home and in the outside world. A woman patient who began to speak well in hospital and joined in a women's group in the speech clinic was transferred to her local hospital for speech therapy when she returned home. Here she was the only patient and her speech steadily regressed; she resorted to a whisper at home and used her voice only in the clinic. Six weeks later she had an appointment to see her surgeon and in the waiting-room met another laryngectomised patient who could talk fluently. To her astonishment, she suddenly found herself speaking with a good oesophageal voice which stayed with her for the rest of that day but was less good the next morning. She now realised that the lack of moral support from other patients was at the root of her difficulties and sensibly asked to be transferred back to group treatment, despite the long journey this necessitated every week. Some patients never overcome their aversion to oesophageal speech, and it is this which accounts for those cases who promise well and are able to obtain a good voice early but never use it outside the speech clinic.

SUGGESTED PLAN OF VOICE PRODUCTION

1. Experiment with vocalising syllables with initial consonants [p], [t] and [k]. The patient must be relaxed, especially in shoulders, neck and jaw. No more effort should be put into articulation than for the normal articulation of these consonants. If the therapist is able to inject air into her own oesophagus and herself demonstrate what is desired this is very helpful. It gives the patient something to imitate and also does much to remove his embarrassment at what he may regard as 'belching'. Every therapist should endeavour to acquire the trick; it is by no means difficult and is an

invaluable aid in teaching. Mimicking oesophageal speech, compressing the lips and cheeks and using an intermittent ventricular band voice may be almost as effective (page 394).

2. Practise a syllable once it is voiced, over and over again until it is achieved easily and effortlessly.

3. Practise different syllables beginning and ending with voiced and voiceless plosives and containing different vowels. It is generally found that various consonant combinations are more helpful than others with individual patients, and assist in the acquisition of the knack of flattening the tongue to the roof of the mouth, and forcing compressed air from the oral cavity into the pharynx and so into the oesophagus. Such consonant combinations as [sk], [tʃ], [skr] may be found helpful, and lists of words beginning with these sounds can be practised. Treatment should be adapted to individual needs. Gradually work through all consonants and vowels obtaining clear and effortless phonation. Crisp articulation renders speech distinct as well as favouring injection. It is in most cases advisable to leave the nasals [m], [n] and [ŋ], till late because they allow the escape of air through the nose and render air compression difficult. The speaker learns, however, to overcome the difficulty by greater elevation of the palate or use of insufflated air only.

The consonant [h] is very difficult as its normal mode of articulation by laryngeal whisper is, of course, no longer possible, and should be taught last, if at all. A good imitation can be produced by lifting the back of the tongue as for the voiceless palatal fricative in 'loch' as suggested by Paget (1930) and Oswald (Hodson and Oswald, 1958). A slight pause before the following vowel is also an effective substitute for [h] (see page 391).

4. Polysyllabic words: contact, scratches, cataract, poppa-cattapettel, double-scotch, butterscotch, biscuits, church gate.

5. Sentences, omitting difficult consonants and words beginning with vowels. 'Bake the cake', 'kick the cat', 'basket of biscuits', not to mention Captain Peter's 'cup of coffee', are easier than 'all men smile easily'.

6. Phrasing. Breathing technique can now be positively linked with speech. Mechanical counting exercises, days of week, A, B, C, etc., or practice of strings of syllables beginning and ending with plosives may be used to extend the length of phrase: e.g. kik-kik-kik, etc. Frequent practice is essential for short periods, throughout the day.

7. Whistling, blowing a mouth-organ in staccato blasts from

the oesophagus by diaphragmatic and thoracic movement are recommended by Oswald.

8. The increase of vocal volume can be obtained by stronger inspiration and expiration and slightly exaggerated articulation which increases the air reservoir and assists in its more forceful ejection. Care must be taken to avoid forcing the voice and the development of tension and blowing from the tracheostoma.

9. Improvement of tone and pitch.

(*a*) Production of vowels with rising and falling intonation.

(*b*) Imitation of short colourful phrases after the therapist with a variety of expressive inflexions.

(*c*) Place the forefinger and thumb on either side of the throat at the level of the pseudo-glottis and experiment with varying pressures and changing tone and pitch of voice, then repeat without external pressure, endeavouring to reproduce the necessary muscular adjustment by ear alone (Stetson, 1937).

(*d*) Practise singing familiar tunes. Although the whole compass of the melody will not be possible the mental concept of the melody inspires pitch change. Five or six notes may be managed and the song be recognisable at first mainly by its rhythm. The effort to sing also develops breathing technique and aspiration.

10. Humming tunes feeling vibration in the nose with fingers.

THE AVOIDANCE OF COMMON FAULTS IN OESOPHAGEAL SPEECH PRODUCTION

The faults and difficulties which commonly arise in learning oesophageal speech are due almost without exception to generalised tension, which interferes with the rhythmic co-ordination of articulation and respiration, and arises out of the excessive effort which the individual in most cases throws into his attempts to vocalise. Relaxation and rhythmic co-ordination, ease and an effortless approach to speech execution must be constantly emphasised in teaching, and mental tension and anxieties as far as possible resolved by explanation and discussion.

1. *Swallowing of Air Inadvertently*

An excessive amount of air may be inspired into the oesophagus and enter the stomach, causing distension of the gas cap. This may cause considerable discomfort and indigestion and the accidental eructation of wind interrupts speech or causes explosive and uncontrolled voicing. The difficulty is more common in patients who have learned air swallowing instead of air injection.

The individual generally learns to adjust the intake of air and prevent its descent into the stomach after a few weeks, but he may be helped by the suggestion that he breathes less forcibly before speaking and also reduces the over-forceful movements of the back of the tongue which are nearly always found to accompany the intake of air in such patients.

2. *Blowing of Chest air from the Tracheal Cannula*

This can be very troublesome and the noise of exhaled air so loud that it drowns the voice. The blowing is generally the result of excessive speech effort in an attempt to eject air from the oesophagus and acquire a louder voice. Tension in the throat and upper thorax are evident, and as muscular tonicity mounts the voice fades and is lost. Relaxation, central breathing, lack of effort and further drills in the easy injection and expulsion of air from the oesophagus must be practised. Practice with an amplifier generally proves most helpful.

Bubbling in the trachea is of course difficult to avoid when bronchial catarrh is present and the treatment of the chest condition is the only remedy. Patients who have learned to speak well often lose their voices with a cold on account of catarrhal complications. This can be readily understood in relation to the importance of breathing in the production of oesophageal voice. When speech deterioration takes place the patient should be reassured by an explanation of its reason and assured of its temporary nature.

3. *Stridor Accompanying Air Intake*

A gulping or clunking sound rather like a noisy swallow often precedes voicing in the initial stages of voice acquisition. The gulp develops in those who rely over much upon tongue movements for air intake. A crowing or squawking sound can occur when relying excessively upon aspiration with excessive glossopharyngeal tension. Such habits can altogether spoil otherwise good speech and must be corrected before they become habitual. When stridor develops emphasis upon relaxation and less pharyngeal tension and greater reliance upon diaphragmatic breathing will be found helpful. Air intake with mouth shut, emphasis upon injection, correction of the common fault of throwing back the head, relaxation and diaphragmatic breathing, and an all-round improvement in speech co-ordination, will be necessary. The voice may be lost or greatly reduced in volume to begin with, but perseverance in improving the method of air intake is well worth a temporary set-back in speech performance, since the oesophageal stridor can become a well-established and ugly fault. Use of an amplifier is recommended.

4. *Grimacing and 'Button-holing'*.

Grimacing due to over-exaggerated articulation is a minor problem which develops through the anxiety to be understood when the voice is weak. An inclination to 'button-hole' the listener and to stand too close for comfort may also develop for the same reasons.

It is sufficient gently to draw the individual's attention to these quite unconscious speech habits for him to correct them.

5. *Failure to Acquire Length in Phrasing*

Proficiency in the ability to obtain and maintain a sufficient air reservoir for phrases of more than a few words is mainly a matter of time. Again, tension, poor co-ordination and poor breathing patterns are the prime causative factors. The inveterate talker is the one who finds the limits imposed by laryngectomy the most frustrating; as he rushes headlong into speech, he gesticulates and tenses and altogether forgets the newly acquired speech technique. Insistence upon slower speech, and the need for patience, are the only means by which such individuals can be helped to adjust to the speech handicap.

Even a slight and transient tension in the throat will render a proficient speaker speechless (Sawkins, 1949). Patients lose their voices when embarrassed or angry, when trying to raise the voice to overtop a noise, to call a dog or a child. Very often tension is quite unconscious but none the less insidious. A patient in a group treatment, for instance, who was making excellent progress, was suddenly unable to voice more than three words at a time in one breath. He was unconsciously tipping back his chair with his heel when speaking. When this was corrected he was able to treble the length of phrase, thus dramatically illustrating the therapist's favourite text, 'no relaxation, no speech'.

6. *Speech Embarrassment*

As speech becomes more fluent many patients remain shy of using oesophageal voice outside the clinic. Some may have great difficulty in overcoming a real dislike of oesophageal speech and this constantly inhibits voice. Speech may fail with strangers and the conviction grow that people are staring at the patient or avoiding him. The sensitive individual often suffers a real post-operative neurosis. Certainly there are difficulties to face—people do not intend to hurt but are often unintentionally tactless through simple embarrassment in face of a misfortune they little understand. Instead of treating the patient normally they may be over-sympathetic or on the other hand apparently callous. A transport driver who was excellently adjusted and spoke well before going back to work, was infinitely depressed by his reception when he resumed his duties. He did not know, he said, which was the harder to bear: the men's ragging him over his belching voice, or the tender sympathy of the girl in the canteen whose eyes filled with tears whenever he asked for a cup of tea. Another annoyance is the tendency of others to shout at the patient as if he were deaf, thinking for some strange reason that the patient cannot understand because he cannot speak. We shout at foreigners in the same way and it is interesting to speculate why this should be.

The patient's family can be advised not to expect too much from the patient's speech at first, to watch his lips and to listen without interruption and to make every endeavour to understand him. Wives must be cautioned not to pursue their household tasks when being addressed. They must encourage speech in every way possible, but the use of a self-erasing pad at first is better than the patient's suffering the exasperation and upset of not being understood. The medical social worker, vicar and local welfare officer can all be asked to help.

Patients should return to work after a suitable period of convalescence: occupation eases financial worries and prevents morbid pre-occupation with health. Speech generally improves greatly when constant demands are made upon the individual to communicate with his companions in the ordinary course of the day's work.

The formation of social clubs for laryngectomised individuals such as the Lost Chord Club and the New Voice Club in America, the Glasgow Club and the Swallow Club in London have proved remarkably successful in helping to effect a better social adjustment in many cases. Regular meetings are held, patients bringing relatives or friends to spend a happy evening playing games and chatting. Speech therapists and members of the nursing and medical staff may join these meetings and are ready to discuss problems and difficulties. Thus, in an atmosphere of sympathy and understanding, in company with fellow sufferers, the fear of speech is soon lost, as is the sense of isolation and social ostracism which so often destroys morale in the early months following laryngectomy.

It is our feeling, however, that a time limit of maybe one year should be placed upon the membership of such clubs or that meetings be held rather irregularly. First, there is the danger that patients may come to rely upon the moral support and shelter the club gives, just as the deaf and stammerers do, and fail to resume a normal social life. Secondly, there is the depressing fact that many members of the club will be back in hospital for further surgery, possibly never to return. All organisers of such clubs know the gloom and exacerbation of fears and depression that the death or absence of a club member engenders. In England these difficulties are undoubtedly greater than in America where no secret is made over the patient having cancer, and a more positive attitude to its cure exists. In England patients are not as a rule informed that they have cancer but a 'growth' over which great care and strong measures must be taken. Patients on the whole accept this explanation. We believe it is more humane to keep an individual ignorant of the worst which the word 'cancer' spells and which, after all, may never transpire. It is often a matter for astonishment that patients accept so readily the naive explanations given. This is presumably on account of an unconscious protective mechanism which suppresses fear and makes acceptable the explanation the patient wants to hear. A laryngectomised patient has said to me in confidence, 'I hear X is in hospital again. They say he's got cancer this time, poor devil'.

This does not mean that patients do not ask questions about their disease. The speech pathologist never takes the responsibility for giving a diagnosis but suggests the patient asks the laryngologist, who exercises his own discretion whether to tell the patient the truth or not. As a general rule, close relatives are informed, possibly not the wife, but a son or daughter.

HOW GOOD CAN SPEECH BECOME?

The oesophageal speaker can become so fluent that strangers do not realise the true nature of the disability and may ask whether the patient has a cold or laryngitis. This is a tribute indeed to the naturalness of the voice which up to this time no artificial larynx has been able to emulate.

The chief handicap in the most excellent speakers is the lack of volume and this is especially felt when speaking against background noise, such as at a party, in the street, in an office or restaurant. Clarke and Hoops (1970) found that laryngectomees' speech deteriorated with increased speech-type background noise, not in intelligibility but in general speech proficiency, with a decrease in phrase length, and increase in lung air-flow.

For public speaking a hand microphone or head-set attached to a transistor-generated table loudspeaker can be used (page 392).

Use of Telephone

Proficient oesophageal speech can be heard quite clearly over the telephone but if volume is insufficient an amplification system can be connected to the telephone by the GPO. Patients often need help and reassurance before using the phone happily. There is also no accounting for the strange misunderstandings which arise on occasion with patients using the simplest equipment, hence the need for constant supervision by speech therapists in the initial stages of treatment. One of our best speakers, who is now a regular stand-by for pre-operative visits to laryngectomees, developed good speech quickly and went back to work, but returned the following week in the greatest depression. He could not use the telephone and without the telephone he could not carry on his business. This was a real puzzle. He was told to telephone the therapist in the adjoining room on the internal circuit. She listened, nothing could be heard. Returning to the patient she asked for a demonstration. He was holding the mouthpiece of the telephone, with bent head and hunched shoulders, as near to the stoma as possible convinced that this was where the voice came from.

We are reminded here that it is not possible to use amplifiers while telephoning and so avoid the expense of installation and rental for a telephone amplifier system. The amplifier loudspeaker can be held over the mouthpiece of the telephone but the microphone picking up speech is necessarily in close proximity, and a feed-back electronic circuit is created with resultant whistle or squeal, as happens always also when the volume of amplification is turned up too high.

Users of electronic vibrators, once they have learned to speak slowly and clearly with them are also easily intelligible over the telephone and many business men are thus able to return to work soon after operation. It is also a great comfort for people living alone to know that they can call for help over the phone in an emergency.

Phrasing

As to length of phrase, this varies considerably. Snidecor and Curry (1960) measured the number of syllables per breath intake of superior laryngeal speakers and found that the mean lowest consecutive sequence consisted of 3·8 syllables and the highest 8·7 with an overall average of 4·98 syllables. The extreme range in these subjects was 22 syllables in one speaker, and Snidecor (1962)

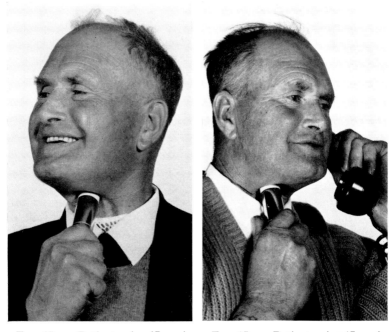

FIG. 45A   Patient using 'Sama' minielectronovox

FIG. 45B   Patient using 'Sama' minielectronovox for telephoning

is of the opinion that 11–12 syllables is a very satisfactory number for superior speakers.

Snidecor and Isshiki (1965) express the opinion that the number of syllables per air charge is not of crucial importance and that speed is a far better criterion of naturalness. A good average rate is 80–120 words per minute although a very superior speaker was found to achieve 153 w.p.m. Snidecor (1962) concluded: 'There is no magic in a long phrase. Clearness, ease of speech and reasonable rate of words per minute should take precedence over any struggle to break records in regard to words per air charge'.

PITCH AND QUALITY OF SUPERIOR OESOPHAGEAL SPEECH

Pitch in oesophageal speech is related to intensity (Snidecor and Curry, 1959). Gimson (1962) states that variations of *intensity* on the same frequency may induce impressions of change of pitch. In order to raise the pitch, greater volume has to be employed necessitating replenishment of the oesophageal reservoir, and for a drop in pitch less intensity must be used. The accomplished speaker may have a pitch range of an octave; the fundamental pitch is much lower than in laryngeal speakers. Damsté (1958) in a study of twenty male patients found a median pitch of 67·5 c.p.s. and Snidecor and Curry (1959), 63·3 c.p.s. Kallen (1934) noted that movements of the head and neck could contribute to pitch change and this aspect might be utilised for emphasis and expressiveness in speech. Stern is quoted as advocating work on inflexion for improvement of naturalness of speech, long after fluency is achieved. Oswald was of this opinion, also, and recommended singing, humming and assiduous practice of reading aloud, which all patients find both difficult and tiring.

The basic tone of oesophageal voice (as distinct from pitch) is rough by reason of the crude vibration and cricopharyngeal muscular recoil. Harmonic analysis by sonograph shows the two vowel formants of oesophageal speech to be 'fuzzy'. Although quality of the vowels may be improved by carefully adjusted articulation and the raising of the resonance pitch, much improvement of the partials is not feasible on account of the poor quality of the fundamental note (Snidecor, 1962).

Case Histories

The following history is presented to demonstrate the modern approach to treatment of cancer of the larynx commencing with deep X-ray and ending with laryngectomy and continuing over a number of years in which the patient is kept well and actively working.

Dr S. developed a carcinoma of one vocal cord at the age of 53 and was treated successfully with radiotherapy. He kept well for six years. His voice had remained rather husky and vocal cords slightly red after radiotherapy. He had to do a considerable amount of talking in his practice and when his voice deteriorated and vocal cords looked swollen it was hoped this was due to vocal strain. A month's vocal rest improved the condition after which he was referred for speech therapy. His breathing was shallow and the voice poorly supported but voice production improved quickly and also the condition of the larynx. A year later he had a recurrence of carcinoma on one cord and a laryngofissure was performed. He acquired a voice which remained severely hoarse and lacked volume due to a laryngeal gap between true and cicatricial cords, but this did not prevent him from returning to work and he experimented with an amplifier but did not really take to it. A year later a further recurrence necessitated a laryngectomy. He quickly obtained a soft voice by using aspiration but the cricopharyngeal sphincter was too slack to get good oesophageal voice and he could not tense the muscle on phonation. Food and liquids were regurgitated if he stooped too soon after a meal. He returned to work, his secretary assisting him as interpreter in the surgery for some six months while he persevered with speech therapy. Then quite suddenly he acquired the knack of co-ordinating pharyngeal tension with speaking and air ejection, and became a fluent and clear speaker. He was able to telephone and stated that he found speech much easier than during the period of laryngofissure. The necessary cricopharyngeal tension for this good performance was achieved by holding the chin up and slightly to one side while speaking—a trick he evolved for himself.

The two case reports below demonstrate some of the difficulties encountered in the treatment of a laryngectomised patient and the possibility of achieving good speech results even in the most difficult and apparently hopeless cases—provided co-operation can be gained and the therapist has the will and inclination to persevere if need be for years, which was a lesson Mabel Oswald taught us.

Mr N., aged 71. Carcinoma of the right pyriform fossa and right vocal fold; voice lost for two months prior to seeking medical advice. A simple total laryngectomy was performed, the hyoid being left undisturbed. The wound healed without any complications. Post-laryngectomy bronchitis developed immediately and continued for six months. Postural drainage only alleviated the condition temporarily, but short-wave electrical treatment twice a week for a month eventually shifted the chronic catarrh and the great London smog did not upset him as much as it did many other old people.

The patient was a spiritualist artist married to a medium and of a very excitable and lively temperament, his mental life engaging contact with an endless procession of spirits, conversation with whom enlivened the duller moments of life, and especially speech therapy. His zest for life and lively sense of humour kept treatment within the bounds of possibility if not always of probability.

The patient's customary speech patterns were in every respect bad. Before laryngectomy, strangers could seldom understand him when excited and even his wife was frequently unable to interpret what he said. He spoke fast and volubly, breathing engaged the upper thorax only, tension was extreme and he was accustomed to resort to wild gesticulation. Articulation was slurred and he had a broad Cork City accent. He was at first hard of hearing and was forcibly supplied with a hearing-aid, but after some months spiritual healing improved sound perception and this difficulty was overcome. He possessed a well-fitting and competent pair of dentures but these he preferred to carry around with him tenderly embedded in cotton wool in a tin, instead of in the oral cavity. For a very long time he could only be persuaded to wear his teeth in the clinic, refusing to do so outside its doors.

He refused to use a vibrator and when persuaded to do so, just to oblige us, was quite incapable of managing it properly, of switching on and off at the appropriate times and of placing it himself correctly against the throat.

Speech progress was naturally very slow. Air swallowing was taught originally but so long as this was relied upon speech remained spasmodic, explosive, altogether uncontrolled, and two words in twenty might be voiced on 'good' days. After two months' treatment, the patient stayed away from the clinic on account of bad weather, colds, moving house and the conviction that speech would progress under the instruction from 'the spirit guides from the other side'. When this proved not to be the case the almoner persuaded him to come for regular weekly individual treatment nine months after laryngectomy. The patient used a pad for all serious communication at this time and had no serviceable or intelligible speech. Relaxation and diaphragmatic breathing were taught, the intake and expulsion of air by change of thoracic pressure was concentrated upon and tongue movement reduced to a minimum. The spirit guides were challenged with their incompetence and withdrew from the arena. From time to time famous singers of days gone by came across to volunteer advice in breathing technique, but since this appeared to be suspiciously akin to the patient's old breathing habits their assistance was rigorously discouraged.

Speech steadily improved, and from 6 to 8 word sentences were achieved if uttered in conjunction with quick rhythmic breathing and practised as exercises. For many months spontaneous speech was disrupted by tension, forcing, and the intense frustration and irritation occasioned by the inability to speak at the old speed. Articulation needed a great deal of correction, drill in the precise tongue movement for all consonants was given, and the need for constant wear of dentures was made clear, and eventually accepted. The dialectal vowel variants were rendered less broad by hearing training. Speech gradually became more intelligible and also more fluent. Two years after laryngectomy this patient was able to take part in discussions and conduct meetings, leading a full and active life, having made a remarkable adjustment to his handicap. It is by no means easy to learn any new skill at the age of seventy-one. This patient had not only to learn anew, but to correct life-long bad speech habits which at the outset threatened to defeat him. It says much for this fine old man's tenacity and courage that they did not do so.

Mr L., aged 47, worked as a milkman and had his own small decorating business. He had always stammered but had improved after leaving school and had only a slight repetitive stammer when he was talking to strangers. When he developed cancer of the larynx he was given radiotherapy but the tumour recurred 8 months later so that a laryngectomy had to be performed and a unilateral block dissection. He developed a small fistula post-operatively which was slow in healing and after several abortive attempts to close it the plastic surgeon was called in 4 months later, after which the wound healed rapidly. During this healing period speaking was stopped altogether and everything had to be written down. During the time when the patient was wearing a feeding tube he constantly asked to be taught to speak and although it was explained to him why he could not with the tube in his gullet, he was encouraged to whisper which he could do quite effectively. His stammer increased and he became anxious and depressed, fearing he would never escape from hospital. He had an attractive and much younger wife who was a great support to him. They had two children at work and a daughter of 8 years and boy of 9. Mr L. was worried about finance and hated his wife having to go out to work.

Before leaving hospital he was able to get a weak intermittent voice, chiefly by inhalation since he stammered badly when given syllables with plosives or sibilants to aid injection. On being discharged from hospital he asked to attend a speech clinic nearer home and was only seen occasionally and informally when followed up in our ENT out-patients department. For the next few months it was noted that progress with speech was poor, he was being taught to swallow air, he was stammering rather more and in despair about ever speaking. He refused to use a vibrator or an amplifier as he felt this made him more conspicuous. He had always been shy and self-conscious he said and speech with strangers a great effort; but now it was impossible.

Eventually he decided to come back to us for his speech treatment—a long uphill battle commenced. Although his throat was hard and flattened in contour, he was now and then able to produce a quiet voice easily once the swallowing of air was corrected. He returned to work 6 months after his operation since milk delivery did not require much speech. Mostly he missed being able to talk at home, control his two young children, and also carry on his decorating activities which did require talking to customers. His voice became steadily louder and more fluent during his lessons but there was no carry-over outside the clinic and he returned week after week with no voice. His wife reported that he tried very little at home. He was frequently so depressed that he was on the verge of tears and might fail to attend for a month at a time until persuaded to return by the combined efforts of his wife, doctor and ourselves. It was felt that Mr L's failure to speak was chiefly psychological; he constantly affirmed that he was afraid of making an exhibition of himself. Long discussions of this problem took place. A year after his laryngectomy his wife complained that he only whispered at home and was spending too long in the pub instead of coming home to lunch. We had ourselves noticed occasional moods of euphoria. The only progress at this time was that he very gradually lost his stammer. He was now persuaded to wear a throat-contact transducer with an amplifier. This helped his speech but he would only use it at home because he felt it drew attention to his deformed throat and disability. He was next persuaded to wear the contact transducer attached to the bracket of a spectacle frame, as this was found to pick up vibrations from the malar bone excellently. He did not mind wearing this because he thought it looked like some sort of hearing aid. His wife and his work-mates encouraged him to use the device, saying he was much easier to understand. Tension and over-exertion when attempting to produce voice were gradually reduced. At the same time it was noted that the tissues of the neck were becoming softer and more elastic and sensation improving. He was stood down for three months with the amplifier on loan. Two months later he called in to return it as he needed it no longer—his speech was now fluent and audible, the voice pleasing and light and very acceptable to the patient.

SPEECH AFTER PHARYNGOLARYNGECTOMY WITH OR WITHOUT
COLON TRANSPLANTS

In pharyngolaryngectomy, since the upper portion of the oesophagus and the hypopharyngeal muscular tissue have to be excised, the sphincter mechanism which remains after simple laryngectomy is lost. Without the cricopharyngeal pseudo-glottis fluent speech is far more difficult to acquire. However, voice is still possible. Air can be aspirated or injected in exactly the same way as for oesophageal voice and as long as sufficient narrowing and dilatability is obtained in the reconstructed oesophageal and pharyngeal tube, it can be vibrated sufficiently loudly to produce a weak voice. The air charge is, of course, under very little control when speaking and is quickly lost, generally after one or two syllables. As a result, air intake has to be accomplished very frequently and voice is tiring for the individual to maintain. At first, too, the throat muscles may ache with fatigue rather readily. The voice is deeper and less resonant than the oesophageal voice of the laryngectomised and in many cases little more than a strong whisper is ever possible. Since air is aspirated rather than injected there is also a tendency to hyperventilation and giddiness.

Very rarely the reconstructed oesophagus, without causing difficulty in swallowing, presents sufficient narrowing at some point to offer resistance to the outgoing ejected air, so that voice is produced as loud and as fluent as that obtained by the patient who has undergone simple laryngectomy. Only one of our patients has obtained speech of such high standard, but Dornhorst and Negus (1954) state that the difficulty in producing the necessary narrowing of the oesophagus should not be insuperable. Surgical technique may improve so that what is now a matter of chance may in the future become a matter of certainty.

We have had three patients who developed the knack of vibrating air in the oesophagealpharynx on both ingoing and outgoing air. The narrowing of the tube was maintained while air was aspirated and expelled by means of rapid lung inspiration and expiration (chest pulses). No air injection took place. This method of voice production was a great advantage because it doubled the number of syllables for each air charge and speech was rapid and fluent as a result, though the voice was weak. Although this method is a disadvantage and indeed scarcely possible with the laryngectomised, it is possibly by far the best method for the pharyngolaryngectomised. In the patients mentioned above the method was not taught but developed naturally and spontaneously and was encouraged because so much more effective than voicing on outgoing air only.

On account of the difficulties in obtaining fluent and audible speech after pharyngolaryngectomy it is often preferable for the patient to use an artificial larynx if possible.

Rather unexpectedly, colon transplant cases may get a colonic whisper or even an audible voice with little trouble and more easily than in the case of a simple laryngectomy. Lall and Evison (1966) have described 4 cases of colon transplant and cineradiographic examination during speech. Case (1) had a good voice and reservoir of air which moved up with the help of the diaphragm, through an upper narrowed segment of the transplant. The segment was capable of narrowing and expanding. Case (2) had no narrowing, air was shifted by the diaphragm, a soft whisper was possible. Case (3) did not hold air in the column and failed to co-ordinate diaphragmatic movement with voice. Case (4) had an excellent colonic voice, the cervical portion of the column from the level of the 7th cervical vertebrae to the first thoracic was noted to be collapsed at rest and the segment vibrated in phonation.

Patients who can only obtain a soft voice may be helped by an amplifier. Many are unable to use a vibrator if there is an inadequate hypopharyngeal air pocket to act as a resonator to the introduced sound, and sound waves cannot travel up to the mouth and be transformed into speech by articulation. Moreover there may be anaesthesia of the neck. It depends entirely upon the structure of the pharynx. One patient was able to use an Aurex vibrator. Another female who disliked the noisy vibrator, managed to produce an audible hollow whisper using a Washington (Faraday) White noise vibrator, which the majority of British speech therapists judged in trials in 1969 to be too weak to be an effective help to patients. This particular female was upset at being introduced to a proficient laryngectomised speaker before operation by a well-meaning new registrar while the Ward sister and senior therapist were on holiday. She was bitterly disappointed at finding herself quite unable to produce a whisper post-operatively. She used the Washington vibrator until her death two

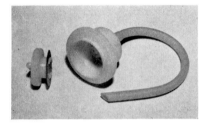

Fig. 46A   Reed-type vibrator (J. J. van Hunen, DSP.8)

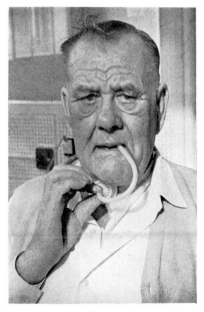

Fig. 46B   Reed-type vibrator in use

years later. Two other male patients liked the Washington very much. (These instruments are no longer marketed.)

Patients who cannot use a vibrator may be able to use devices which introduce sound orally, not pharyngeally. The Tait oral vibrator consists of a transistorised oscillator in a small case with on-off switch, and the frequency can be adjusted to suit the patient. It is attached by a lead into the mouth to a sealed vibrator unit which is attached to a dental plate or purpose-made plate. The disadvantages of this apparatus are the lead hanging out of the mouth, the need to remove the plate when eating (though swallowing fluids is possible with the plate in position) and the difficulty orthodontists inexperienced in this particular work have in fitting the vibrator unit into the plate satisfactorily.

Oral reed vibrators were the first instruments ever to be devised. Gussenbaumer designed one in 1874 (Levin, 1962a). They are virtually never used in Britain and America and are more popular in Spain and other European countries. They are cheaper than electronic aids, cannot develop faults and do not consume batteries. They consist essentially of a tube which must be fitted into or over the tracheal stoma; a vibratory reed is inserted in the pipe which is vibrated by the patient's exhaled breath. The other end of the pipe is held in the mouth and sound is shaped by the articulatory movements as with the Tait oral vibrator. The Dutch polythene reed-type vibrator, H. J. Van Hunen, DSP. 8, is easy to sterilise and use, having few technicalities to confuse elderly patients. A hand is needed to hold the instrument in place and a disc over the oral end of the tube makes it possible to hold the tube in the mouth without its slipping through the teeth. The Bell Telephone Laboratories also make a reed vibrator. Cooper-Rand produce an electronic version designed along the same lines. A vibrator unit with tube attached to introduce sound into the mouth is attached by a lead to a pocket oscillator with an on-off switch.

To be or not to be allowed to use an artificial larynx

A deep-rooted prejudice unfortunately prevails in the minds of many speech therapists and surgeons against the use of the vibrator or 'artificial larynx'. Why this should be so is inexplicable unless it is due to a subconscious feeling that recourse to an artificial and mechanical device is to denigrate the professional skill of the surgeon and therapist. We believe that the patient should be allowed to try out instruments, be shown how to use them to best advantage and decide for himself whether he wants one or not. The majority of patients prefer oesophageal voice and dislike the bizarre and unnatural noise of an electronic aid, and also the inconvenience and constant reminder it provides of disability. On the other hand there is no doubt that a vibrator is often a necessary crutch in the early stages of treatment and to some it makes life literally worth while. It is necessary to draw attention to the fact that in all surveys of unselected laryngectomee populations, only a third of the total acquire serviceable speech.

Failure to acquire some sort of pseudo-voice is very generally assumed to be due to 'psychological' factors (Diedrich and Youngstrom, 1968) but insufficient attention in our opinion is paid to the physiological equipment of the patient. Scarring and post-radiation induration may render voice quite impossible despite the most stable personality and determination to overcome difficulties. It may take two years for the muscular structures to become fully mobile and elastic, during which time speech improves gradually owing to improved conditions which are physiological not mental.

It is usual to find that laryngectomees with difficulty in producing oesophageal voice also have difficulty with using a vibrator and for the same reasons of poor pharyngeal structure. One of the chief and immediate post-operative troubles is anaesthesia of the neck so that it is difficult to place the vibrating head of the instrument on the exactly right spot each time and also to hold it flat against the skin. Failure to use a vibrator successfully may discourage the patient and also the therapist from using one again, but it must be borne in mind that when the throat has improved in mobility and sensation the use of a vibrator may be perfectly possible. The instrument should be tried out at intervals of perhaps 3 months up to a period of 2 years if a patient is still without adequate speech and would obviously benefit from being able to use a vibrator if he could do so successfully.

Insufficient appreciation of the real need for many patients to be equipped with vibrators is demonstrated vividly by the fact that although artificial aids to hearing, seeing, chewing, walking and many other functions are available free of charge as a matter of legal right through the British National Health service, aids to such a crippling handicap as surgically acquired aphonia are not. The relevant section of the National Health Service regulations concerning appliances not subject to central contract are given below since it seems they are not generally known to speech therapists.

Appliances not subject to Central Contract

Section 66. If a consultant prescribes for the treatment of a patient of an appliance or article, other than those mentioned in paragraphs 17 and 22, and which is not available under the

Ministry's central contracts (e.g. crutches, oxygen equipment, tracheotomy equipment, low visual aids, etc.) hospitals should make their own arrangements for the purchase of the item and issue it to the patient on loan for as long as it is required. Hospital authorities are responsible for the installation and or maintenance of such items where necessary. When the patient has no further need for the appliance it should, if suitable, be taken back into stock for re-issue to another patient.

Section **67**. Where articles are loaned to patients difficulty is sometimes experienced in recovering them. This difficulty may be reduced by:

(*a*) Marking such articles—'This is the property of the . . . Hospital and should be returned to this hospital when no longer required'.

(*b*) Obtaining the patient's signature to an undertaking: 'I acknowledge that the . . . received by me at the . . . Hospital is the property of the . . . Hospital and only supplied to me for the purpose of medical treatment. I undertake to return it to the . . . Hospital when required to do so or when it is no longer in use.

'I understand that failure to return the . . . in good condition may render me liable to pay the cost of repair or replacement of the. . . .'

(From 'National Health Service. Provision of Medical and Surgical Appliances'. Enclosure to HM (65) 11, page 10.)

When difficulty is encountered in persuading a consultant to prescribe or a hospital management committee to supply the necessary funds for speech aids, an appeal can be made to the Cancer Society, but this is best done by the medical social worker. The Hospital League of Friends is another possible source of funds, and a generous one in cases of need.

Quite apart from the physical impossibility or otherwise of a patient being able to produce audible voice, some patients have a personal preference for using an artificial larynx and dislike oesophageal voice intensely, and this attitude should be respected. The therapist should not adopt an attitude of disapproval or entertain any secret feeling that the patient lacks proper moral fibre. Sometimes, moreover, the therapist is under the impression that the patient's speech is perfectly adequate for his needs when it is not, sincerely believing it to be better when produced naturally than when using an artificial sound source. She may however be unwittingly influenced in her judgement by the professional bias of her training, besides professional skill in interpreting very mediocre speech production. McGrosky and Mulligan (1963) in rating the relative intelligibility of oesophageal speech and artificial larynx discovered that naive listeners rated the artificial larynx of higher intelligibility, while students and therapists rated oesophageal speech higher.

As we have said, not all patients can use vibrators and, to summarise, the following list of factors militating against successful use of a throat vibrator is given:

(*a*) Inadequate pharyngeal air-filled space for picking up vibrations from vibrator.

(*b*) Anaesthetic throat and induration which is responsible for patient's inability to hold vibrating head flat against the skin and avoid tipping it so causing ambient noise, and to find quickly the best spot for placement.

(*c*) Hearing impairment and inability to monitor artificial voice produced. Hearing needs to be tested and hearing aid provided, although this may not help patients to monitor speech any better when using vibrator.

(*d*) Nervousness with a noisy gadget and in the elderly reactions too slow to manipulate an on-off switch between phrases.

(*e*) Poor articulation and utter incompetence over adjusting degree and speed of oral movements to pick up vibrations. Speakers endeavour to use voice and cannot understand that mouthing is all that is necessary.

(*f*) A determination not to speak audibly on any account and to avoid returning to work. Patients in low socio-economic circumstances are often financially better off on sick benefit and national assistance.

(*g*) Preference for a whisper which is adequate for a retired patient's domestic needs.

We must reiterate here that when the induration and anaesthesia of the throat resolves, a patient may be able to use a vibrator successfully even if earlier he failed. He should be encouraged, therefore, to try again later on. Also with patience and determination the most incredibly inept patient can be taught to use a vibrator. For example, we had a patient (an old man of 72) who had spent his life on the railways as a workman. He was cheerful, philosophical and uninhibited, button-holing one in the hospital 'Out-patients', gesticulating and mouthing enormously, blowing from his stoma and nearly falling over one in his efforts to be heard.

He was practically edentulous except for 2 fangs of eye teeth but refused to be fitted with dentures. Speech therapy produced absolutely no results and his speech remained voluble, unintelligible and much the same as the day his feeding tube was removed. He was also totally incapable of using a vibrator, although he was happy to try. We gave up and discharged him, only to have him referred back to us by his surgeon with instructions to *teach* him to use a vibrator. His wife and perhaps the surgeon were being driven frantic by inability to understand him, for he was unable to write. This time we had a little better success and sufficient to warrant loan of a Mark 5 Western Electric larynx to be used under instruction from his local speech therapist. She persevered with the infinite patience of the dedicated young and he now uses his vibrator with great care and caution, pausing between each word; communication is slow but clear and everybody shares his delight.

Case histories illustrating that electronic vibrators can be real lifesaving devices:

Mrs V. was a beautiful woman of 45 with an attractive low and melodious voice. Laryngectomy is a terrible blow to a sensitive and attractive woman and she was profoundly depressed when she returned home. There were no children to hold the marriage together and her husband who was horrified by his wife's developing cancer, her operation and loss of voice, deserted her. She was able to obtain a quiet oesophageal voice intermittently but detested it. She persevered with her speech therapist but became increasingly desperate and threatened suicide. Somehow she heard of Dr Watson's work (Watson, 1967) and wrote to him. He showed her how to use the Aurex vibrator and designed a battery charger unit for her use; he also played speech recordings accompanied by coloured slides of a gracious Canadian laryngectomee who had visited us the year before. Mrs V. began to change her attitude to a vibrator, which she had rejected at first. A male therapist—he need not be a speech therapist—is a real morale-booster at times like these and Greene remained in the background in handling this case. Almost two years later Mrs V. wrote to Watson asking whether he would help another laryngectomised woman she had met quite by chance. She had been out walking with her dog by the sea and had called him, using her vibrator. She was heard by the mother of a laryngectomee who immediately approached her and confided her great anxiety over her daughter, a woman of 48 who had undergone a simple laryngectomy 3 months previously. She was under a young speech therapist but was making slow progress and was desperately unhappy.

This time Greene dealt with the problem. Mrs R. arrived with her mother. She was in a distraught state. It appeared everybody —her mother, grown-up daughter and friends—could understand her but her husband of 57 would not try. They had been the happiest of couples and she worshipped him, but now they were drifting apart. He had been very upset by his wife's operation, and he now could not bear to look at her and try to understand her. He was spending every evening away from home.

Mrs R. spoke very fast but was able to produce a voice when she calmed down, and relaxed. She was inappropriately dressed. Although the fashion was for high-necked dresses, she wore a particularly low-cut dress completely exposing the unstitched bib of white medical gauze which flapped up and down as she spoke. Her mother on the other hand was tastefully dressed in a high-necked blouse and strings of pearls. Attention was drawn to the matter of dress and it was suggested that her husband perhaps was not so unreasonable in not wanting to look at her or take her out. She was quite astonished, this having not occurred to her. She was given an Aurex vibrator to use. At first, in her agitation, she went on talking waving it in the air switched on. Gradually she was persuaded to use it properly and convinced that if she relaxed and used the vibrator there was no need to panic. It was further suggested that she should not use the instrument with her husband until she had practised with her speech therapist and gained greater confidence and expertise. She was assured that natural speech would develop in time if she followed her speech therapist's instruction in relaxation, quiet breathing and slow speech. Furthermore, since batteries of the Aurex would need recharging and Mrs V. had the battery charger unit, she would have to go and see her when batteries ran down. Thus she could discuss her difficulties with an experienced laryngectomee.

Two months later Mrs R. wrote to say that things were going much better and her husband, whom we had promised to see if necessary, was far more co-operative. A month after this she returned the vibrator with the news that she no longer needed it. Her speech was now excellent and she and her husband were fully reconciled.

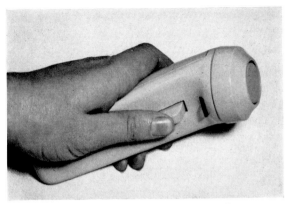

Fig. 47a   Mark 5 Western electric vibrator

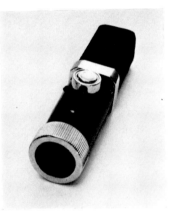

Fig. 47b   Aurex 'Neovox'

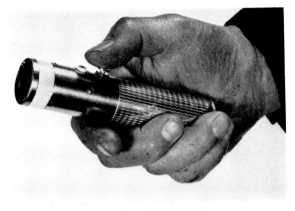

Fig. 47c   'Sama' minielectronovox

LIST OF SPEECH AIDS

Amplifiers

S. G. Brown Ltd., King George's Avenue, Watford, Herts., England.

> 'Therapeutic Speech Amplifier.' (Developed in collaboration with St. Bartholomew's Hospital Departments of Medical Electronics and Speech Therapy, on hospital research grant.)
> Hand microphone, No B 104162.
> Pacific Head-set microphone, No B 103778.
> Throat microphone, No B 104361.
> Table loudspeaker, No C 104131.

Lustraphone Ltd., St. George's Works, Regent's Park Road, London, NW1, England.

> Amplifier, LSA/620.
> Contact transducer, CDA/72.
> Crystal microphone, LC/620M.

'Sama', Via Saluzzo 98, 10126 Torino, Italy.

> 'Sama' amplifier and battery charger unit, separate off-on and volume-control switches.
> Supplier in Britain: Londesborough Instruments Ltd., Scientific Instruments Division, 43 York Road, King's Heath, Birmingham 14, England.

Smye-Rumsby Engineering Co. Ltd., 2 Queen Street, Dover, England.

> Amplifier and hand microphone, battery type, PP3.

Cooper-Rand Development Corporation, 13600 Deise Avenue, Cleveland, Ohio, USA.

> Voice amplifier and hand microphone.

Electronic Vibrators

> 'Sama' Minielectronovox, Rc 815.
> Suppliers: *see* under Sama, above.

Aurex Corporation, 315 West Adams Street, Chicago, Illinois; Down Bros., and Mayer and Phelps, Ltd., Church Path, Mitcham, Surrey, England.

> Aurex 'Neovox'. Serial No 6757.

Bell Laboratories Developments, USA; and Down Bros., and Mayer Phelps, Ltd. (as above).
　　Western Electric Mark 5, artificial larynx.

Dr Kuhn and Company. Grub H., 5 Köln-Merheim, Ostmerheviner 198, Germany.
　　Servox Speech Aid.

Washington, Blue Town, Sheerness, Kent, England.
　　Washington Speech Aid Unit (white noise vibrator).

Kett Engineering Company, 920 Santa Monica Buildings, Santa Monica, California, USA.
　　Kett Mark III electro-larynx.

Fortiphone Ltd., 125–9 Middlesex Street, London, E1, England.
　　Tait oral vibrator.

Bell Laboratories Developments, USA.
　　Artificial larynx (reed type).

Cooper-Rand Development Corporation (as above).
　　Cooper-Rand electrolarynx (reed type).

Air-activated Vibrator
H. J. van Hunen, Technisch Bureau, Memacon, Postbus 56, Velp, Holland.
　　Artificial larynx (reed type), DSP. 8.

Bibliography

Abercrombie, D. (1968) 'Paralanguage'. *Brit. J. Dis. Comm.*, **3**, 55.

Aikin, W. A. (1951) *The Voice.* 2nd Edition Ed. H. St J. Rumsey. Longmans Green, London.

Akin, J. (1958) *Voice and Articulation.* Prentice Hall, London.

Alvin, J. (1961) 'Music therapy and the cerebral palsied child'. *Cerebral Palsy Bull.*, **3**, 255.

Allan, C. M., Turner, J. W., Gadea-Ciria, M. (1966) 'Investigations into speech disturbances following stereotaxic surgery for Parkinsonism'. *Brit. J. Dis. Comm.*, **1**, 55.

Allan, C. M. (1970) 'Treatment of non-fluent speech resulting from neurological disease—treatment of dysarthria'. *Brit. J. Dis. Comm.*, **5**, 1.

Amado, J. H. (1953) 'Tableau général des problèmes posés par l'action des hormones sur le développement du larynx'. *Ann. Otolaryng.* Paris, **70**, 117.

Andrews, G., Harris, M. (1964) *The Syndrome of Stuttering.* William Heinemann Medical Books, London; and Spastics Society Medical, Education and Information Unit.

Aranson, A. E., Brown, J. R., Litin, E. M., Pearson, J. S. (1968) 'Spastic dysphonia. I. Voice, neurologic and psychiatric aspects'. *J. Speech Dis.*, **33**, 203.

Aranson, A. E., Brown, J. R., Litin, E. M., Pearson, J. S. (1968a) 'Spastic dysphonia. II. Comparison with essential (voice) tremor and other neurologic and psychogenic disorders'. *J. Speech Dis.*, **33**, 219.

Ardran, G. M., Kemp, F. H. (1966) 'The mechanism of the larynx Part I. The movements of the arytenoid cartilages'. *Brit. J. Radiol.*, **39**, 641.

Ardran, G. M., Kemp, F. H. (1967) 'The mechanism of the larynx Part II. The epiglottis and closure of the larynx'. *Brit. J. Radiol.*, **40**, 372.

Arnold, G. E. (1957) 'Vocal rehabilitation of paralytic dysphonia, III. Present concepts of laryngeal paralysis'. *Arch. Otolaryng.*, **65**, 317.

Arnold, G. E. (1958) 'Dysplastic dysphonia'. *Laryngoscope*, **68**, 142.

Arnold, G. E., Heaver, L. (1959) 'Spastic dysphonia'. *Logos*, **2**, 3.

Arnold, G. E. (1960) 'Studies in tachyphemia, I: Aetiology'. *Logos*, **3**, 25.

Arnold, G. E. (1962) 'Vocal nodules and polyps: laryngeal tissue reaction to habitual hyperkinetic dysphonia'. *J. Speech Dis.*, **27**, 205.

Arnold, G. E. (1962a) 'Vocal rehabilitation of paralytic dysphonia. VIII'. *Arch. Otolaryng.*, **72**, 76.

Arnold, G. E. (1964) 'Further experiences with intracordal teflon injection'. *Laryngoscope*, **74**, 802.

Ascher, E. (1959) 'Motor symptoms of functional or undetermined origin' in *American Handbook of Psychiatry*, Vol I Chap X. Ed. S. Arieti. Basic Books, New York.

Baf, C. L., Ingram, T. T. S. (1955) 'Problems in the classification of cerebral palsy in childhood'. *Brit. Med. J.*, **2**, 163.

Baker, D. C., Savetsky, L. (1966) 'Congenital partial atresia of the larynx'. *Laryngoscope*, **77**, 616.

Bangs, J. L., Freidinger, A. (1950) 'A case of hysterical dysphonia in an adult'. *J. Speech Dis.*, **15**, 316.

Barlow, W. (1952) 'Postural Homeostasis'. *Ann. Phys. Med.*, **1**, 77.

Barlow, W. (1954) 'Posture and the resting state'. *Ann. Phys. Med.*, **2**, 113.

Barlow, W. (1955) *Modern Trends in Psychosomatic Medicine*, Chap 17. Ed. D. O'Neill. Butterworth, London.

Barlow, W. (1959) 'Anxiety and muscle tension pain'. *Brit. J. Clin. Prac.*, **13**, 339.

Barrett, H. (1968) *Practical Methods in Speech*. 2nd Edition. Holt, Rhinehart.

Barton, R. T. (1965) 'Life after laryngectomy'. *Laryngoscope*, **75**, 1408.

Bastiaans, J., Groen, J. (1955) *Psychogenesis and Psychotherapy in Psychosomatic Medicine*. Chap 15. Ed. D. O'Neill. Butterworth, London.

Bateman, G. H., Dornhorst, A. C., Leathart, G. L. (1952) 'Oesophageal speech'. *Brit. Med. J.*, **2**, 1177.

Bateman, G. H., Negus, V. E. (1954) *Speech After Laryngectomy. British Surgical Progress*. Butterworth, London.

Baynes, R. A. (1966) 'An incidence study of chronic hoarseness in children'. *J. Speech Dis.*, **31**, 172.

Bell Telephone Laboratories (1937) *High Speed Motion Picture of Vocal Cords*. New York Bureau of Publications.

Berry, M. F., Eisenson, J. (1962) *Speech Disorders. Principles and Practices of Therapy*. Owen, London.

Birch, D. (1948) *The Art of Good Speech*. Hutchinson.

Birrell, J. F. (1954) 'Hoarseness in childhood'. *Speech*, **18**, 40.

Bloch, P. (1965) 'Neuro-psychiatric aspects of spastic dysphonia'. *Folia Phoniat*, **17**, 30.

Bloomfield, L. (1933) *Language*. Holt, New York.

Bobath, B. (1963) 'Control of postures and movements in the treatment of cerebral palsy'. *J. Physiotherapy*, **39**, 99.

Bohme, G. (1968) 'Stammering and cerebral lesions in early childhood'. *Folia Phoniat*, **20**, 239.

Boone, D. R. (1966) 'Treatment of functional aphonia in a child and an adult'. *J. Speech Dis.*, **31**, 69.

Bosma, J. F. (1953) 'Studies of disability of the pharynx resultant from poliomyelitis'. *Ann. Otol. (St. Louis)*, **62**, 529.

Braithewaite, F., Morley, E. M. (1963) 'Cleft palate'. *Speech Path. and Therap.*, **6**, 1.

Brewer, D. W., Briess, F. B., Faaborg-Anderson, K. (1960) 'Phonation:

clinical testing versus electromyography'. *Ann. Otol. (St. Louis)*, **69**, 781.

Briess, F. B. (1959) 'Voice therapy, Part II: Essential treatment phases of specific laryngeal muscle dysfunction'. *A.M.A. Arch. Otolaryng.*, **69**, 61.

Briess, F. B. (1964) *Voice Diagnosis and Therapy. Research Potentials in Voice Physiology.* Ed. D. W. Brewer. State University, New York.

Broad, D. J. (1968) 'Kinematic considerations for evaluating laryngeal cartilage motions'. *Folia Phoniat.*, **20**, 269.

Broadbent, T. R., Swinyard, C. A. (1959) 'The dynamic pharyngeal flap'. *Plast. Reconstr. Surg.*, **23**, 301.

Brodnitz, F. S. (1953) *Keep Your Voice Healthy.* Harper, New York.

Brodnitz, F. S. (1959) 'Vocal rehabilitation in a child with oesophageal voice'. *Proceedings of XIth Speech and Voice Therapy Conference.* Karger, Basel.

Brodnitz, F. S. (1961) 'Contact ulcer of the larynx'. *Ann. Otol. (St. Louis)*, **74**, 90.

Brodnitz, F. S. (1962) 'The voice of the speaker and singer', in *Voice and Speech Disorders: Medical Aspects.* Chap 12. Ed. N. M. Levin. Thomas, Illinois.

Brodnitz, F. S., Conley, J. J. (1967) 'Vocal rehabilitation after reconstructive surgery for laryngeal cancer'. *Folia Phoniat.*, **19**, 89.

Brodnitz, F. S. (1969) 'Functional aphonia'. *Ann. Otol. (St. Louis)*, **78**, 1244.

Brown, I. (1949) *Shakespeare.* Collins, London.

Burkowsky, M. R. (1968) 'Vocal ulcers in a seventy-one-year-old male'. *J. Speech Dis.*, **33**, 268.

Butfield, E. (1961) 'Dysarthria'. *Speech Path. and Therap.*, **4**, 74.

Byrne, M. C. (1959) 'Speech and language development of athetoid and spastic children'. *J. Speech Dis.*, **24**, 231.

Bzoch, K. (1964) 'The effects of a specific pharyngeal flap operation upon the speech of 40 cleft palate persons'. *J. Speech Dis.*, **29**, 264.

Calnan, J. (1953) 'Movements of the soft palate'. *Brit. J. Plast. Surg.*, **5**, 286.

Calnan, J. (1954) 'The error of Gustav Passavant'. *Plas. Reconstr. Surg.*, **13**, 275.

Calnan, J. (1955) 'Diagnosis, prognosis and treatment of "palato-pharyngeal incompetence" with special reference to radiographic investigations'. *Plast. Reconstruct. Surg.*, **16**, 352.

Calnan, J., Renfrew, C. E. (1961) 'Blowing tests and speech'. *Brit. J. Plast. Surg.*, **13**, 340.

Canter, J. G. (1963) 'Speech characteristics of patients with Parkinson's disease: I. Intensity, pitch, duration'. *J. Speech Dis.*, **28**, 221.

Canter, J. G. (1965) 'Speech characteristics of patients with Parkinson's disease: II. Physiological support for speech'. *J. Speech Dis.*, **30**, 44.

Canter, J. G. (1965a) 'Speech characteristics of patients with Parkinson's disease: III. Articulation, diadochokinesis and over-all speech adequacy'. *J. Speech Dis.*, **30**, 217.

Capps, F. C. W. (1958) 'The Semon Lecture: "Abductor paralysis" in theory and practice since Semon'. *J. Laryng.*, **72**, 1.

Cavanagh, F. (1955) 'Vocal palsies in children'. *Speech*, **10**, 45, and *J. Laryng.*, **69**, 399.

Cherry, J., Delahunty, J. E. (1968) 'Experimentally produced vocal cord granulomas'. *Laryngoscope*, **78**, 1941.

Cherry, J., Margulies, S. I. (1968) 'Contact ulcer of the larynx'. *Laryngoscope*, **78**, 1937.

Clarke, W. M., Hoops, H. R. (1970) 'The effect of speech-type background noise on oesophageal speech production'. *Ann. Otol. (St. Louis)*, **79**, 653.

Clerf, C. H. (1950) 'The surgical treatment of bilateral posticus paralysis of the larynx'. *Laryngoscope*, **60**, 142.

Clerf, C. H., Baltzell, W. H. (1953) 'Re-evaluation of Semon's hypothesis'. *Laryngoscope*, **58**, 693.

Conley, J. J. (1962) 'Rehabilitation of the airway system by neck flaps'. *Ann. Otol. (St. Louis)*, **71**, 924.

Cooper, I. S. (1962) 'Cryogenic surgery of the basal ganglion'. *J. Amer. Med. Assn.*, **181**, 600.

Cooper, M., Nahum, A. M. (1967) 'Vocal rehabilitation for contact ulcer of the larynx'. *Arch. Otolayrng.*, **85**, 41.

Cotton, E. (1965) 'The institute for movement therapy and school for "conductors", Budapest, Hungary. A report on a study visit'. *Develop. Med. Child Neurol.*, **7**, 437.

Craddock, W. H. (1949) 'Perennial nasal allergy'. *Ann. Otol. (St. Louis)*, **58**, 671.

Critchley, M. (1949) 'Observations on essential voice tremor'. *Brain*, **72**, 113.

Curran, D., Guttman, E. (1949) *Psychological Medicine: A Short Introduction*. Livingstone, Edinburgh.

Curry, E. T. (1940) 'The pitch characteristics of the adolescent male voice'. *Speech Monographs* (Research Annual), **7**, 48.

Curry, E. T. (1949) 'Hoarseness and voice change in male adolescents'. *J. Speech Dis.*, **14**, 23.

Curry, E. T. (1949b) 'Voice breaks and pathological larynx conditions'. *J. Speech. Dis.*, **14**, 356.

Curry, R. (1940) *Mechanism of the Voice*. Churchill, London.

Dalcroze, J. (1930) *Eurythmics: Art and Education*. Chatto and Windus, London.

Damsté, P. H. (1958) *Oesophageal Speech*. Hoitsema, Gröningen.

Damsté, P. H. (1959) 'The glosso-pharyngeal press'. *Speech Path. Ther.*, **2**, 70.

Damsté, P. H. (1962) 'Congenital short palate without cleft'. *Proceedings of 12th International Speech and Voice Therapy Conference, Padua*. Eds. L. Croatto, C. Croatto-Martolini.

Damsté, P. H. (1964) 'Virilisation of the voice due to anabolic steroids'. *Folia Phoniat.*, **16**, 10.

Damsté, P. H. (1967) 'Voice change in adult women caused by virilizing agents'. *J. Speech Dis.*, **32**, 126.

Dawson, J. (1902) *The Voice of the Boy*. Kellog, New York.

De Ajurriaguerra, J., Stamback, M. (1955) 'L'évolution des syncinésies chez l'enfant. Place des syncinésies dans le cadre de la débilité motrice'. *Extrait de la Presse Médicalle, 63e Année*, No. **39**, 817.

Dekelbaum, A. M. (1965) 'Papillomas of the larynx'. *Arch. Otol. (St. Louis)*, **81**, 390.

Delahunty, J. E., Ardran, G. M. (1970) 'Globus hystericus—a manifestation of reflex oesophagitis'. *J. Laryng.*, **84**, 1049.

Delattre, P. C. (1955) 'Acoustic loci and transitional cues for consonants'. *J. Acoust. Soc. Amer.*, **27**, 769.

Di Carlo, L. M., Amster, W. W., Herer, G. R. (1955) *Speech after Laryngectomy*. Syracuse University Press.

Diedrich, W. M., Youngstrom, K. A. (1966) *Alaryngeal Speech*. Thomas, Springfield.

Diehl, C. F., White, R., Burck, K. W. (1959) 'Voice quality and anxiety'. *J. Speech Dis.*, **2**, 282.

Dixon, F. W., Hoerr, N. L., McCall, J. W. (1949) 'The nasal mucosa in the laryngectomized patient'. *Ann. Otol. (St. Louis)*, **58**, 535.

Dornhurst, A. C., Negus, V. E. (1954) 'Speech after removal of the oesophagus and the larynx and part of the pharynx'. *Brit. Med. J.*, **2**, 16.

Dowie, L. N. (1965) 'Functional dysphonia'. *Speech Path. Ther.*, **8**, 18.

Doyle, P. J., Brummett, R. E., Everts, E. C. (1967) 'Results of surgical section and repair of the recurrent laryngeal nerve'. *Laryngoscope*, **77**, 1245.

Draper, M. H., Ladefoged, P., Whitteridge, D. (1959) 'Respiratory muscles in speech'. *J. Speech Res.*, **2**, 16.

Duff, J. (1968) 'Laryngeal trauma'. *J. Laryng. (St. Louis)*, **82**, 825.

Dunker, E., Schlosshauer, B. (1964) 'Irregularities of the laryngeal vibratory pattern in healthy and hoarse persons'. *Research Potentials in Voice Physiology*. Ed. D. W. Brewer. State University, New York.

Edwards, T. M. (1952) 'Progress in the surgical treatment of bilateral laryngeal paralysis'. *Ann. Otol. (St Louis)*, **61**, 159.

Ellis, M. (1952) 'Acute diseases of the larynx' in *Diseases of Ear, Nose and Throat*, Chap 29. Ed. W. G. Scott-Brown. Butterworth, London.

Ellis, M. (1952b) 'Chronic specific laryngitis' in *Diseases of the Ear, Nose and Throat*, Chap 31. Ed. W. G. Scott-Brown. Butterworth, London.

Emil-Behnke, K. (1938) *The Technique of Good Speech*. Curwen, London.

Emil-Behnke, K. (1955) *Singers' Difficulties*. Chappell, London.

English, D. T., Blevins, C. E. (1967) 'Motor units of laryngeal muscles'. *Arch. Otolaryng.*, **89**, 778.

Evans, M. F. (1947) 'Problems in cerebral palsy'. *J. Speech Dis.*, **12**, 29.

Everett, J. D. (1907) *Deschanel's Natural Philosophy*. Blackie, London.

Ewing, A. W. G. (1930) *Aphasia in Children*. Oxford University Press.

Eysenck, H. J. (Ed.) (1960) *Behaviour Therapy and the Neuroses*. Pergamon.

Faaborg-Anderson, K. (1957) 'Electromyographic investigation of intrinsic laryngeal muscles in humans'. *Acta. Physiol. Scand. (Suppl.)*, **41**, 140.

Faaborg-Anderson, K. (1964) 'Electromyography of the laryngeal muscles in man'. *Research Potentials in Voice Physiology*. Ed. D. W. Brewer. State University, New York.

Faaborg-Anderson, K., Nykøbing, F. (1965) 'Electromyography of laryngeal muscles. Technics and results' in *Aktuelle Probleme in Phoniatrics and Logopedics*, Vol. 3. Karger, Basel.

Fairbanks, G. (1942) 'An acoustical study in the pitch of infant wails'. *Child Develop.*, **13**, 227.

Fairbanks, G., Herbert, E. L., Hammond, J. M. (1949) 'An acoustical study of vocal pitch in seven- and eight-year-old girls'. *Child. Develop.*, **20**, 71.

Fairbanks, G., Wiley, J. H., Lassman, F. M. (1949) 'An acoustical study of vocal pitch in seven- and eight-year-old boys'. *Child Develop.*, **20**, 63.

Fairbanks, G. (1960) *Voice and Articulation Drill Book*. 2nd Edit. Harper, New York.

Fairman, H. D., John, H. T. (1966) 'Treatment of cancer of the pharynx and cervical oesophagus'. *J. Laryng.*, **80**, 1091.

Fawcus, M. (1964) 'Group therapy for aphasic patients'. *Speech Path. Ther.*, **7**, 30.

Fawcus, R. (1964a) 'The speech therapist in the geriatric unit'. *Speech Path. Ther.*, **7**, 37.

Ferenczi, S. (1926) *Further Contributions to the Theory and Technique of Psycho-Analysis*. Kegan Paul, London.

Ficarra, B. J. (1960) 'Myxoedematous hoarseness'. *Arch. Otolaryng.*, **72**, 75.

Figi, F. A. (1953) 'Hemilaryngectomy with immediate skin graft for the removal of carcinoma of the larynx'. *Ann. Otol. (St. Louis)*, **62**, 400.

Fink, D. H. (1943) *Release from Nervous Tension*. Simon and Schuster, New York.

Fisch, L., Bach, D. E. (1961) 'The assessment of hearing in young cerebral palsied children'. *Cerebr. Palsy Bull.*, **3**, 145.

Flach, M., Schwickardi, H., Simon, R. (1969) 'What influence do menstruation and pregnancy have on the trained singing voice?' *Folia Phoniat.*, **21**, 199.

Flatau, T. S., Gutzmann, H. (1907) 'Die Singstimme des Schulkindes'. *Archiv. Laryng. Rhin.*, **20**, 185.

Fontaine, A., Mitchell, J. C. E. (1960) 'Oesophageal voice: a factor of readiness'. *J. Laryng.*, **74**, 870.

Formby, D. (1967) 'Maternal recognition of infant's cry'. *Develop. Med. Child Neurol.*, **9**, 293.

Fothergill, P., Harrington, R. (1949) 'The clinical significance of the stretch reflex in speech re-education for the spastic'. *J. Speech Dis.*, **14**, 353.

Fox, D. R. (1969) 'Spastic dysphonia: a case presentation'. *J. Speech Dis.*, **34**, 275.

Frank, F. (1969) 'Beweglichkeit des Gaumensegels vor und nach Tonsillektomie'. *Folia Phoniat.*, **21**, 47.

Freud, S. (1938) *The Basic Writings of Sigmund Freud*. Book 3, 'Three contributions to the theory of sex'. Modern Library, New York.

Freud, S. (1943) *A General Introduction to Psycho-Analysis*. Garden City, New York.

Friedman, S., Goffin, F. B. (1966) 'Abductor vocal weakness in myasthenia gravis'. *Laryngoscope,* **77,** 1520.

Fritzell, B. (1960) 'Speech improvement following palatoplasty with elongated flap'. *Folia Phoniat.,* **2,** 118.

Fritzell, B. (1969) 'The velopharyngeal muscles in speech. An electromyographic and cineradiographic study'. *Acta Otolaryng.,* Supplement 250. Göteborg, Sweden.

Froeschels, E., Jellinek, A. (1941) *Practice of Voice and Speech Therapy.* Expression, Boston.

Froeschels, E. (1948) *Twentieth Century Voice Correction,* Chap V. Philosophical Library, New York.

Froeschels, E. (1948a) 'Should the speech therapist be a voice therapist?' *J. Speech Dis.,* **13,** 346.

Froeschels, E. (1957) 'The question of the origin of the vibrations of the vocal cords'. *Arch. Otolaryng.,* **66,** 512.

Froeschels, E. (1957a) 'Nose and nasality'. *Arch. Otolaryng.,* **66,** 629.

Fry, D. B. (1948) 'An experimental study of tone deafness'. *Speech,* **12,** 4.

Fry, D. B. (1957) 'Speech and language'. *J. Laryng.,* **71,** 434.

Fry, D. B. (1963) 'Coding and decoding in speech' in *Signs, Signals and Symbols,* Chap 7. Ed. S. Mason. Methuen, London.

Fry, D. B. (1968) 'Prosodic phenomenon' in *Manual of Phonetics.* Ed. B. Malmberg. North Holland, Amsterdam.

Garfield-Davies, D. (1969) 'Fibrosarcoma and pseudosarcoma of the larynx'. *J. Laryng.,* **83,** 423.

Gedda, L., Fiori-Ratti, L., Bruno, G. (1960) 'La voix chez les jumeaux monozygotique'. *Folia Phoniat.,* **12,** 81.

Gimson, A. C. (1962) *An Introduction to the Pronunciation of English.* Arnold, London.

Goda, S. (1966) 'Speech therapy with selected patients with congenital velo-pharyngeal inadequacy'. *Cleft. Pal. J.,* **3,** 268.

Goff, W. F. (1969) 'Teflon injection for vocal cord paralysis'. *Arch. Otolaryng.,* **90,** 98.

Grady, P. (1958) 'The treatment of dysarthria in cases of congenital suprabulbar paresis'. *Speech Path. Ther.,* **2,** 51.

Gray, H. (1949) *Anatomy: Descriptive and Applied.* 30th Edit. Ed. T. B. Johnston, J. Whillis. Longmans, London.

Greene, M. C. L. (1955) 'Puberphonia'. *Report on the British Conference on Speech Therapy, April* 1952. College of Speech Therapists, London.

Greene, M. C. L. (1957) 'Speech of children before and after removal of tonsils and adenoids'. *J. Speech Dis.,* **22,** 361.

Greene, M. C. L., Canning, A. (1959) 'The incidence of nasal and lateral defects in cleft palate'. *Folia Phoniat.,* **11,** 208.

Greene, M. C. L. (1960) 'Speech analysis of 263 cleft palate cases'. *J. Speech Dis.,* **25,** 144.

Greene, M. C. L. (1960a) *Learning to Talk: A Guide to Parents.* Harper, New York, Heinemann, London.

Greene, M. C. L. (1961) 'Problems involved in the speech and language training of the partially deaf child'. *Speech Path. Ther.,* **4,** 22.

Greene, M. C. L. (1962) 'Possible areas of co-operation between speech therapists and teachers of the deaf'. *Speech Path. Ther.,* **5,** 57.

Greene, M. C. L., Conway, J. (1963) *Learning to Talk: A Study in Sound of Infant Speech Development*. Folkways Records (New York) FX 6271.

Greene, M. C. L. (1964) *The Voice and its Disorders*. 2nd Edit. Pitman, London.

Greene, M. C. L. (1967) 'Management of aphonia after surgical treatment of carcinoma of the larynx, pharynx and oesophagus'. *Brit. J. Dis. Comm.*, **2**, 30.

Greene, M. C. L. (1967a) 'Speechless and backward at three. What the speech therapist can do about it'. *Brit. J. Dis. Comm.*, **2**, 134.

Greene, M. C. L. (1968) 'Vocal disabilities of singers'. *Proc. Roy. Soc. Med.*, **61**, 1147.

Greene, M. C. L., Watson, B. W. (1968) 'The value of speech amplification in Parkinson's Disease patients'. *Folia Phoniat.*, **20**, 250.

Grewel, F. (1957) 'Classification of dysarthrias'. *Acta Psych. Neurol. Scand.*, **32**, 325.

Grewel, F. (1959) 'How do children acquire the use of language?' *Phonetica*, **3**, 193.

Grewel, F. (1960) 'Speech, language and hearing disorders in encephalopathy'. *Folia Phoniat.*, **12**, 282.

Grewel, F., Greene, M. C. L. (1968) 'Diagnosis and treatment of speaking and language disorders following cerebral injury in old age'. *Psychiat. Neurol. Neurochir.*, **71**, 469.

Grossberg, J. M. (1965) 'Successful behaviour therapy in a case of speech phobia'. *J. Speech Dis.*, **30**, 285.

Grossman, M. (1897) 'Experimentelle Beitrage zur Lehre von der "Posticuslähmung" '. *Arch. Laryng. u. Rhin.*, **6**, 282 and 339.

Guthrie, D. (1952) *Logan Turner's Diseases of the Nose, Throat and Ear*. 5th Edition. Wright, Bristol.

Guthrie, D. (1966) 'Forty-two years survival after laryngectomy'. *J. Laryng.*, **80**, 851.

Hahn, E., Lomas, C. W., Hargis, D. E. Vandraegen, D. (1952) *Basic Voice Training for Speech*. McGraw-Hill, New York.

Hall, I. S., (1954) 'Laryngeal abnormalities and their surgical correction'. *Speech*, **18**, 33.

Hamlen, M. (1967) *Speech Assessment Following Palatopharyngeal Flap Procedures and Speech Therapy*. British College of Speech Therapists Fellowship Thesis (unpublished), London.

Hanley, T. D., Thurman, W. L. (1962) *Developing Vocal Skills*. Holt, Rheinhart and Winston, New York.

Hardy, J. C., Rembolt, R. R., Spriestersbach, D. C., Jayapathy, B. (1961) 'Surgical management of palatal paresis and speech problems in cerebral palsy: a preliminary report'. *J. Speech Dis.*, **26**, 320.

Hardy, J. C., Netsell, R., Schweiger, J. W., Morris, H. L. (1969) 'Management of velopharyngeal dysfunction in cerebral palsy'. *J. Speech Dis.*, **34**, 123.

Harmer, W. D., (1919) 'Warfare injuries of the larynx'. *J. Laryng.*, **34**, 2.

Harpman, J. A. (1952) 'On the management of bilateral paralysis of the vocal cords following operations on or disease of the thyroid gland'. *J. Laryng.*, **66**, 599.

Harris, H. H., Ainsworth, J. Z. (1965) 'Immediate management of laryngeal and tracheal injuries'. *Laryngoscope*, **75**, 1103.

Harrison, D. F. N. (1964) 'Pharyngo-esophageal replacement in post cricoid and esophageal carcinoma'. *Ann. Otol. (St. Louis)*, **73**, 1026.

Head, H. (1925) *Aphasia and Kindred Disorders of Speech*. Cambridge University Press.

Heaver, L. (1958) 'Psychiatric observations on the personality structure of patients with habitual dysphonia'. *Logos*, **1**, 21.

Heaver, L. (1962) 'Psycho-semantic aspects of non-verbal communication'. *Logos*, **5**, 60.

Heaver, L., Arnold, G. E. (1962) 'Rehabilitation of alaryngeal aphonia'. *Post Grad. Med.*, **32**, 11.

Heinemann, M. (1969) 'Myxoedem und Stimme'. *Folia Phoniat.*, **21**, 55.

Henderson, D., Gillespie, R. D. (1950) *A Text Book of Psychiatry for Students and Practitioners*. Oxford University Press.

Henderson, R. (1954) *Kathleen Ferrier*. Hamilton, London.

Hess, D. A. (1959) 'Pitch, intensity and cleft palate voice quality'. *J. Speech Res.*, **2**, 113.

Hildernisse, L. W. (1956) 'Voice diagnosis'. *Acta Physiol. Pharmacol. Neerl.*, **5**, 73.

Hirano, M., Koike, Y., Von Leden, H. (1968) 'Maximum phonation time and air usage during phonation'. *Folia Phoniat.*, **20**, 185.

Hiroto, I., Hirano, M., Tomita, H. (1968) 'Electromyographic investigation of human vocal cord paralysis'. *Ann. Otol. (St. Louis)*, **77**, 296.

Hobbs, R. C., Mullard, K. (1966) 'The treatment of post cricoid carcinoma by single stage pharyngo-laryngectomy and colon transplant'. *J. Laryng.*, **80**, 1193.

Hodson, C. J., Oswald, M. V. O. (1958) *Speech Recovery after Total Laryngectomy*. Livingstone, Edinburgh.

Holl-Allen, R. T. J. (1967) 'Laryngeal nerve paralysis and benign thyroid disease'. *Arch. Otolaryng.*, **85**, 335.

Holland, B. C., Ward, R. S. (1959) 'Homeostasis and psychosomatic medicine'. *American Handbook of Psychiatry*, Vol III Chap 10. Ed. S. Arieti. Basic Books, New York.

Hollien, H. (1960) 'Some laryngeal correlates of vocal pitch'. *J. Speech Res.*, **3**, 52.

Hollinger, P. H. (1959) *Treatment of Cancer and Allied Diseases*, Vol 3 Chap 34. Ed. G. T. Pack and I. M. Ariel. Pitman, London.

Hollinger, P. H., Schild, J. A., Maurizi, D. G. (1968) 'Internal and external trauma to the larynx'. *Laryngoscope*, **78**, 1.

Hutzinga, E. (1966) 'Historical Vignette. Sir Felix Semon'. *Arch. Otolaryng.*, **84**, 473.

Hunt, R. B. (1964) 'Rehabilitation of the laryngectomee'. *Laryngoscope*, **74**, 382.

Hynes, W. (1954) 'The primary repair of clefts of the palate'. *Brit. J. Plast. Surg.*, **7**, 242.

Ingram, T. T. S. (1960) 'Paediatric aspects of developmental dysphasia, dyslexia and dysgraphia'. *Cerebr. Palsy Bull.*, **2**, 254.

Ingram, T. T. S., Barn, J. (1961) 'A description and classification of common speech disorders associated with cerebral palsy'. *Cereb. Palsy Bull.*, **3**, 57.

Isshiki, N., Von Leden, H. (1964) 'Hoarseness: aerodynamic studies'. *Arch. Otolaryng.*, **70**, 206.

Isshiki, N. (1965) 'Vocal intensity and air flow rate'. *Folia Phoniat.*, **17**, 19.

Isshiki, N. (1968) *Airflow in Esophageal Speech*, 2nd Edition Chap 9: 'Speech rehabilitation of the laryngectomised'. Ed. J. C. Snidecor. Thomas, Illinois.

Isshiki, N., Okamura, H., Tanabe, M., Morimoto, M. (1969) 'Differential diagnosis of hoarseness'. *Folia Phoniat.*, **21**, 9.

Isshiki, N., Honjow, I., Morimoto, M. (1969) 'Cine-radiographic analysis of movement of the lateral pharyngeal wall'. *Plas. Reconstr. Surg.*, **44**, 357.

Jackson, C. (1940) 'Myasthenia laryngis. Observations on the larynx as an air column instrument'. *Arch. Otolaryng.*, **32**, 434.

Jackson, C., Jackson, C. L. (1935) 'Contact ulcer of the larynx'. *Arch. Otolaryng.*, **22**, 1.

Jackson, C., Jackson, C. L., Editors. (1945) *Diseases of the Nose, Throat and Ear*. Saunders, Philadelphia and London.

Jacobson, E. (1929) *Progressive Relaxation*. University of Chicago Press.

James, J. A. (1952) 'Acute rhinitis and rhinorrhoea' in *Diseases of the Ear, Nose and Throat*, Vol 1, Chap 7. Ed. W. G. Scott-Brown. Butterworth, London.

Janet, P. (1920) *The Major Symptoms of Hysteria*. Macmillan, New York.

Jasienska, A., Kuzniarz, J. (1964) 'Avelli's syndrome with underlying herpes zoster'. *Otolaryng. Polska*, **18**, 287.

Jenkins, J. C. (1967) 'Preliminary report on the treatment of multiple papillomata by ultrasound'. *J. Laryng.*, **81**, 385.

Johnson, W., Darley, F. L., Spriesterbach, D. C. (1963) *Diagnostic Methods in Speech Pathology*. Harper, New York.

Jones, A. M. (1949) 'African Music'. *Occasional Papers of The Rhodes-Livingstone Museum*, No 4. Livingstone, Edinburgh.

Jones, D. (1947) *An Outline of English Phonetics*. Heffer, Cambridge

Kallen, L. A. (1934) 'Vicarious vocal mechanisms'. *Arch. Otolaryng.*, **20**, 460.

Kiml, J. (1965) 'Recherches expérimentales de la dysphonie spastique'. *Folia Phoniat.*, **17**, 241.

King, B. T., Gregg, R. L. (1948) 'An anatomical reason for the various behaviours of paralysed vocal cords'. *Ann. Otol.* (*St. Louis*), **57**, 925.

King, E. B. (1953) 'Bilateral abductor paralysis'. *Ann. Otol.* (*St. Louis*), **62**, 196.

Kingdon-Ward, W. (1941) *Stammering: A Contribution to the Study of its Problems and Treatment*. Hamish Hamilton, London.

Kinsey, A. C., Pomeroy, W. B., Martin, C. (1948) *Sexual Behaviour in the Human Male*. Sanderson, Philadelphia.

Kirchner, J. A., Wyke B. D. (1965) 'Articular reflex mechanisms in the larynx'. *Ann. Otol.* (*St. Louis*), **74**, 749.

Kirchner, J. A. (1966) 'Atrophy of laryngeal muscles in vagal paralysis'. *Laryngoscope*, **77**, 1753.

Kirchner, F. R., Toledo, P. S., Stroboda, D. J. (1966) 'Studies of the larynx after teflon injection'. *Arch. Otolaryng.*, **83**, 350.

Kirikae, H., Hirose, H., Kawamura, S., Sawashima, M., Kobayashi, T., (1962) 'An experimental study of central motor innervation of the laryngeal muscles in the cat'. *Ann. Otol. (St. Louis)*, **71**, 222.

Kirsch, D. (1962) 'Radiotherapy in laryngeal malignancy', in *Voice and Speech Disorders: Medical Aspects.* Ed. N. M. Levin Thomas, Springfield.

Kleinsasser, O. (1968) *Microlaryngoscopy and Endolaryngeal Microsurgery.* Translated by P. W. Hoffman. Saunders, London.

Koike, Y., Hirano, M., Von Leden, H. (1967) 'Vocal initiation: acoustic and aerodynamic investigations in normal subjects'. *Folia Phoniat.*, **19**, 173.

Kremer, M., Russell, W. R., Smith, G. E. (1947) 'A mid-brain syndrome following head injury'. *J. Neurol. Neuro-Surg. Psych.*, **10**, 49.

Labarraque, M. L. (1952) 'Les phonophobies'. *Ann. D'Otolaryng.* (Paris), **69**, 200.

Lacina, O. (1968) 'Der Einfluss der Menstruation auf die Stimme der Sängerinnen'. *Folia Phoniat.* **20**, 13.

Ladefoged, P. (1960) 'The regulation of sub-glottal pressure'. *Folia Phoniat.*, **12**, 169.

Ladefoged, P. (1962) *Elements of Acoustic Phonetics.* Oliver and Boyd, London.

Ladell, R. M. (1940) *The Stammerer Unmasked.* Pitman, London.

Laguaite, J. K., Waldrop, W. F. (1963) 'Acoustical analysis of fundamental frequency of voices before and after therapy'. *N.Z. Speech Ther. J.*, **18**, 23.

Lall, M., Evison, G. (1966) 'Voice production following laryngo-pharyngo-oesophagectomy'. *J. Laryng.*, **80**, 1208.

Lange, M. J. (1953) 'Thyroidectomy: a review of 1,000 consecutive cases'. *Brit. J. Surg.*, **40**, 544.

Last, R. J. (1960) *Anatomy Regional and Applied.* Churchill, London.

Lauder, E. (1965) 'The role of the laryngectomee in post-laryngectomy voice instruction'. *J. Speech Dis.*, **30**, 145.

Lauder, E. (1968) 'The laryngectomee and the artificial larynx'. *J. Speech Dis.*, **33**, 147.

Lauder, E. (1968a) *Self Help for the Laryngectomee.* From the author: 6334 Dove Hill Drive, San Antonio, Texas, 78238, USA.

Laver, J. D. M. (1968) 'Voice quality and indexical information'. *Brit. J. Dis. Comm.*, **3**, 43.

Lawrence, T. E. (1941) *Selected Letters of T. E. Lawrence.* Ed. David Garnett. World Books, London.

Lebo, C. P., Oliphant, K. P. (1968) 'Music as a source of acoustic trauma'. *Laryngoscope*, **78**, 1211.

Lederer, F. L. (1948) 'Present concepts of laryngeal disease'. *J. Speech Dis.*, **13**, 11.

Lederman, M., Dalley, V. M. (1965) 'The treatment of glottic cancer. The importance of radiotherapy to the patient'. *J. Laryng.*, **79**, 767.

Lell, W. A. (1941) 'Diagnosis and direct laryngoscopy treatment of functional aphonia'. *Arch. Otolaryng.*, **34**, 141.

Lennenberg, E. H., Rebelsky, F., Nichols, I. (1965) 'The vocalisation of infants born to deaf and hearing parents'. *Human Develop.*, **8**, 23.

Lenz, M., Okrainetz, C., Berne, A. S. (1959) 'Radiotherapy of the larynx' in *Surgical Progress*, Vol 3, Chap 36. Ed. G. T. Pack and I. M. Ariel. Pitman, London.

Levin, N. M. (1952) 'Speech rehabilitation after total removal of larynx'. *J. Amer. Med. Assn.*, **149**, 1281.

Levin, N. M. (1962) 'Surgery of the larynx, trachea and neck' in *Voice and Speech Disorders: Medical Aspects*, Chap 9. Ed. N. M. Levin. Thomas, Illinois.

Levin, N. M. (1962a) 'Esophageal speech' in *Voice and Speech Disorders: Medical Aspects*, Chap 10. Ed. N. M. Levin. Thomas, Illinois.

Levitt, S. (1962) *Physiotherapy in Cerebral Palsy*. Thomas, Illinois.

Lewis, M. M. (1951) *Infant Speech*. Routledge, London.

Lewy, R. B. (1966) 'Responses of laryngeal tissue to granular teflon in situ'. *Arch. Otolaryng.*, **83**, 355.

Liberman, A. M. (1957) 'Some results of research on speech perception'. *J. Acoust. Soc. Amer.*, **29**, 117.

Lieberman, P. (1967) *Intonation, Perception and Language*. Research Monograph No 38. M.I.H. Press, Cambridge, Mass.

Linden, J. W., Hill, B. J., Waldrop, W., Monroe, C. (1968) 'Voice changes following adenotonsillectomy: a study of velar function by cinefluorography and video-tape'. *Laryngoscope*, **78**, 1.

Linford Rees, W. L. (1969) (*a*) 'Psychiatric examination'. Chap 14. (*b*) 'Psychosomatic disorders'. Chap 18. (*c*) 'Affective disorders'. Chap 22. (*d*) 'Hysteria'. Chap 23. (*e*) 'Obsessional states'. Chap 24. (*f*) 'Behaviour therapy'. Chap 31. (*g*) 'Sexual disorders'. Chap 26, in *A Short Textbook of Psychiatry*. English University Press, London.

Linford Rees, W. L. (1970) *Personal Communication*.

Ling, D. (1963) 'The use of hearing and the teaching of speech'. *Teacher of Deaf*, **61**, 59.

Lubit, E. C., Larson, R. E. (1969) 'The Lubit palatal exerciser: a preliminary report'. *Cleft Pal. J.*, **6**, 425.

Luchsinger, R. (1953) 'Physiologie der Stimme'. *Folia Phoniat.*, **5**, 58.

Luchsinger, R., Dubois, C. (1956) 'Phonetische und Stroboskopische Untersuchungen an einem Stimmphänomen'. *Folia Phoniat.*, **8**, 201.

Luchsinger, R. (1962) 'Voice disorders on an endocrine basis' in *Voice and Speech Disorders: Medical Aspects*. Ed. N. M. Levin. Thomas, Illinois.

Luchsinger, R., Arnold, G. E. (1965) (*a*) 'Physiology of respiration'. Chap I. (*b*) 'Pathology of respiration'. Chap II. (*c*) 'Physiology of laryngeal function'. Chap V. (*d*) 'The qualities of voice'. Chap VI. (*e*) 'Professional use of the voice'. Chap IX. (*f*) 'Primary dysphonia and secondary laryngitis'. Special Part Chap II. (*g*) 'Endocrine dysphonia'. Chap III, in *Voice, Speech and Language*. Constable, London.

Luria, A. R. (1961) *The Role of Speech in the Regulation of Normal and Abnormal Behaviour*. Pergamon, Oxford.

Luria, A. R. (1963) *The Mentally Retarded Child*. Pergamon, Oxford.

Luria, A. R. (1966) *Higher Cortical Functions*. Tavistock, London.

McAllister, A. H. (1952) *A Year's Course in Speech Training*. University of London Press.

McCroskey, R. L., Mulligan, M. (1963) 'The relative intelligibility of esophageal speech and artificial larynx'. *J. Speech Dis.*, **16**, 9.

McDonald, E. T., Baker, H. K. (1951) 'Cleft palate speech: an integration of research and clinical observation'. *J. Speech Dis.*, **16**, 9.

McGlone, R., Hollien, H. (1963) 'Vocal pitch characteristics of aged women'. *J. Speech Res.*, **6**, 164.

McWilliams, B. J. (1960) 'Cleft palate management in England'. *Speech Path. Ther.*, **3**, 3.

McWilliams, B. J., Bradley, D. P. (1965) 'Ratings of velopharyngeal closure during blowing and speech'. *Cleft. Pal. J.*, **2**, 46.

Makuen, G. H. (1911) 'Relation of the tonsil operation to the soft palate and the voice'. *Trans. Amer. Laryng. Assn.*, 223.

Malcolmson, K. G. (1968) 'Globus hystericus vel pharyngis'. *J. Laryng.*, **82**, 219.

Marland, P. M. (1949) 'A direct method of teaching voice after total laryngectomy'. *Speech*, **13**, 4.

Marland, P. M. (1952) 'The treatment of dysphonia due to recurrent laryngeal nerve palsies'. *College of Speech Therapists Oxford Conference Report*.

Marland, P. M. (1953) 'Speech therapy for cerebral palsy based on reflex inhibition'. *Speech*, **17**, 65.

Marres, E. H. M. A., Wentges, R. T. R., Brinkman, W. F. B. (1966) 'Cryosurgical treatment of juvenile papillomatosis'. *Laryngoscope*, **77**, 1979.

Mason, M. (1950) 'The rehabilitation of patients following surgical removal of the larynx'. *J. Laryng.*, **64**, 759.

Massengill, R., Bryson, M. (1967) 'A study of velopharyngeal function as a cinéfluorographic television monitor'. *Folia Phoniat.*, **19**, 45.

Michel, J., Hollien, H., Moore, P. (1966) 'Speaking fundamental characteristics of 15-, 16- and 17-year-old girls'. *Language and Speech*. **9**, 46.

Millar, H. (1969) 'Pathology of vocal cord paralysis'. *J. Otolaryng. Soc. Aust.*, **2**, 56.

Millard, D. R. (1963) 'The island flap in cleft palate surgery'. *Surg. Gynec. Obstet.*, **116**, 297.

Miller, A. H. (1967) 'First experience with the Asai technique for vocal rehabilitation after total laryngectomy'. *Ann. Otol. (St. Louis)*, **76**, 829.

Miller, A. H. (1968) 'First experience with the Asai technique for vocal rehabilitation after total laryngectomy' in *Speech Rehabilitation of the Largyngectomised*, Chap 3. 2nd Edition. Ed. J. C. Snidecor. Thomas, Illinois.

Miller, R. (1970) 'Verdict on the million pound voices'. *Mirror Magazine*, March 7th.

Mills, W. (1906) *Voice Production in Singing and Speaking Based on Scientific Principles*. Curwen, London.

Mitchell, S. W. (1908) 'Treatment by rest, seclusion etc. in relation to psychotherapy'. *J. Amer. Med. Assn.*, **50**, 2033.

Monrad-Krohn, G. H. (1947) 'Dysprosody or altered "melody of language" '. *Brain*, **70**, 405.

Monrad-Krohn, G. H. (1947) 'The prosodic quality of speech and its disorders'. *Acta Psychiatrica et Neurologica*, **22**, 255.

Moolenaar-Bijl, A. (1952) 'The importance of certain consonants in esophageal voice after laryngectomy'. *Ann. Otol. (St. Louis)*, **62**, 979.

Moolenaar-Bijl, A. J. (1953) 'Connection between consonant articulation and the intake of air in oesophageal speech'. *Folia Phoniat.*, **5**, 212.

Moolenaar-Bijl, A. J. (1956) 'Voice correction under pathological conditions'. *Acta Physiol. Neerl.*, **5**, 85.

Moore, W. E. (1939) 'Voice quality and anxiety'. *J. Speech Dis.*, **4**, 33.

Moore, P. (1962) 'Observations on the physiology of hoarseness'. *Proceedings of the 4th International Congress of Phonetic Sciences*, page 92. Mouton, The Hague.

Moravek, M., Langova, J. (1962) 'Some electrophysiological findings among stutterers and clutterers'. *Folia Phoniat.*, **14**, 305.

Morley, M. E. (1966) *Cleft Palate*. Livingstone, Edinburgh.

Morrison, W. W. (1931) 'The production of voice and speech following total laryngectomy'. *Arch. Otolaryng.*, **14**, 413.

Morrison, L. F. (1948) 'The "reverse King operation". A surgical procedure for restoration of phonation in cases of aphonia due to unilateral cord paralysis'. *Ann. Otol. (St. Louis)*, **57**, 945.

Morrison, L. F. (1952) 'Recurrent laryngeal nerve paralysis'. *Ann. Otol. (St. Louis)*, **61**, 567.

Moses, P. J. (1954) *The Voice of Neurosis*. Grune and Stratton, New York.

Moses, P. J. (1958) 'Rehabilitation of the post-laryngectomised patient'. *Ann. Otol (St. Louis)*, **67**, 538.

Moses, P. J. (1959) 'The vocal expression of emotional disturbances'. *Kaiser Foundation Med. Bull.*, **7**, 107.

Moses, P. J. (1960) 'The psychology of the castrato voice'. *Folia Phoniat.*, **12**, 204.

Munro-Black, J. I., Jackson, J. M., Holti, G. (1964) 'A hoarse voice and a red face'. *J. Laryng.*, **78**, 924.

Murphy, G. E., Bisna, A. L., Ogura, J. H. (1964) 'Determinants of rehabilitation following laryngectomy'. *Laryngoscope*, **74**, 1535.

Musgrove, J. (1952) 'Nervous diseases of the larynx' in *Diseases of the Ear, Nose and Throat*, Vol 1 Chap 28. Ed. W. G. Scott-Brown. Butterworth, London.

Myerson, M. C. (1952) 'Smoker's larynx'. *Ann. Otol. (St. Louis)*, **59**, 541.

Mysak, E. D. (1959) 'Pitch and duration characteristics of older males'. *J. Speech Res.*, **2**, 46.

Mysak, E. D. (1959a) 'Significance of neuro-physiological orientation to cerebral palsy habilitation'. *J. Speech Dis.*, **24**, 221.

Mysak, E. D. (1959) 'A servo model for speech therapy'. *J. Speech Dis.*, **24**, 144.

Nahum, M. C. (1967) 'Vocal rehabilitation for contact ulcer of the larynx'. *Arch. Otolaryng.*, **85**, 41.

Naidr, J., Zboril, N., Ševčik, K. (1965) 'Die pubertalen Veränderungen der Stimme bei Jungen im verlauf von 5 Jahren'. *Folia Phoniat.*, **17**, 1.

Negus, V. E., Neil, E., Floyd, W. F. (1957) 'The mechanisms of phonation'. *Ann. Otol. (St. Louis)*, **66**, 817.

Negus, V. E. (1931) 'Observations on Semon's Law derived from evidence of comparative anatomy and physiology'. *J. Laryng.*, **46**, 1.

Negus, V. E. (1949) *The Comparative Anatomy and Physiology of the Larynx.* Heinemann Medical, London.

Negus, V. E. (1950) 'Radiotherapy in cancer of the larynx'. *J. Laryng.*, **64**, 731.

Negus, V. E. (1957) 'The mechanism of the larynx'. *Laryngoscope*, **67**, 1961.

Negus, V. E. (1957a) 'The function of the paranasal sinuses'. *Arch. Otolaryng.*, **66**, 430.

New, G. B., Devine, K. D. (1949) 'Contact ulcer granuloma'. *Ann. Otol. (St. Louis)*, **58**, 548.

Oliver, R. T. O. (1961) *Conversation: The Development and Expression of Personality.* Thomas, Illinois.

Osgood, C. E. (1953) *Method and Theory in Experimental Psychology.* Oxford Press.

Ostwald, P. F., Freedman, D. G., Kurtz, J. H. (1962) 'Vocalisation in infant twins'. *Folia Phoniat.*, **14**, 1.

Oswald, M. V. O. (1949) 'Oesophageal voice following total laryngectomy'. *College of Speech Therapists Conference Report.* Tavistock, London.

Owsley, J. O., Lawson, L. I., Miller, E. R., Blackfield, H. M. (1966) 'Experience with high attached pharyngeal flaps'. *Plas. Reconstr. Surg.*, **38**, 232.

Paget, R. (1930) *Human Speech.* Kegan Paul, London.

Palmer, M. F. (1947) 'Studies in clinical techniques, normalisation of chewing, sucking and swallowing reflexes'. *J. Speech Dis.*, **12**, 415.

Palmer, M. F. (1949) 'Studies in clinical techniques, IV'. *J. Speech Dis.*, **14**, 20.

Pantoja, E. (1968) 'The laryngeal cartilages'. *Arch. Otolaryng.*, **87**, 416.

Peacher, W. G., Hollinger, P. H. (1947) 'Contact ulcer of the larynx. The role of vocal re-education'. *Arch. Otolaryng.*, **46**, 617.

Peacher, W. G. (1949) 'The neurological evaluation of delayed speech'. *J. Speech Dis.*, **14**, 344.

Peacher, W. G. (1949a) 'Neurological factors in the etiology of delayed speech'. *J. Speech Dis.*, **14**, 147.

Peacher, W. G. (1950) 'The etiology and differential diagnosis of dysarthria'. *J. Speech Dis.*, **15**, 252.

Peacher, G. M. (1961) 'Vocal therapy for contact ulcer—a follow up of 70 patients'. *Laryngoscope*, **71**, 37.

Pear, T. H. (1931) *Voice and Personality.* Chapman and Hall, London.

Pearce, E. C. (1959) *Anatomy and Physiology for Nurses.* 13th Edition. Faber and Faber, London.

Pepinsky, A. (1942) 'The laryngeal ventricle considered as an acoustical filter'. *J. Acoust. Soc. Amer.*, **14**, 32.

Perello, J. (1954) 'Le traitement de la voix bandes ventriculaires'. *Folia Phoniat.*, **6**, 42.

Perello, J. (1962) 'La disfonia premenstrual'. *Acta O.R.L. Iber-Amer.*, **13**, 561.

Perello, J. (1962a) 'Dysphonies Fonctionelles'. *Folia Phoniat.*, **14**, 150.

Peterson, G. E. (1954) *Phonetics, Phonemics and Pronunciation.* Georgetown Mon. Series, Language and Linguistics, No 6.

Pfau, W. (1954) 'Tonsilectomy and voice'. *J. Laryng.*, **33**, 39.

Piaget, J. (1952) *Play, Dreams and Imitation in Childhood.* Translated by C. Gattegno and M. E. Hodgson. Heinemann, London.

Pollack, D. (1952) 'Post arytenoidectomy voice therapy'. *Speech*, **16**, 4.

Portmann, G., Robin, J., Laget, P., Husson, R. (1956) 'La myographie des cordes vocales'. *Acta Otolaryng.*, **46**, 250.

Postman, L., Rosenweig, M. R. (1957) 'Perceptual organisation of words'. *J. Speech Dis.*, **22**, 245.

Potter, R. K., Kopp, G. A., Green, H. C. (1947) *Visible Speech.* van Nostrand, New York.

Pressman, J. J. (1954) 'Cancer of the larynx: Laryngoplasty to avoid laryngectomy'. *Arch. Otolaryng.*, **59**, 395.

Pressman, J. J., Bailey, B. J. (1968) 'The surgery of cancer of the larynx with special reference to subtotal laryngectomy' in *Speech Rehabilitation of the Laryngectomized*, Chap II. 2nd Edition. Ed. J. C. Snidecor. Thomas, Illinois.

Punt, N. A. (1967) *The Singer's and Actor's Throat.* 2nd Edition. Heinemann, London.

Punt, N. A. (1968) 'Applied laryngology: singer and actors'. *Proc. Roy. Soc. Med.*, **61**, 1152.

Putney, F. J. (1952) 'Hematoma of the larynx from external trauma'. *Ann. Otol. (St. Louis)*, **61**, 452.

Putney, F. J. (1958) 'Rehabilitation of the post-laryngectomised patient'. *Ann. Otolaryng.*, **67**, 544.

Rabbett, W. F. (1965) 'Juvenile laryngeal papillomatosis. The relation of irradiation and malignant degeneration'. *Ann. Otol. (St. Louis)*, **74**, 1149.

Reidy, J. P. (1958) '370 personal cases of cleft lip and palate'. *Ann. Surg.*, **23**, 341.

Renfrew, C. E., Mitchell, J. C. E., Wallace, A. R. (1957) 'Listening'. *Speech*, **21**, 34.

Réthi, A. (1963) 'L'innervation du larynx'. *Acta O.R.L. Ibero-Amer.*, **2**, 43.

Rigby, R. G. (1952) 'The present status of globus hystericus'. *Laryngoscope*, **62**, 401.

Ridrodsky, S., Morrison, E. B. (1970) 'Speech changes in Parkinsonism L-Dopa therapy: preliminary findings'. *J. Amer. Geriat. Soc.*, **18**, 142.

Rippon, T. S., Fletcher, P. (1940) *Reassurance and Relaxation.* Routledge, London.

Ritter, F. N., (1967) 'The effects of hypothyroidism upon the ear, nose and throat'. *Laryngoscope*, **77**, 1427.

Robe, E. Y., Moore, P., Andrews, A. H., Hollinger, P. H. (1956) 'A study of the role of certain factors in the development of speech after laryngectomy. 1. Type of operation. 2. Site of pseudoglottis. 3. Co-ordination of speech with respiration'. *Laryngoscope*, **66**, 173, 382, 481.

Robe, E. Y., Moore, P., Brumlik, J. (1960) 'A study of spastic dysphonia'. *Laryngoscope*, **70**, 219.

Robe-Finkbeiner, E. Y. (1968) 'Surgery and speech, the pseudoglottis and respiration in total standard laryngectomy' in *Speech Rehabilitation of the Laryngectomised*, Chap 4. 2nd Edition. Ed. J. C. Snidecor. Thomas, Illinois.

Roy, A. D., Gardiner, R. H., Niblock, W. M. (1956) 'Thyroidectomy and the recurrent laryngeal nerves'. *Lancet*, June, 988.

Rubin, H. J. (1960) 'The neurochronaxic theory of voice production—a refutation'. *Arch Otolaryng.*, **71**, 913.

Rubin, H. J., Hirt, C. C. (1960) 'The falsetto: a high speed cinematographic study'. *Laryngoscope*, **70**, 1305.

Rubin, H. J. (1965) 'Pitfalls in treatment of dysphonia by intracordal injections of synthetics'. *Laryngoscope*, **75**, 1381.

Rubin, H. J., LeCover, M., Vennard, W. (1967) 'Vocal intensity, subglottic pressure and air flow in relationship to singers'. *Folia Phoniat.*, **19**, 393.

Russell, G. O. (1931) *Speech and Voice*. Macmillan, New York.

Ruesch, J. (1959) 'General theory of communication in psychiatry' in *American Handbook of Psychiatry*, Chap 5 Vol I. Ed. S. Arieti. Basic Books, New York.

Rutherford, B. (1944) 'A comparative study of rate, force, pitch, rhythm and quality in speech of children handicapped with cerebral palsy'. *J. Speech Dis.*, **9**, 263.

St. Onge, K. R., Calvert, J. J. (1959) 'The brain stem damage syndrome; speech and psychological factors'. *J. Speech Dis.*, **24**, 43.

Sawkins, J. (1949) 'Voice without a larynx'. *Med. Press.* **222**, 193.

Saxman, J. H., Burk, K. W. (1967) 'Speaking fundamental frequency characteristics of middle aged females'. *Folia Phoniat.*, **19**, 167.

Schilling, R. (1925) 'Untersuchungen über die Atembewegungen beim Sprechen und Singen'. *Mschr. Ohrenheilk.*, **59**, 51.

Schlosshauer, B., Möckel, G. (1958) 'Auswertung der Röntgentonfilmaufnahmen von Speiseröhrensprechern'. *Folia Phoniat.*, **10**, 154.

Scholes, P. A. (1950) *The Oxford Companion to Music*. Oxford University Press.

Sedláčkova, E. (1960) 'Les dysphonies hypercinétiques des enfants causées par surmenage vocal'. *Folia Phoniat.*, **12**, 48.

Seeman, M. (1922) 'Speech and voice without larynx. An experimental and clinical study of the development of speech without larynx.' *Čas. Lék. Čes.*, **41**, 369.

Seeman, M. (1959) *Sprachstörungen bei Kindern*. Marhold Saale.

Sessions, D. G., Maness, G. M., McSwain, B. (1965) 'Laryngofissure in the treatment of carcinoma of the vocal cord: a report of 40 cases and review of the literature'. *Laryngoscope*, **75**, 490.

Seth, G., Guthrie, D. (1935) *Speech in Childhood*. Oxford University Press.

Shakespeare. W. (1924) *Plain Words in Singing*. Putnam, London.

Shaw, H. J., Friedman, I. (1962) 'Diffuse keratosis of the larynx with multicentric malignant change and metastatic neuropathy'. *J. Laryng.*, **78**, 757.

Shaw, H. J., (1966) 'Partial laryngectomy'. *J. Laryng.*, **80**, 839.

Shaw, H. J. (1966a) 'Glottic cancer'. *J. Laryng.*, **80**, 1238.

Shepherd, G. (1960) 'Studies in tachyphemia. 2: Phonetic description of cluttered speech'. *Logos.*, **3**, 73.

Shepperd, H. W. H. (1966) 'Androgenic hoarseness'. *J. Laryng (St. Louis)*, **80**, 403.

Sherrington, C. (1947) *The Integrative Action of the Nervous System.* Cambridge University Press.

Shinn, M. W. (1909) 'The development of the senses in the first three years of childhood' in *Notes on the Development of a Child*, Vol 4. Berkeley University, California, Publications in Education.

Shumrick, D. A. (1967) 'Trauma of the Larynx'. *Arch. Otolaryng.*, **86**, 691.

Siegel, G. M. (1969) 'Vocal conditioning in infants'. *J. Speech Dis.*, **34**, 3.

Siegler, J. (1967) 'Rehabilitation of voice after recurrent laryngeal nerve paralysis using teflon suspension'. *J. Laryng.*, **81**, 1121.

Simpson, I. C. (1971) 'Dysphonia: the organisation and working of a dysphonia clinic'. *Brit. J. Dis. Comm.*, **6**, 70.

Smith, J. K., Rise, E. N., Gralnek, D. E. (1966) 'Speech recovery in laryngectomized patients'. *Laryngoscope*, **77**, 1540.

Smith, S. (1957) 'Chest register versus head register in the membrane cushion model of the vocal cords'. *Folia Phoniat.*, **9**, 32.

Smurthwaite, H. (1919) 'War neurosis of the larynx and speech mechanism'. *J. Laryng.*, **34**, 13.

Snidecor, J. C. (1943) 'A comparative study of pitch and duration characteristics of impromptu speaking and oral reading'. *Speech Monogr.*, **10**, 50.

Snidecor, J. C. (1948) 'The speech correctionist and the cerebral palsy team'. *J. Speech Dis.*, **13**, 67.

Snidecor, J. C., Curry, E. T. (1959) 'Temporal pitch aspects of superior oesophageal speech'. *Ann. Otol. (St. Louis)*, **68**, 623.

Snidecor, J. C., Curry, E. T. (1960) 'How effectively may the laryngectomee speak?' *Proceedings of the 11th International Speech and Voice Therapy Conference.* Ed. L. Stein. Karger, New York.

Snidecor, J. C. (1962) *Speech Rehabilitation of the Laryngectomized.* Chap 7. Ed. J. C. Snidecor. Thomas, Illinois.

Snidecor, J. C., Isshiki, N. (1965) 'Air volume and air flow relationships of 6 male oesophageal speakers'. *J. Speech Dis.*, **30**, 205.

Snidecor, J. C. (1968) *Speech Rehabilitation of the Laryngectomised.* 2nd Edition Chap 13. Ed. J. C. Snidecor. Thomas, Illinois.

Sokolowksy, R. R., Junkermann, E. B. (1944) 'War aphonia'. *J. Speech Dis.*,' **9**, 193.

Sonninen, A. (1960) 'Laryngeal signs and symptoms of goitre'. *Folia Phoniat.*, **12**, 41.

Sonninen, A. (1968) 'The external frame function in the control of pitch in the human voice'. *Ann. N.Y. Acad. Sciences*, **155**, 68.

Soper, P. L. (1963) *Basic Public Speaking.* 3rd Edition. Oxford University Press.

Spiegel, R. (1959) 'Specific problems of communication in psychiatric conditions' in *American Handbook of Psychiatry*, Vol 1 Chap 46. Ed. S. Arieti. Basic Books, New York.

Stark, R. B., DeHaan, C. R. (1960) 'The addition of a pharyngeal flap to a primary palatoplasty'. *Plas. Reconstr. Surg.*, **26**, 378.

Stark, R. B., DeHaan, C. R., Frileck, S. P., Burgess, P. D. (1969) 'Primary pharyngeal flap'. *Cleft Palate J.*, **6**, 381.

Stein, L. (1949) *The Infancy of Speech and the Speech of Infancy.* Methuen, London.

Stetson, R. H. (1937) 'Esophageal speech for any laryngectomised patient'. *Arch. Otolaryng.*, **26**, 132.

Strauss, A. A., Lehtinen, L. E. (1947) *Psychopathy and Education of the Brain-Injured Child.* Grune and Stratton, New York.

Strauss, A. A., Kephart, N. C. (1955) *Psychopathology and Education of the Brain-Injured Child.* Grune and Stratton, New York.

Stroud, M. H., Zwiefach, E. (1956) 'The mechanism of the larynx'. *J. Laryng.*, **70**, 86.

Stuart, D. W. (1966) 'Surgery in cancer of the cervical oesophagus: plastic tube replacement'. *J. Laryng.*, **80**, 382.

Tarneaud, J. (1961) *Traité Pratique de Phonologie et de Phoniatrie.* Libraire Maloine, Paris.

Taylor, F. S. (1949) *Science Past and Present.* Heinemann, London.

'Terminology for Speech Pathology' (1960). *Speech Path. and Therap.*, **3**, 35.

Terracol, J., Guerrier, Y., Camps, F. (1956) 'Le sphincter glottique; étude anatomo-clinique'. *Ann. Otolaryng* (Paris), **73**, 451.

Thomson, S., Negus, V. E., Bateman, G. H. (1955) *Diseases of the Nose and Throat,* 6th Edition. Cassell, London.

Thurburn, G. L. (1939) *Voice and Speech.* Nisbet, London.

Valanne, E., Vuorenkoski, V., Partanen, T. J., Lind, J., Wasz-Höckert, O. (1967) 'The ability of human mothers to identify the hunger cry signals of their own newborn infants during lying-in period'. *Experientia*, **23**, 768.

Van den Berg, J. W. (1955) 'On the role of the laryngeal ventricle in voice production'. *Folia Phoniat.*, **7**, 57.

Van den Berg, J. W. (1958) 'On the myoelastic-aerodynamic theory of voice production'. *The Bulletin, Nat. Assn. Teachers of Singing,* **14**, 6. (No 4.)

Van den Berg, J. W. (1962) 'Modern research in experimental phonetics'. 12th International Congress of Logopedics and Phoniatrics Report. *Folia Phoniat.*, **14**, 81.

Van den Berg, J. W. (1964) 'Some physical aspects of voice production'. *Research Potentials in Voice Physiology.* Ed. D. W. Brewer. State University, New York.

Van Michel, C. (1967) 'Morphologie de la courbe glottographique dans certains troubles fonctionnels du larynx'. *Folia Phoniat.*, **19**, 192.

Van Riper, C., Irwin, J. V. (1958) *Voice and Articulation Drill Book.* Prentice Hall, New York.

Van Thal, J. H. (1934) *Cleft Palate Speech.* Allen and Unwin, London.

Van Thal, J. H. (1956) 'The value of empirical contributions to speech pathology and therapeutics'. *Speech*, **1**, 19.

Van Thal, J. H. (1961) 'Dysphonia'. *Speech Path. and Therap.*, **4**, 11.

Van Thal, J. H. (1962) 'Four generations of aphonia'. *Report of 12th Congress of Int. Soc. Logopedics and Phoniatrics. I.A.L.P.* Report. Karger, Zurich.

Van Thal, J. H. (1969) *Elements of Logopedics. A Handbook for Students of Speech Therapy.* Kaye and Ward, London.

Vennard, W., Von Leden, H. (1967) 'The importance of intensity modulation in the perception of a trill'. *Folia Phoniat.*, **19**, 19.

Vermeuling, V. R. (1966) 'Laryngeal carcinoma in the young'. *Laryngoscope*, **77**, 1724.

Von Leden, H., Moore, P. (1960) *Contact Ulcer of the Larynx.* Motion Picture Voice Research Lab., Northwestern Medical School, Chicago.

Von Leden, H. (1961) 'The mechanism of phonation'. *Arch. Otolaryng.*, **74**, 660.

Von Leden, H., Moore, P. (1961) 'The mechanics of the cricoarytenoid joint'. *Arch. Otolaryng.*, **73**, 541.

Von Leden, H., Isshiki, N. (1966) 'An analysis of cough at the level of the larynx'. *Arch. Otolaryng.*, **83**, 616.

Von Leden, H., Yanagihara, N., Werner-Kukuk, E. (1967) 'Teflon in unilateral vocal cord paralysis'. *Arch. Otolaryng.*, **85**, 666.

Von Michel, C. (1967) 'Morphologie de la courbe glotto-graphique dans certains troubles fonctionnels du larynx'. *Folia Phoniat.*, **19**, 192.

Vrtička, K., Svoboda, M. (1961) 'A clinical and X-ray study of 100 laryngectomised speakers'. *Folia Phoniat.*, **13**, 174.

Vrtička, K., Svoboda, M. (1963) 'Time changes in the X-ray picture of the hypopharynx, pseudoglottis and esophagus in the course of vocal rehabilitation in 70 laryngectomised speakers'. *Folia Phoniat.*, **15**, 1.

Waldrop, W. F., Gould, M. A. (1956) *Your New Voice.* American Cancer Soc.

Walshe, F. M. R. (1952) *Diseases of the Nervous System.* Livingstone, Edinburgh.

Walter, G. W. (1953) *The Living Brain.* Duckworth, London.

Warburton, J. W. (1967) 'Depressive symptoms in Parkinson's disease referred for thalamotomy'. *J. Neurochem. Neurosurg. Psychiat.*, **30**, 368.

Wasz-Höckert, O., Lind, J., Vuorenski, V., Partanen, T. J., Valanne, E. (1968) *The Infant Cry: A Spectrographic and Auditory Analysis.* Clinics in Developmental Medicine No 29. Spastics International Medical Publication in association with Heinemann Medical.

Watson, B. W. (1967) 'Progress in artificial voice aids'. *Med. Biol. Illust.*, **17**, 158.

Watson, B. W., Greene, M. C. L. (1968) 'A speech aid for the laryngectomy patient'. *Brit. J. Dis. Comm.*, **3**, 111.

Wattles, M. (1949) 'Bilateral granuloma of the larynx following intratracheal anesthesia'. *Ann. Otol. (St. Louis)*, **58**, 873.

Weiss, D. A. (1950) 'The pubertal change of the human voice (mutation)'. *Folia Phoniat.*, **2**, 126.

Weiss, D. A. (1955) 'The psychological relations to one's own voice'. *Folia Phoniat.*, **7**, 209.

Weiss, D. A. (1959) 'Discussion of the neurochronaxic theory (Husson)'. *Arch. Otol.*, **70**, 607.

Weiss, D. A. (1960) 'Therapy of cluttering'. *Folia Phoniat.*, **12**, 217.

Weiss, D. A. (1964) *Cluttering.* Prentice Hall, New York.

Werner-Kukuk, E., Von Leden, H., Yanagihara, N. (1968) 'The effects of radiation therapy on laryngeal function'. *J. Laryng.*, **82**, 1.

West, R. (1957) *The Rehabilitation of Speech. Part* 1. 3rd Edition. Eds. R. West, M. Ansberry, A. Carr. Harper, New York.

White, E. G. (1938) *Science and Singing*. Dent, London.

Willmore, L. (1959) 'The role of speech therapy in voice cases'. *J. Laryng.*, **73**, 104.

Wilson, C. P. (1952) 'Trauma, stenosis and benign tumours of the larynx' in *Diseases of the Ear, Nose and Throat*, Vol 1. Chap 32. Ed. W. G. Scott-Brown. Butterworth, London.

Winckel, F. (1952) 'Elektroakustische Untersuchungen an der Menschlichen Stimme'. *Folia Phoniat.*, **4**, 93.

Wittkower, E. D., Mandelbrote, B. M. (1955) *Thyrotoxicosis in Psychosomatic Medicine*, Chap 13. Ed. D. O'Neill, Butterworth, London.

Wohl, M. T. (1968) 'The electronic metronome. An evaluation study'. *Brit. J. Dis. Comm.*, **3**, 89.

Wohl, M. T. (1970) 'The treatment of non-fluent utterance. A behavioural approach'. *Brit. J. Dis. Comm.*, **5**, 66.

Wolf, S. G. (1952) 'Causes and mechanisms in rhinitis'. *Laryngoscope*, **62**, 601.

Wolfsohn, A. (1956) *Vox Humana*. Folkways Records, New York. EXP 123 A.

Wolman, L., Darke, C. S., Young, A. (1965) 'The larynx and rheumatoid arthritis'. *J. Otolaryng.*, **79**, 403.

Wolpe, J. (1958) *Psychotherapy by Reciprocal Inhibition*. Stanford University Press, California.

Wolski, W., Wiley, J. (1965) 'Functional aphonia in a 14-year-old boy. A case report'. *J. Speech Dis.*, **30**, 71.

Wolski, W. (1967) 'Hypernasality as a presenting symptom of myasthenia gravis'. *J. Speech Dis.*, **32**, 36.

Woodman, De G. (1946) 'A modification of the extralaryngeal approach to arytenoidectomy for bilateral abductor paralysis'. *Arch. Otolaryng.*, **43**, 63.

Woodman, De G. (1948) 'The open approach to arytenoidectomy for bilateral abductor paralysis with a report of 23 cases'. *Ann. Otol. (St. Louis)*, **57**, 695.

Woodman, De G., Pollack, D. (1950) 'Bilateral abductor paralysis. The post operative care and speech therapy following arytenoidectomy'. *Laryngoscope*, **60**, 832.

Woodman, De G. (1953) 'Bilateral abductor paralysis. A survey of 521 cases of arytenoidectomy via the open approach as reported by ninety surgeons'. *Arch. Otolaryng.*, **58**, 150.

Worster-Drought, C. (1953) 'Dysarthria'. *Speech*, **17**, 48.

Wyke, B. (1967) 'Recent advances in the neurology of phonation and reflex mechanisms in the larynx'. *Brit. J. Dis. Comm.*, **2**, 1.

Wyke, B. (1969) 'Deus ex machina vocis. An analysis of laryngeal reflexes in speech'. *Brit. J. Dis., Comm.* **4**, 1.

Wyke, B. (1970) 'Neurological mechanisms in stammering: an hypothesis'. *Brit. J. Dis. Comm.*, **5**, 6.

Wyllie, J. (1894) *The Disorders of Speech*. Oliver and Boyd, London.

Wynn-Williams, D. (1958) 'Congenital supra bulbar paresis'. *Speech Path. Ther.*, **1**, 3.

Yanagihara, N., Koike, Y. (1967) 'The regulation of sustained phonation'. *Folia Phoniat.*, **19**, 1.

Yellowlees, H. (1932) *Clinical Lectures on Psychological Medicine.* Churchill, London.

Young, E. H., Hawk, S. S. (1955) *Children with Delayed or Defective Speech: Motokinaesthetic Factors in their Training.* Stanford University Press, California and Milford, London.

Zaliouk, A. (1960) 'Falsetto voice in deaf children' in *Aktuelle Probleme der Phoniatrie und Logopedie*, Vol 1. Karger, Zurich.

Zaliouk, A. (1963) 'The tactile approach to voice placement'. *Folia Phoniat.*, **15**, 147.

Zenker, W. (1964) 'Vocal muscle fibres and their motor end-plates' in *Potentials in Voice Physiology.* Ed. D. Brewer. State University Press, New York.

Zenker, W. (1964a) 'Questions regarding the function of external laryngeal muscles' in *Research Potentials in Voice Physiology.* Ed. D. W. Brewer. State University Press, New York.

Zilstorff, K. (1968) 'Vocal disabilities of singers'. *Proc. Roy. Soc. Med.*, **61**, 1147.

Author Index

Abercrombie, D., 5
Aikin, W. A., 26, 27, 72
Ainsworth, J. Z., 346
Akin, J., 156
Allan, C. M., 294, 295
Alvin, J., 307
Amado, J. H., 102, 104, 219
Amster, W., 365, 373, 383, 390, 394, 397
Andrews, A. H., 365, 383, 386
Andrews, G., 295
Ansberry, M., 225
Ardran, G. M., 34, 38, 42, 45, 52, 115, 181, 228, 260
Arnold, G. E., 46, 48, 52, 81, 123, 126, 209, 210, 214, 219, 220, 225, 228, 295, 314, 321, 323, 329, 344, 374, 385, 390
Aranson, A. E., 208, 209, 210, 211, 297
Ascher, E., 213

Bach, D. E., 302
Baf, C. I., 302
Bailey, B. J., 362
Baker, D. C., 220
Baker, H. K., 242
Baltzell, W. H., 320
Bangs, J. L., 195
Barlow, W., 157
Barn, J., 302
Barrett, H., 156
Barton, R. T., 373, 374, 375
Bastiaans, J., 119, 120, 210
Bateman, G. H., 352, 365, 369, 377, 380, 383
Baynes, R. A., 118
Berry, M. F., 277, 299
Berne, A. S., 359

Birch, D., 73, 156
Birrel, J. F., 351
Bisna, A. L., 375, 437
Blackfield, H. M., 247
Blevins, C. E., 54
Bloch, P., 209
Bloomfield, L., 4
Bobath, B., 305
Böhme, G., 295
Boone, D. R., 127
Bosma, J. F., 309, 311, 380
Bradley, D. P., 242
Brain, W. R., 297
Braithewaite, F., 59, 245, 246, 248
Brewer, D. W., 53
Briess, F. B., 53, 115, 150, 153, 164
Brinkman, W. F. B., 352
Broad, D. J., 42
Broadbent, T. R., 246
Brodnitz, F. S., 77, 124, 132, 137, 139, 144, 146, 149, 164, 201, 202, 352, 362
Brown, I., 222
Brown, J. R., 208, 209, 210, 211, 297
Brumlik, J., 210
Brummett, R. E., 317
Bruno, G., 5
Burgess, P. D., 246
Burk, K. W., 105
Burkowsky, M. R., 140
Butfield, E., 280, 282, 283, 291, 292
Byrne, M. C., 303
Bzoch, K., 247

Calnan, J., 61, 62, 68, 73
Calvert, J. J., 300

Camps, F., 93
Canning, A. C., 248
Canter, J. G., 286, 287, 288, 291, 294
Capps, F. C. W., 314, 316
Carr, A., 225
Cavanagh, F., 312
Cherry, J., 141
Clarke, W. M., 405
Clerf, C. H., 320, 336
Conley, J. J., 361, 362
Conway, J., 92, 95
Cooper, I. S., 288
Cooper, M., 140, 164
Cotton, E., 307
Craddock, W. H., 272
Critchley, M., 211, 297
Curran, D., 189
Curry, E. T., 101, 118, 226, 353, 406, 407
Curry, R., 98

Dalley, V. M., 359
Damsté, P. H., 236, 249, 365, 373, 378, 382, 394, 407
Darke, C. S., 343
Darley, F. L., 111, 164
Dawson, J., 47, 99
De Ajuriaguerra, J., 84
De Haan, C. R., 246
Dekelbaum, A. M., 350
Delahunty, J. E., 181
Delattre, P. C., 239
Devine, K. D., 138
Di Carlo, L. M., 365, 373, 383, 390, 394, 397
Diedrich, W. M., 376, 377, 383–5, 390, 394, 416
Dixon, F., 370
Dornhorst, A., 412
Dowie, L. N., 112, 123, 184
Doyle, P. J., 317
Draper, M. H., 22
Dubois, C., 100
Duff, J., 346
Dunker, E., 117

Edwards, T. M., 330
Eisenson, J., 277, 299

Ellis, M., 115, 118, 343
Emil-Behnke, K., 163
English, D. T., 54
Evans, M. F., 307
Everett, J. D., 13
Everts, E. C., 317
Evison, G., 368, 369, 413
Ewing, A. W. G., 55
Eysenck, H. J., 158, 213

Faaborg-Anderson, K., 37, 52, 53, 314
Fairbanks, G., 89, 90, 94, 98, 111, 151
Fairman, H. D., 368
Ferenczi, S., 221, 223
Fawcus, M., 282
Fawcus, R., 282
Ficarra, B. J., 237
Figi, F. A., 361
Fink, D. H., 158
Fiori-Ratti, L., 242
Fisch, L., 302
Flach, M., 103, 234
Flatau, T. S., 119
Fletcher, P., 158
Floyd, W. F., 50
Fontaine, A., 373, 374
Formby, D., 5, 95, 381
Fothergill, P., 307
Fox, D. R., 212
Frank, F., 250
Freedman, D. G., 5
Freidinger, A., 195
Freud, S., 188, 195, 207, 221, 222, 223
Friedman, I., 359
Friedman, S., 347
Frileck, S. P., 246
Fritzell, B., 59, 61, 62, 248
Froeschels, E., 51, 149, 172, 173, 230, 238, 307, 332
Fry, D. B., 4, 89, 280

Gadea-Ciria, M., 294
Garcia, M., 71
Gardiner, R. H., 316
Garfield-Davies, D., 358
Gedda, L., 5

Gillespie, R., 180
Gimson, A. C., 15, 72, 407
Goda, S., 242
Goff, W. F., 329
Goffin, F. B., 347
Grady, P., 253
Gralnek, D. E., 366
Gray, H., 42, 55, 82, 83, 309
Green, H. C., 13
Greene, M. C. L., 62, 89, 92, 93, 95, 96, 97, 119, 130, 225, 243, 248, 250, 270, 282, 286, 288, 292, 307, 308, 360
Gregg, R. L., 314, 318
Grewel, F., 282, 286, 299, 302, 305, 306
Groen, J., 119, 120, 210
Grossberg, J. M., 213
Guerrier, Y., 92
Guthrie, D., 118, 225, 231, 341, 342, 360
Guttman, E., 189
Gutzmann, H., 119, 229

Hahn, E., 69, 156
Hall, I. S., 345
Hammond, J. M., 98
Hanley, T. D., 156
Hardy, J. C., 253
Harmer, W. D., 338
Harpman, J. A., 317
Harrington, R., 307
Harris, H. H., 346
Harris, M., 295
Harrison, D. F. N., 366, 367, 368
Hawk, S. S., 306
Head, H., 296
Heaver, L., 123, 208, 209, 210, 214, 374, 385, 390
Heinemann, M., 237
Henderson, D., 180
Henderson, R., 81
Herer, G., 365, 373, 383, 390, 394, 397
Herbert, E. L., 98
Hess, D. A., 244
Hildernisse, L. W., 103, 227
Hill, B. J., 250
Hirano, M., 24, 46, 315
Hiroto, I., 315

Hirt, C. C., 48, 77, 229
Hobbs, R. C., 368
Hodson, C. J., 365, 381, 383, 386, 394
Hoerr, N., 370
Holl-Allen, R. T. J., 321
Hollien, H., 102, 105
Hollinger, P. H., 80, 138, 346, 352, 365, 383, 386
Holti, G., 116
Hoops, H. R., 405
Hunt, R. B., 366
Husson, R., 50, 51, 54
Hutzinga, E., 313, 382
Hynes, W., 246, 249

Ingram, T. T. S., 302, 304
Irwin, J. V., 172, 177, 224
Isshiki, N., 24, 111, 165, 247, 253, 380, 384, 397, 406

Jackson, C., 121, 135, 136, 158, 194, 358, 361
Jackson, J. M., 116
Jacobson, E., 158, 160
James, J. A., 273
Janet, P., 189, 195
Jasienska, A., 312
Jayapathy, B., 253
Jellinek, A., 149, 173
Jenkins, J. C., 351
John, H. T., 368
Johnson, J., 111, 164
Jones, A. M., 72
Jones, D., 72
Junkerman, E. B., 193, 194

Kallen, L. A., 374, 378, 407
Kemp, F. H., 34, 38, 42, 45, 52, 115, 228, 260
Kephart, N., 303
Kilner, T. P., 343, 346
Kiml, J., 208
King, B. T., 314, 318, 330
Kingdon-Ward, W., 212
Kinsey, A. C., 223
Kirchener, J. A., 53, 315, 329, 330

Kirsch, D., 360
Kleinsasser, O., 123, 130, 136, 137, 346, 347, 349, 353, 356
Koike, Y., 23, 24, 46, 165
Kopp, G. A., 13
Kremer, M., 300
Kurtz, J. H., 5
Kuzniarz, J., 312

Labbarraque, M. L., 194, 339
Lacina, O., 103
Ladefoged, P., 12, 22
Ladell, R. M., 158
Laget, P., 50
Laguaite, J., 171
Lall, M., 368, 369, 413
Lange, M. J., 322
Langova, J., 295
Larson, R. E., 254
Lassman, F. M., 98
Last, R. J., 26, 28, 37, 39, 60
Lauder, E., 371, 390, 394, 395
Laver, J. D. M., 5
Lawson, L. I., 247
Leatheart, G. L., 412
Lebo, C. P., 129
Le Cover, M., 78
Lederer, F. L., 144
Lederman, M., 24, 359
Lehtinen, L., 303
Lell, W. A., 193, 194, 195
Lennenberg, E. H., 94
Liberman, A. H., 296
Lieberman, P., 29
Lind, J., 94
Linden, J. W., 250
Linford-Rees, W. L., 123, 157, 182, 184, 188, 197, 212
Lenz, M., 359
Levitt, S., 304, 307
Lewis, M. M., 96
Lewy, R. B., 329
Ling, D., 90
Litin, E. M., 208, 209, 210, 211, 297
Lubit, E. C., 254
Luchsinger, R., 27, 28, 46, 48, 52, 69, 77, 78, 99, 104, 123, 177, 219, 225, 228
Luria, A. R., 287, 307, 308

McAllister, A., 91, 156
McCall, J. W., 370
McDonald, E. T., 242
McGlone, R., 102, 105
McGrosky, R. L., 418
McSwain, B., 361
McWilliams, B. J., 242, 245
Makuen, G. H., 119
Malcolmson, K. G., 181, 195
Mandelbrote, B. M., 321, 323
Maness, G. M., 361
Margulies, S. I., 141
Marland, P. M., 306, 332, 381
Marres, E. H. M. A., 352
Mason, M., 365
Massengil, R., 58
Michel, J., 102
Millar, H., 315, 316
Millard, D. R., 258
Miller, A. H., 129, 367
Miller, E. R., 247
Mills, W., 75, 162
Mitchell, J. C. E., 110, 243, 373, 374
Mitchell, S. W., 157
Mockel, G., 383
Monrad-Krohn, G. H., 92, 302
Monroe, C., 250
Moolenaar-Bijl, A., 382, 390, 394
Moore, P., 42, 48, 102, 117, 139, 210, 365, 383, 386
Moravek, M., 295
Morley, M. E., 59, 239, 245
Morris, H. L., 253
Morrison, E. B., 290
Morrison, L. F., 314, 317, 343
Morrison, W. W., 377, 379, 388
Moses, P. J., 5, 93, 99, 113, 181, 219, 220, 224, 233
Mullard, K., 368
Mulligan, M., 418
Munro-Black, J. L., 116
Murphy, G. E., 375
Musgrove, J., 312, 313, 318
Myerson, M. C., 138
Mysack, E. D., 105, 280, 306

Nahum, M. C., 140, 164
Naidr, J., 102

Negus, V. E., 18, 34, 38, 42, 43, 47, 51, 63, 65, 72, 93, 136, 210, 311, 313, 317, 319, 352, 359, 365, 367, 369, 377, 381, 383
Neil, E., 50
Netsell, R., 253
New, G. B., 138
Niblock, W. H., 316
Nichols, I., 94
Nykøbing, F., 37, 314

Ogura, J. H., 375
Okrainetz, C., 359
Oliphant, K. P., 129
Osgood, C. E., 94
Ostwald, P. F., 5
Oswald, M. V. O., 365, 373, 377, 378, 381, 382, 383, 385, 386, 388, 390, 394, 399, 407, 408
Owsley, J. O., 247

Paget, R., 70, 73, 75, 238, 240, 296, 399
Palmer, M. F., 230, 307
Pantoja, E., 104
Partanen, T. J., 94, 96, 99, 117
Peacher, G. M., 139
Peacher, W. G., 138, 277, 280, 299, 302
Pear, T. H., 4
Pearce, E. C., 30
Pearson, J. S., 208, 209, 210, 211, 297
Pepinsky, A., 63
Peréllo, J., 103, 112, 115, 203, 323
Peterson, G. E., 16
Pfau, W., 119
Piaget, J., 96
Pollack, D., 331, 332
Portmann, G., 50
Postman, L., 296
Potter, R. K., 13
Pressman, J. J., 362
Punt, N. A., 121, 131, 132
Putney, J. F., 338, 366

Rabbett, W. F., 350, 351, 358
Reidy, J. P., 243

Rembolt, R. R., 253
Renfrew, C. E., 110, 243, 244
Réthi, A., 234, 330
Richardson, M., 96
Rigby, R. G., 189
Rigrodsky, S., 290
Rippon, T. S., 158
Rise, E. N., 366
Ritter, F. N., 237
Robe-Finkbeiner, E. Y., 210, 365, 383, 385, 386
Robin, J., 50
Rosenweig, M. R., 296
Roy, A. D., 316
Rubin, H. J., 24, 48, 51, 77, 165, 229, 329
Ruesch, J., 5, 198
Russell, G. O., 61
Russell, W. R., 300
Rutherford, B., 303

St. Onge, K. R., 300
Sawkins, J., 378, 380, 402
Savetsky, L., 220
Saxman, J. H., 105
Schlosshauer, B., 383
Sedláčkova, E., 119, 123, 127
Seeman, M., 123, 365, 379
Sessions, D. G., 361
Seth, G., 225, 231
Ševčic, K., 102
Siegel, G. M., 94
Siegler, J., 329, 337
Simon, R., 103, 234
Simpson, I. C., 128
Schild, J. A., 346
Schilling, R., 78
Scholes, P. A., 79, 86
Schweiger, J. W., 253
Schwickardi, H., 103, 234
Shakespeare, W., 74
Shaw, H. J., 347, 359, 362
Shepherd, G., 295
Shepperd, H. W. H., 236
Sherrington, C., 83, 85
Shinn, M. W., 88
Shumrick, D. A., 346
Smith, G. E., 300
Smith, J. K., 366
Smith, S., 48, 366

Smurthwaite, H., 191, 193, 194, 195, 341
Snidecor, J. C., 105, 305, 377, 380, 390, 406, 407
Sokolowsky, R., 193, 194
Sonninen, A., 37, 49, 131, 312, 322, 323
Soper, P. L., 156
Spiegel, R., 189, 190, 213
Spriestersbach, D. C., 111, 164, 253
Stamback, M., 84
Stark, R. B., 246
Stein, L., 87, 228
Stetson, R. H., 379, 380, 382, 400
Strauss, A. A., 303
Stroboda, D. J., 329
Stroud, M. H., 39, 41, 314
Stuart, D. W., 367
Svoboda, M., 365, 383, 386, 394

Tarneaud, J., 26, 28, 69, 97, 227, 234
Taylor, F. S., 311
Teledo, P. S., 329
Terracol, J., 93
Thomson, S., 113, 136, 210, 211, 319, 341, 345
Thurburn, G. L., 74, 86, 89, 91
Thurman, W. L., 156
Tomita, H., 315
Turner, J. W., 294

Uris, D., 5, 156

Valanne, E., 5, 94, 95, 96, 99, 117
Vallancien, B., 48, 52
Van den Berg, J. W., 25, 48, 51, 63, 70, 71, 73, 110, 115, 238, 239, 242, 282
Van Michel, C., 52
Van Riper, C., 172, 177, 224
Van Thal, J., 208, 266, 313, 332
Veau, V., 68
Vennard, W., 78
Vermeuling, V. R., 351, 358
Vesalius, A., 312

Von Leden, H., 24, 25, 42, 46, 51, 78, 93, 139, 165, 329
Vrtička, K., 365, 383, 386, 394
Vuoreneski, V., 94, 96, 99, 117

Waldrop, W. F., 171, 250
Wallace, A., 110, 243
Walshe, F. M. R., 309, 311
Walter, G. M., 29, 88
Warburton, J. W., 291
Wardill, T. P., 59, 245, 246, 248
Wasz-Höckert, O., 94, 96, 99, 117
Watson, B. W., 286, 288, 292, 419
Wattles, M., 137
Weiss, D. A., 51, 97, 98, 99, 173, 226, 227, 295
Wentges, R. T. R., 352
Werner-Kukuk, E., 25, 329
West, R., 65, 225, 240, 242
White, R., 75
Whitteridge, D., 22
Wiley, J., 98, 221
Willmore, L., 156
Winckel, F., 77, 80, 89
Wittkower, E. D., 323, 324
Wohl, M. T., 295
Wolf, S. G., 273
Wolfsohn, A., 100
Wolman, L., 343
Wolpe, J., 158
Wolski, W., 221, 254
Woodman, D. G., 330, 331, 335, 343
Wyke, B. D., 26, 53, 54, 83, 117
Wyllie, J., 5
Wynn-Williams, D., 253, 279

Yanagihara, N., 23, 80, 165, 329
Yellowlees, H., 189
Young, A., 343
Young, E. H., 306
Youngstrom, K. A., 376, 377, 383, 384, 390

Zaliouk, A., 80, 171
Zboril, N., 102
Zenker, W., 34, 53, 104
Zilstorff, K., 113, 121, 125
Zwiefach, E., 39, 41

Subject Index

Adenoidectomy, 119, 243, 249, 255, 260, 272, 275, 344
Adenoids, 241, 247, 272
Adenoma, 322, 326
Adolescence, 219, 323
  voice mutation, 222
Air flow rate, 23–6, 165
  swallowing, *see* Oesophageal voice
Amplification value in therapy, 140, 143, 150, 152, 215, 283, 292, 296, 349, 363, 368
Amplifiers, 292–3, 326, 368, 376, 387, 391–3, 401, 411
  advisory services, 294
  electronic feed-back, 405
  manufacturers, 422
  telephone, 294, 331, 405
  throat microphone, 293, 331, 363
Amplitude of voice, 8, 9, 16, 23, 25, 46, 72, 78, 171, 177
Anarthria, 277, 298, 300
Anastomosis, recurrent laryngeal nerve, 317
  faciohypoglossal, 301
Androgeus, 218, 235–6
Ankylosis, arytenoid joint, 343; *see* Arthritis
Anxiety state, 5, 85, 112, 114, 118, 120, 123, 139, 145, 157, 158, 180–8, 304, 325, 346, 356, 375, 410
  hysterical, 190, 208
  personality, 182, 211
  prognosis, 184
Aorta, 310
Aortic aneurysm, 311

Aphasia, 196, 280, 296, 300–1, 320
Aphonia, 109, 142, 185, 191–2, 195–6, 202, 204, 221, 292, 313, 325, 336, 342, 416
Arteriosclerosis, 278, 285, 301
Arthritis, 182, 190, 191, 195, 334, 342
Articulation, 12, 13, 55–81, 92, 196, 296
  in cerebral palsy, 305, 307
  in cleft palate, 239, 242, 246–8, 264–70
  in hysteria, 234
  in oesophageal speech, 380, 389, 396–7
  in phonetics, 296
  in singing, 175
  in speech development, 96
  in speech monitoring, 296
  in vocal training, 75, 175, 270, 277
  organs of, 55
Artificial larynx, *see* Vibrators
Arytenoid cartilages, 33, 118, 135, 139, 141, 315
Arytenoidectomy, 320, 330–1
Aryepiglottic folds, 42, 48, 63, 240, 345, 356
Asai operation, 367
Asthenic voice, 120, 181–2, 323
  therapy, 177–9, 185, 202, 212, 223, 301, 312, 339, 353
Asthma, 27, 119, 124, 158, 189, 190, 272, 371
Ataxia, 297, 299
Athetosis, 283, 302
Auditory feedback, *see* Ear training

Babbling in cerebral palsy, 305
  in deaf children, 306
  in normal children, 305–6
Balanced tone, 76, 151
Baranyi boxes, 194, 206, 339
Behaviour therapy, 158, 213
Bell's palsy, 301
Block dissection, 359
Bowing cords, *see* Internal tensor
  weakness
Breathing, 19–29, 75, 162
  central method, 26, 162, 333
  clavicular, 27, 166, 207, 275
  diaphragmatic intercostal, 26,
      169, 292, 330, 344, 382,
      384
  disorders, 116, 120, 139, 162,
      175, 209, 279, 303, 333
  dual control, 29–30
  exercises, 165–72, 194
  in asthma, 27, 120
  in laryngofissure, 363
  in oesophageal speech, 370,
      380, 382–5
  in reverse, 306, 330, 332, 336
  in singing, 76, 99
  muscles, 20–22
  techniques, 26, 29, 164, 169
Bronchitis, 369, 408
Buccal whisper, 352, 387, 389
Bulbar palsy, 210, 297, 309,
      311
  poliomyelitis, *see* Poliomyelitis

Cancer, *see* Carcinoma
Carcinoma, 125, 144, 182, 235,
      see Laryngectomy
  laryngeal, 196, 347, 351, 358,
      364
  post-cricoid, 360, 366
Castrati singers, *see* Singing
Cerebellar ataxia, 197, 297, 299
Cerebral palsy, 25, 278, 284, 302–
      308
Chewing therapy, 149, 164
Chorea, 284
Cleft palate, 62, 424
  blowing exercises, 242, 265, 270
  congenital short palate, 249,
      259

Cleft palate (*continued*)
  Hynes pharyngoplasty, 62,
      246–9, 261, 264
  palatoplasty, 246, 248–9
  pharyngeal flap, 253–8
  phonetic assessment, 269
  pitch, 244–9
  Rosenthal pharyngoplasty,
      253, 279
  speech therapy, 265–70
  sub-mucous cleft, 248
  surgery, cosmetic, 245, 261,
      270
Climacteric, 235, 323, 351
Cluttering, 287, 295, 299, 303
Conductor therapy, 308
Conus elasticus, 38, 44, 47, 48,
      54
Co-ordination, 82, 83, 87
  in breathing and phonation,
      101, 154, 169, 175, 241,
      304
  in cerebral palsy, 307
  in movement, 98, 157, 210
  in oesophageal speech, 380,
      382, 384–5, 397
Communication, 4, 89, 180, 280,
      371, 374
Contact ulcers, 135–43, 137, 165,
      356
  surgery, 136
  vocal symptoms, 138, 348
Coughing, 120, 124, 127, 139, 149,
      192, 194, 200, 209, 314, 358,
      369, 372, 375
Covered singing, 49, 78
Cranial trauma, 300
Cricoarytenoid joint, 342–3
  muscle, 42, 315
Cricoid cartilage, 36, 345, 364
Cricopharyngeus muscle (sphinc-
      ter), 34, 364, 365, 367, 376–9,
      381, 389, 390, 407–8, 412
Cricothyroid muscle, 38, 48,
      228–9, 310, 315, 319
Crico-vocal membrane, *see* Conus
      elasticus
Crying infant, 84, 94–6, 119, 306,
      345
Cryogenic surgery, 352
Cuneiform cartilage, 33, 44

Deafness, 59, 90, 129, 144, 171, 246, 255, 282, 306–7, 390, 404
in athetosis, 302
in cleft palate, 247, 249, 266
in vocal strain, 115, 147, 348, 409, 418
Decortication, 130
Depression, 182, 218, 235, 270, 282, 291, 324, 372–6
Diaphragm, 21–3, 26–8, 44, 209
Diplophonia, 129, 193, 326
Diphtheria, 254, 301, 312
Disseminated sclerosis, 210, 297, 299
Drop shoulder, 370
Drug therapy, 103, 145, 156, 184, 198, 217–18, 285, 287, 290, 297
Dysarthria, 84, 90
dyspraxic, 258, 295
hysterical, 196, 252
in lower motor neurone lesion, 298–309
in upper motor neurone lesion, 30, 277–83
scanning, 196–7, 280
striatal, 258, 295
Dysarthrophonia, 277–308
in cerebral palsy, 252, 253, 303
in striatal lesions, 283
treatment, 281
Dysgraphia, 302
Dyslexia, 302
Dysphasia, 282, 288, 302
Dysphonia, 84, 92, 196
causes, 111–12, 137, 144
definition, 109–10, 117
dysplastic, 344
endocrine, 103, 196
functional, 112, 199, 206
hyperkinetic, 54, 112, 127, 155–79, 208
hypokinetic, *see* Asthenic voice
hysterical, 213
laryngeal palsy, 316, 323, 327
nasal, *see* Nasality
Dyspnoea, 318, 342, 345, 351, 364
Dyspraxia, 258, 295, 302
Dysprosody, 92, 302

Ear, 140
anatomy, 7
diagnosis by, 25, 50, 53, 78, 94, 110–11, 141, 239
hearing, 129, 274
training, 74, 80, 152, 159, 194, 228, 241, 243, 274, 296, 353, 410
Endocrine disorders, 103, 183, 196, 219–20, 234, 321, 323
Electroglottograph, 52
Electromyograph, 23, 37, 52, 53, 59, 151, 246, 314, 320
Electrostroboscope, 128
Epiglottis, 33, 43, 48–9, 63, 72, 81, 240, 310, 345, 356

Faciohypoglossal surgery, 301
False cords, *see* Ventricular folds
Falsetto, 47–9, 77, 100, 193, 201, 214, 219–20, 226, 228, 325
Faradic treatment, 194, 201, 243
Fistula, *see* Laryngectomy
Flap valve cannula, 318, 331, 343
Forcing exercises, 178, 328, 331, 336, 362
Frequency, *see* Pitch
Frog speech, 353
Functional voice disorder, 112, 186, 196, 206, 218, 231, 236, 297, 301, 320, 323, 336, 339, 341
Fundamental pitch, 16, 49, 69, 71–2, 75, 102, 140, 226, 244, 325
oesophageal, 378

Geriatrics, 282
Globus hystericus, 181, 195, 334–5, 358
Glo sopharyngeal nerve, 309
press, 383
Glottal roll, 117
tension, 120, 165, 181, 208–10, 292, 332
Glottis, 24–5, 38, 44, 46, 49, 54, 78, 93, 100, 115, 118, 137, 314, 318
Goitre, 321, 322

Grammar, *see* Linguistics
Grave's disease, 321

Habitual dysphonia, *see* Dysphonia, hyperkinetic
Hearing training, *see* Ear training
Helmholz resonators, 12
Hemilaryngectomy, 361
Hoarseness, 117, 125, 214
  in adolescence, 101
  in asthma, 27, 119
  in children, 95, 118–19, 127, 272, 344
  in endocrine disorder, 102
  in laryngeal palsy, 316
  in laryngofissure, 363
  in senescence, 103, 105
Homeostasis, 156, 180, 201
Homosexuality, 222, 233
Husson theory, 50–1, 54
Hyoid bone, 56, 365
Hyperthyroidism, 196, 236
  personality, 321
Hyperventilation, 30, 168, 412
Hypopharynx, 353, 360, 365
  as resonator, 366, 378, 382, 386
Hypothyroidism, *see* Myxoedema
Hysteria, 133, 180, 188–97
  anxiety, 190, 208
  aphonia, 192, 202, 204, 234, 314, 324
  conversion symptoms, 188, 189, 192, 208, 211, 216, 217, 338
  dysarthria, 197
  personality, 190, 197
  treatment of, 194–5, 197, 199

Image intensifier, 51, 68
Implosion, *see* Oesophageal injection
Inferior constrictor, 364, 377; *see* Cricopharyngeus muscle
Inflection, 84, 88, 92, 143, 176, 198, 305
Influenza virus, 116, 148, 182, 221, 301, 306, 312, 337

Injection, *see* Oesophageal
Insufficient nasality, *see* Nasality
Insufflation, *see* Oesophageal aspiration
Intelligence, 247, 249, 262, 280, 302
Intonation, 4, 89, 154
Interarytenoid muscle, *see* Transverse arytenoid
Intercostal muscles, 20–3, 26
Internal tensor weakness, 39, 104, 115, 120, 121, 181, 186, 194, 203, 213
Intratracheal intubation, 137–8

Keratosis, 346, 356
Kinaesthetic feed-back, 74, 88, 90, 165, 230, 266, 281, 305, 363, 395–6
King operation, 330, 343
Kleinsasser microsurgery, 130, 134, 136, 165, 347–8, 353

Language laboratory, 89, 172, 283
Laryngeal palsy, 18
  childhood, 313
  flaccid lower motor neuron, 300, 309
  hysterical adductor, 189, 191, 202, 314
  peripheral, 313, 317
  spastic upper motor neuron, 277–9
  teflon injection, 329
  thyroidectomy, 315, 317, 321
  traumatic, 300, 346
  viral, 221, 312
Laryngectomy, 88, 262, 358–9, 364, 367
  anaesthetic throat, 366, 413, 416, 418
  clubs, 372, 403
  fistula, 366, 369, 377, 388
  partial, 358–9
  post-operative progress, 370, 373
  psychology, 372–6, 385, 403–4, 410, 414, 416, 420

Laryngectomy (*continued*)
  speech rehabilitation, 18
  supra-glottic surgery, 362
Laryngis sicca, 355, 359
Laryngitis, 101, 112–17, 124, 211,
    221, 329, 332
  chronic, 128, 50, 208, 364,
    408
  psychosomatic, 114, 191, 193
  radiation, 359
  vocal abuse, 75, 103, 112, 191,
    178
Laryngofissure, 345, 359–64, 408
  granuloma, 361
Laryngologist, 112, 114, 126, 128,
    131, 184, 215, 227
  role of, 144–5, 198, 313, 346
Laryngoscopy, 47, 7, 81, 104,
    121, 125, 151
  direct, 114, 145–6, 204, 220
  indirect, 114, 192–3, 209, 390
Laryngostroboscope, 52
Larynx, 32, 35, 44
  embryology, 362
  cartilages, 32–4, 40–1, 43, 78,
    101
  cavity, 43
  congenital anomalies, 220, 344
  functions, 18, 93
  growth, 93, 101, 219, 227
  muscles extrinsic, 32, 34, 37,
    49, 64, 165, 227, 240
  muscles intrinsic, 32, 38, 40–1,
    53, 151
  nerve supply, 36, 234, 309–10
  sinus, 43, 44, 71
  stenosis, 342, 345–6, 350
  trauma, 312, 338, 341, 345
  webbing, 220, 341, 344–5
Lateral crico-arytenoid muscle,
    41
Lateral X-ray photography, 67,
    68, 71, 79, 238, 246, 249, 256,
    263, 365, 379, 381, 389
Leukoplakia, 116, 346
Levator palati muscle, 60
Linguistics, 3, 87, 89, 110, 209,
    241, 281, 303, 306
Lips, 55
Litigation, 130, 326, 328, 346
Lungs, 20, 22–3, 165–6

Lymphatic glands, 362
  block dissection, 359, 366
  metastasis, 358, 362

Malignancy, 52, 322, 329, 350,
    352; *see* Carcinoma
Malingering, 188, 203
Mechanoreceptor reflex, 53–4,
    127, 165, 355
Medical social worker, 341, 417
Medulla oblongata, 277, 309
Menstruation, 103, 123, 133, 183,
    234, 321, 323
Metalanguage, 6, 198
Minor's disease, *see* Tremor
Monitoring, *see* Ear Training
Musical instruments, 7, 10, 16,
    17, 81, 86
Mutation, vocal: boys, 97, 102,
    128; girls, 102; *see* Puber-
    phonia
Myasthenia gravis, 121, 254, 301
  laryngis, 120
Myoelastic theory, 50
Myopathy, 341
Myxoedema, 196, 236
  deafness, 237

Nasal cavity, 56, 65
  escape, 56, 61, 62, 239, 249,
    254, 279
  grimace, 243, 255, 265, 267
  obstruction, 65, 240, 271, 274,
    275
  speech, 238–76
Nasality, 67, 73, 76, 78, 94, 239
  acoustic structure, 239
  causes, 244–55
  excessive, 238, 245, 247
  insufficient, 119, 238, 243,
    246–7, 271–5
  mixed, 239
  palatal paralysis, 252–4, 259,
    298
Nasopharyngeal incompetence,
    244–76, 259, 262
Nasopharynx, 56, 61, 68, 73
Neuritis, palatal, 254
  rheumatic, 300, 336–8

Neurochronaxic theory, 50, 51, 54
Neurosis, *see* Psychoneurosis

Obturator, 245, 248, 253, 258
Oesophageal sphincter, *see* Cricopharyngeal sphincter
Oesophageal voice, 366, 370, 376, 378, 416
  air flow, 380, 386
  air reservoir, 379–80, 402, 406
  air swallowing, 377, 385, 394, 400, 409, 411
  aspiration method, 365, 380, 382–3, 394, 396
  assessment, 396
  breathing, 380, 387, 397
  difficulties, 391, 403
  faults, 400–2
  implosive method, *see* injection
  injection, 380, 382–3, 388, 394–397
  pitch resonance, 407
  resonator, 413
  speech exercises, 398–400
  speech therapy, 388
Oesophago-pharyngo-laryngectomy, 360, 368
Oesophagus, 58, 310–11, 364, 366, 379
Orbicularis muscle, 55
Oscilloscope, 10, 14, 23, 53, 98
Osteoarthritis, 182

Pachydermia, 136, 139, 346–7
Palatoglossal muscle, 59
Palatopharyngeal sphincter, 60–62, 65, 67, 73, 76, 238, 241
Palatoplasty, *see* Cleft palate
Papillomata, 346, 350–6, 358
Parkinson's disease, 210, 283, 284–96, 352
  speech, 286–8, 292, 294
  speech therapy, 295–6
  surgery, 288
  writing, 285, 295
Paranasal sinuses, *see* Resonators
Passavant's ridge, 60, 62
Peptic acid reflux, 141

Peripheral nerve palsy, 300, 336–8
Peto method, 307
Personality, 120, 211, 261
  in cleft palate, 261–2, 266, 270
  in laryngectomy, 373–6
  Parkinsonism, 289, 290–1
  thyrotoxicosis, 323–4
Pharyngoplasty, *see* Cleft palate
Pharyngeal flaps, 62, 242, 253, 258
  voice, 376, 378, 381
Pharyngolaryngectomy, 360, 366, 377, 412, 413
Pharynx, 58, 61, 320
  as resonator, 64, 240
  dimensions, 245, 248, 252, 260
Phonasthenia, *see* Asthenic voice
Phonation, 18, *see* Voice
Phthisis laryngea, 341, 417
Physiotherapy, 280, 288, 292, 302, 304, 366, 370, 408
Pillars of the fauces, 59–61, 73, 76, 241, 245, 267, 378
Pitch, 4, 8–10, 16, 24, 34, 47, 63
  breaks, 95, 98, 172, 221, 316
  disorders, 122, 135, 219, 221, 233, 237
  exercises, 229
  fundamental, 69
  nasality, 244
  optimum, 70, 80
  psychopathologic, 75, 328
Plicae ventricularis, 348
Poliomyelitis, 243, 253, 256, 259, 298, 380
Pollution, 115, 125, 130, 347
Polyp, 130, 132, 134, 241, 272, 346, 349
Pop singers, *see* Singing
Posterior cricoarytenoid, 39, 41, 48, 83, 315, 318, 370
Posture, 85, 157, 164, 183, 232, 397
Pregnancy, 103, 284, 351
Prosody, 4, 92
Pseudo-bulbar palsy, *see* Suprabulbar palsy
Pseudo-glottis, *see* Cricopharyngeus muscle
Pseudo-voice, *see* Oesophageal

Psychiatric chemotherapy, 350, 375
Psychiatrist, role of, 190–1, 195, 198, 201, 208, 213, 215, 224
Psychoneurosis, 123–4, 126–7, 173, 192, 209, 327
Psychosomatic symptoms, 183, 190, 210, 221, 223, 232, 291, 324, 372
Psychotherapy, 221, 304
Puberphonia, 75, 193, 221, 244, 345
    predisposition, 225
    treatment, 227, 229
    vocal symptoms, 225
Puberty, 97–102, 220, 351
Pushing exercises, *see* Forcing
Pyriform fossa, 408

Quality of voice, *see* Resonance

Radiotherapy, 322, 351, 358–60, 368–9, 372, 389, 407–8
    ischemia, 366
    induration, 418
Recording of speech, 130–1, 140, 142, 150, 153, 206, 228, 231, 233, 244, 259, 283, 349
Recurrent laryngeal nerves, 310, 321
    oesophageal branch, 377, 379
Registers, *see* Singing
Relaxation, 73–5, 77, 165, 275
    basis of co-ordination, 82
    controlled, 84, 157
    exercises, 160
    in dysarthrophonia, 280, 304–5
    in laryngectomee, 363, 385, 400, 402
    in suggestion, 161, 172
    in therapy, 120, 156–62, 184, 202, 211, 230, 240, 265, 330, 333, 344
Resonance, 12, 16, 28, 63, 69
    cul-de-sac, 65, 76, 240
    disorders of nasality, 238–75
    forward tone, 69
    head, 67, 76

Resonance (*continued*)
    optimum, 70, 75, 79, 141
    pharyngeal, 366, 407
    physics, 10–16
Resonator scale, 76
Resonators, anatomy, 63, 101
    paranasal sinuses, 69, 75
    subglottic, 63, 228
    supraglottic, 63, 69, 70, 366
Respiration, 19–29
    dual control, 29–30
Reverse King operation, 343
Rheumatic arthritis, *see* Arthritis
Rhinitis, *see* Vasomotor
Rhythm, 47, 79, 82, 85–90
    in dysarthria, 90, 280, 306
    in oesophageal speech, 400
    in Parkinsonism, 284, 295
    in speech development, 92, 306
Rosenthal pharyngoplasty, 253, 279

Salpingopharyngeus muscle, 58, 246
Schizophrenia, 181
Semon's law, 313
Senescence, 92, 103–5, 183, 350, 357–8, 363, 415, 418
Singing, 25, 28–9, 37, 54, 72, 74
    castrati, 219, 232
    contrasted with speaking, 77–81
    children, 86, 88, 97, 99, 102, 306
    endocrine disorder, 103, 183, 219
    exercises, 174
    laryngeal palsy, 316, 318
    pop, 77, 121, 129, 130, 133, 146, 148
    registers, 47–9, 67, 79, 94, 113
Sinus of larynx, 43–4, 63, 104, 240–2
Sinuses, *see* Resonators
Sinusitis, 144
Sinus tone, 75
Smoking, 115, 125, 134, 136, 138, 142, 145, 149, 151, 172, 177, 196, 217, 347, 370

Sound, 13–18
Spastic dysphonia, 208–18, 211, 215–16
Speaking tube, 318
Spectrograph, 14–15, 72–3, 80, 94–6, 110, 238, 407
Speech therapist's role, 115, 118–19, 130–1, 136, 140, 146, 151, 153–5, 179, 184, 190, 198, 203, 212, 245, 294, 300, 376, 381, 405, 409
Stammer, 90, 91, 173, 181, 192, 195, 210, 212, 230–1, 255, 257, 284, 296, 404, 410
Stereotactic surgery, 288
Strap muscles, 36
Striatal lesions, 283
Suggestion, 197–200
Sulcus glottides, 128
Superior constrictor muscle, 58, 60–2
laryngeal nerve, 309–11, 320
Supra-bulbar palsy, 196, 278–9, 297
Synkinesis, 84
Syphilis, 136, 342

Tactile feed-back, 74, 90, 266, 281, 363, 395
Team approach, 304, 308
Teflon injection, 329
Telephone, 280–1, 294, 331, 405
Tension, *see* Relaxation
Tensor palati muscle, 58–9
Thalamotomy,
stereotactic, 288–9
cryogenic, 288–9
Thorax, 19, 228
Thymectomy, 254
Thyroarytenoid muscle, 38–9, 41, 43, 47–8, 53, 93, 120, 193, 315, 320, 361
Thyroid cartilage, 33, 36, 40, 178, 220, 229, 345, 361
calcification, 104
Thyroid gland, 101, 195, 236, 312, 317, 321
pressure symptoms, 322
Thyroidectomy, 314, 321–3, 334
laryngeal palsy, 163, 316–19

Thyroidectomy (*continued*)
psychosomatic symptoms, 324
voice disorder, 237, 316
Thyrotoxicosis, 312, 321
Thyroxine, 321, 323
Tics, 209, 212
Tomograph, 47, 51
Tone, 11; *see* Resonance
Tongue, 55–7
articulation, 72
dysarthria, 281, 288
laryngectomy, 366, 378, 383, 385, 388, 396
Tonsils, 119, 130
Trachea, 25, 43, 78, 311
Tracheal cannula, 318, 351, 369
stoma, 364, 370–2, 385, 396, 401
Tracheotomy, 318, 331, 335, 343, 346, 351, 364
Transverse arytenoid muscle, 42, 315, 319
Tremolo, 78
Tremor familial, 211, 218
Parkinsonian, 284, 297
senile, 297
Trill, 78
Twins, 5, 124, 190, 215
Tuberculosis, 136, 341

Ultrasonic therapy, 351–2

Vagus nerve, 309
Vasomotor disorder, 183, 189
rhinitis, 195, 207, 234, 271, 273
Velum, 58
Ventricle (Morgagni), *see* Larynx
Ventricular voice, 115, 192–3, 208, 333, 335, 337, 348, 394
folds, 4, 44, 77, 104, 115, 240, 356, 360
Vestibule of larynx, 78
Vibrators, 368, 374, 376, 387, 404, 413, 414, 416, 419, 421
difficulties, 418
intelligibility, 418
manufacturers, 422
National Health supply, 417

Vibrators (*continued*)
  objections to, 415
  telephoning, 289, 294, 405–6
Virilisation, 235
Virus infection, 312, 336, 350–1, 355
Vocal abuse, 75, 99, 112, 117, 129, 139, 146, 208, 211, 347, 356, 359
  aids, *see* Amplifiers, Vibrators
  assessment, 113, 150–1
  cords, 38–50, 78, 79
    anatomy and physiology, 33, 38, 41–2, 45, 49, 53–4, 71
    atrophic changes 128
    bowing, 39, 121
    breathing, 45
    congenital anomalies, 129–220
    growth, 93, 101–2
    mechanoreceptors, 53–4, 127, 165
    phonation, 17, 45
    pitch, 34, 46, 48
    positions in paralysis, 315–319
    scarring, 130, 342, 345
    stripping, 116, 127, 130, 134, 136, 237, 345, 347–8
    ulceration, 342, 348
    vibration, 77–8, 117
  fold, *see* Vocal cords
  fry, 117
  ligament, *see* Vocal cord
  nodules, adult, 122–3, 165, 349

Vocal nodules (*continued*)
  children, 92, 115, 117, 119, 123, 126–9, 172, 226
  surgery, 116, 175, 127, 165, 346
  process, *see* Arytenoid
  rest, 313, 341, 343
  strain, 6, 27, 52, 54, 79, 91, 99–115, 132, 156, 195, 201, 235
Vocalis muscle, *see* Thyroarytenoid muscle
Voice, 1–4, 18
  exercises, 174–8
  expression of personality, 1, 6, 95, 100, 110, 117, 123, 147, 156, 180, 231, 233, 373
  in infancy, 83–4, 87, 92, 96
  production, 73, 131, 147, 195, 224
Volume, *see* Amplification
Vowels, 1, 61, 68, 69, 73
  formants, 12, 55, 70, 110
  in nasality, 58, 239
  in oesophageal voice, 407

Wasserman, 342
Whispering, 4, 45, 74–5, 125, 134, 138, 170, 185, 192, 152–3, 320, 368, 389
White noise vibrator, 413
Woodman operation, 320, 330, 335
Wrisberg cartilage, *see* Cuneiform cartilage

Yodelling, 79